# Dominant Exudative Vitreoretinopathy and other Vascular Developmental Disorders of the Peripheral Retina

# Monographs in Ophthalmology 5

Dr  W. JUNK PUBLISHERS THE HAGUE/BOSTON/LONDON

C.E. van NOUHUYS

# Dominant Exudative Vitreoretinopathy and other Vascular Developmental Disorders of the Peripheral Retina

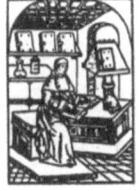

Dr W. JUNK PUBLISHERS THE HAGUE/BOSTON/LONDON

Distributors:

*for the United States and Canada*
Kluwer Boston Inc.
190 Old Derby Street
Hingham, MA 02043
USA

*for all other countries*
Kluwer Academic Publishing Group
Distribution Center
P.O. Box 322
3300 AH Dordrecht
The Netherlands

ISBN-13:978-94-009-8023-5       e-ISBN-13:978-94-009-8021-1
DOI: 10.1007/978-94-009-8021-1

# PREFACE

Dominant exudative vitreoretinopathy (DEVR) is an eye disease which has only recently received wider attention. In 1969 Criswick and Schepens used the designation "familial exudative vitreoretinopathy" to describe a syndrome they observed in six patients belonging to two families. The condition was characterized by several symptoms involving the vitreous and retina, e.g. "posterior vitreous detachment, organized vitreous membranes, heterotopia of the macula, retinal neovascularizations, subretinal and intraretinal exudates, and localized retinal detachment". The clinical features impressed the authors as strongly reminiscent of retrolental fibroplasia, but none of the patients had a record of premature birth or postnatal oxygen administration.

In 1971 Gow and Oliver described the same syndrome in several members of one family. They considered their findings to be compatible with autosomal dominant transmission. Canny and Oliver (1976) were the first to demonstrate the fluorescein-angiographic changes of DEVR in four members of the abovementioned family. The most striking finding was "abrupt cessation of the capillary network in a scaloped edge near the equator". Fluorescein was seen to leak from the retinal vessels localized in this marginal zone, and in some eyes from massive fibrovascular lesions as well. Similar fluorescein-angiographic changes have been described in recent years in other reports on families with DEVR (Nijhuis et al., 1979; Slusher and Hutton, 1979; Dudgeon, 1979; Ober et al., 1980; Laqua, 1980).

In 1979 I commenced a clinical study of this still little-known condition at the Nijmegen University Institute of Ophthalmology (The Netherlands). This venture was prompted by the fact that two families with DEVR had been known for some time at this institute. The study led to identification of the disease in seven more families. The findings obtained in this total of nine families are presented and discussed in this thesis.

Part I briefly reviews the normal development and anatomy of the retinal vasculature, more specifically in the peripheral fundus.

Part II discusses the pathology of (peripheral) retinal vascular development. In addition to DEVR there are other eye diseases or general syndromes in which fundus changes are based on disturbed development of the peripheral retinal vasculature, or in which such a pathogenesis is considered not to be improbable. Moreover, other conditions whose primary lesions are not based on disturbed vascular development can be incidentally associated with symptoms suggestive of a disorder in the vasculogenesis of the peripheral retina. The selection of the conditions discussed in part II is based partly on a study of the literature and partly on personal observations, some of which have been presented in previous publications.

Apart from DEVR, I have not attempted to discuss all the features of the various other diseases but always accentuated the aspect of disturbed retinal vascular development.

Both the literature and the histories of our patients show that DEVR very frequently causes diagnostic confusion. This is why I have given ample attention to differential diagnosis. With regard to diseases in which retinal vascular developmental disorders play a role, the differential diagnosis is discussed in part II. For other diseases this is done in part III.

C.E. VAN NOUHUYS

*Afdeling Oogheelkunde*
*Canisius-Wilhelmina Ziekenhuis*
*St.Annastraat 289*
*6500 GS Nijmegen*
*The Netherlands*

# ACKNOWLEDGEMENTS

Several persons have given me the benefit of their assistance in my research and in the preparation of this publication.

I am indebted to Mr A.L. Aan de Kerk for his competent help in photographing the peripheral eye fundus in a large number of patients.

The ophthalmological study of several members of the A family by Dr F.A. Nijhuis has been of essential importance to me in the early phase of this study.

Dr A. Hamburg of the Eye Clinic of the University of Utrecht was kind enough to send me several histological specimens.

I thank my colleagues of the Department of Ophthalmology of the Canisius-Wilhelmina Hospital, Nijmegen, for their kindness in supplying me with clinical data on their patients.

The expert criticism I received from Prof. J.J.de Laey of Ghent (Belgium) and from Prof. S.J. Geerts of Nijmegen proved to be very valuable to me.

The photomicrographs and the line drawings were prepared by the audio-visual service of the St. Radboud Hospital and by Mrs Th. Hermans Den Brok, Nijmegen.

My wife José typed the manuscript in her limited spare time and collated the bibliography.

The English translation was made by Mr Th. van Winsen.

# CONTENTS

PART I

THE NORMAL VASCULATURE OF THE PERIPHERAL RETINA

# CHAPTER 1

# DEVELOPMENT AND ANATOMY OF THE NORMAL VASCULATURE OF THE PERIPHERAL RETINA

Developmental disorders of the retinal vasculature can be studied only in relation to the normal embryonic vascular development. Structural changes in the vasculature of the peripheral retina can be identified only by differentiating them from the normal vascular pattern.

This is why this chapter discusses some aspects of the normal embryology and anatomy of the retinal vasculature which may be of importance for this study.

## 1.1 Definitions of anatomical boundaries

To indicate regions and their boundaries in the fundus, I use the system described by Rutnin (1967).

The fundus is divided into a posterior and a peripheral fundus, the boundary between these two being formed by an imaginary circle through the posterior extremities of the vortex veins. These demarcations are as a rule readily distinguishable at ophthalmoscopy.

The peripheral fundus is divided into an equatorial region and an ora serrata region. The former is bisected by the equator, which takes its course slightly peripheral to the ampullae of the vortex veins. The boundary between the equatorial and the ora serrata region is formed by the midline between the equator and the ora serrata.

For a more detailed account of this division of the normal ocular fundus, I refer to Rutnin (1967).

## 1.2 Development and regression of the hyaloid vessels and the primary vitreous

Very early in the course of embryonic development, shortly after invagination of the optic vesicle, mesodermal tissue enters the newly formed optic cup along with the primitive hyaloid artery, via the foetal fissure. In the fibrillar tissue localized between the lens vesicle and the inner layer of the optic cup, blood vessels arise from the hyaloid artery to form the foetal intraocular blood system. This consists of a network of vessels on the posterior surface of the lens, the tunica vasculose lentis, and the ramifications localized more posteriorly in the primary vitreous: the hyaloid vasa propria. On the posterior side of the lens the two vascular systems anastomose and, anteriorly along the equator of the lens, form anastomoses with vessels of mesenchymal tissue outside the optic cup. The latter anastomoses develop to capsulopupillary vessels which are to drain the blood from the vessels of the hyaloid system to the annular vessel near the anterior rim of the optic cup. This drainage is necessary because the hyaloid artery is not accompanied by a venous system.

The hyaloid vasa propria attain their maximal development at about the 40 mm stage (10th week), and in this period extend throughout the optic cup, but without direct contact with the retinal surface (Mann, 1964). In this phase the neuroretina seems to depend mainly on diffusion from the outer ramifications of the hyaloid viasa propria. The network of delicate fibrillar structures which fills the optic cup and encompasses the hyaloid vessels is known as primary vitreous. These delicate fibrils in the foetal eye are found, at light-microscopic examination, to show connections with the superficial ectoderm of the lens vesicle, the neuroectoderm of the inner layer of the optic cup, and the mesenchymal tissue surrounding the hyaloid artery, respectively. This observation suggests that the primary vitreous is a joint product of these three structures (Mann, 1964).

The retrogression of the foetal hyaloid system begins at about the 50 mm stage with gradual atrophy of the proximal segment of the hyaloid vasa propria, which lose their connection with the hyaloid artery close to the point of ramification. Regression of the tunica vasculosa lentis and the hyaloid artery follows later in the course of development, but remnants of these vessels as a rule persist until the final months of intrauterine development, and sometimes even until after birth.

Hyaloid remnants are therefore often found in premature neonates (Jones, 1963), and the same applies to remnants of the anterior portion of the tunica vasculosa lentis (Gans, 1959).

## 1.3 Development of the choroid of the peripheral fundus

According to Heimann (1972), the pigmented epithelium in the human embryo is covered at the end of the second month by a dense capillary network: the primitive choriocapillaris. This network comprises meridionally arranged capillaries which, in the course of further foetal development, gradually move towards the surface of the choroid and thus allow the underlying network of the definitive choriocapillaris to close. This is a gradual process, from the posterior parts of the choroid in anterior direction, and in fact the definitive choriocapillaris near the posterior portion of the ciliary body does not develop until the final months of intrauterine development.

The primordial layer of large vessels which ultimately becomes Haller's layer, develops mainly in the 4th month. Sattler's layer, which is made up of smaller vessels and localized between Haller's layer and the choriocapillaris, develops somewhat later, approximately during the 5th month (Heimann, 1972). It is not until very late in the course of development (between the 6th and the 10th month) that the recurrent ciliary arteries develop; they usually arise from the major arterial circle of the iris and grow in posterior direction to be ultimately connected with previously established parts of the choroid. Some authors believe that these vessels also form direct arterial anastomoses with the posterior choroidal arteries (Wybar, 1954; Ring and Fujino, 1967; Krey, 1981), but others have been unable to identify such anastomoses (Heimann, 1972).

## 1.4 Development of the retinal vasculature

According to Versari (1904), the development of the retinal vasculature begins at the 70 mm stage with the formation of vascular buds from the hyaloid artery at the site of the papilla. At the 100 mm stage (4th month), small vessels are visible which are in connection with the hyaloid artery and form delicate ramifications entering the nerve fibre layer of the retina near the papilla. These vessels constitute the primordium of the arterial ramifications of the future central retinal artery. Ashton (1954, 1957) maintained that this ingrowth of retinal vessels occurs, not through a process of budding from the hyaloid artery but by preliminary invasion of primitive mesenchymal cells.

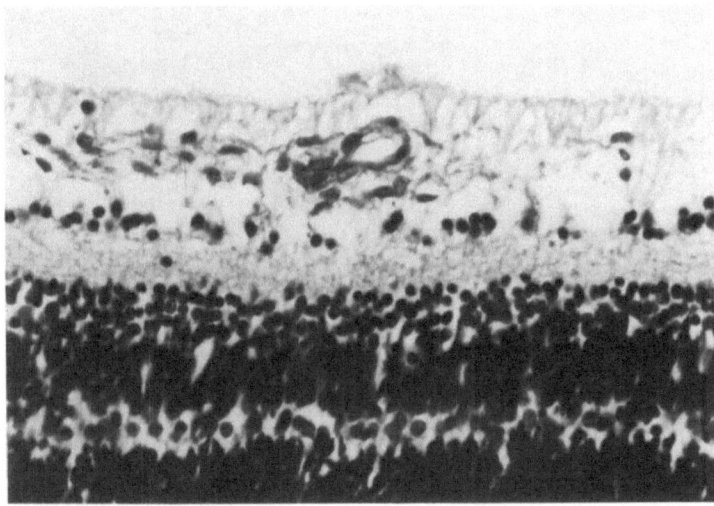

Figure 1a. Cross-section through the neuroretina of a 7-month foetus posterior to the equator. Small blood vessels are present in the nerve fibre layer (PAS, × 50).

6

As these advance into the retina, they gradually differentiate into endothelial cells and form a capillary network from which the adult retinal vessels evolve.

A network of primitive capillaries grows centrifugally from the papilla into the nerve fibre layer of the retina, and the outer zone of advancing capillaries is surrounded by the abovementioned mesenchymal cells (Figure 1a).

In histological specimens, PAS-positive granules can be found in association with this outer zone of growing vessels and the surrounding mesenchymal cells (Figure 1b). Serpell (1954) identified these granules histochemically as glycogen. Another histochemical property was demonstrated by Nilausen (1958): the presence of the enzyme alkaline phosphatase in association with the mesenchymal cell formation at the periphery of the advancing vascular system, the endothelium of the peripheral capillaries and the cells scattered between the vessels. These findings are consistent with Ashton's hypothesis that the mesenchymal cells in question are precursors of the endothelial cells of the immature, newly formed capillaries.

In man, solid cords are first formed. crevices form between these cords and a polygonal network develops as the cords become canalized to capillaries (De Oliveira, 1968; Ashton, 1970). Blood cells appear in the newly formed capillaries at an early stage. This primitive network of small retinal vessels is gradually subject to substantial changes, and finally attains the adult configuration of blood vessels.

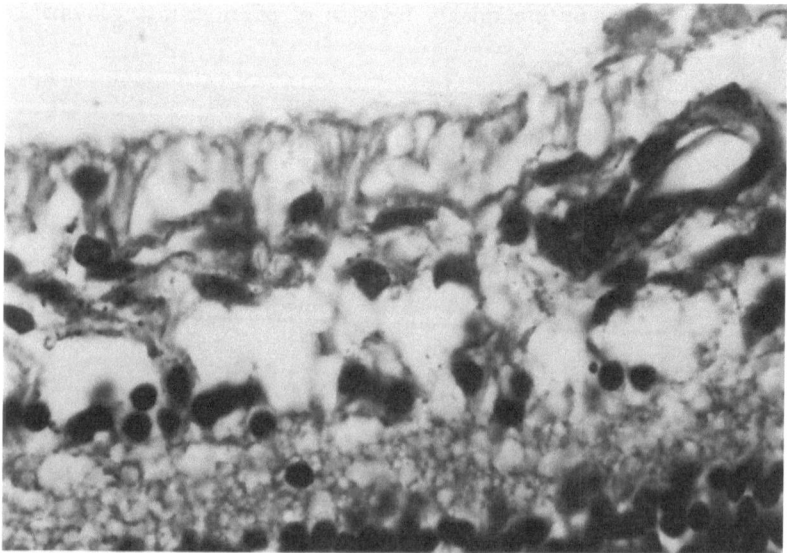

Figure 1b. The same section as in Figure 1a, at higher magnification. Several nuclei of mesenchymal cells are localized in the nerve fibre layer in the zone of growing vessels, along with a large number of PAS-positive granules (× 110)

Retraction of many newly formed capillaries is an important component of this transformation. This regression and disappearance of elements of the immature vascular system is not specific for the retina but a well-known phenomenon of vasculogenesis in numerous tissues (Clark, 1918; Wolff et al., 1975).

In particular the trypsin digest technique, which makes it possible to study the retinal vasculature in flat specimens after enzymatic removal of the other retinal structures (Kuwabara and Cogan, 1960), has contributed substantially to our knowledge of the foetal development of the vascular system. The retraction of immature capillaries was readily demonstrable by this technique (Cogan, 1963; Ashton, 1970).

Studies of the development of the retinal vasculature in cats and rats, in which most of the retina is not vascularized until after birth, have demonstrated a similar phenomenon of retraction and disappearance of parts of the immature vasculature (Engerman and Meyer, 1965; Lemmingson, 1966; Henkind and De Oliveira, 1967). Some adjacent vessels are separated by strands of tissue which Kuwabara and Cogan (1960) described as intercapillary bridges; these are probably remnants of degenerated primitive vessels (Engerman and Meyer, 1965). However, the latter authors hold that, at least in the rat retina, capillaries also disappear without leaving such intercapillary bridges.

Whereas some parts of the newly formed vascular bed degenerate and disappear, other vessels increase in luminal width and are tranformed into vascular branches which come to play a role in the supply or drainage of blood to and from various more peripheral capillaries. The mechanism underlying this transformation of some primitive capillaries into venules and arterioles is obscure, but it seems likely that this process is determined by haemodynamic as well as by biochemical factors.

It is certain that arterial and venous vessels develop from primitive capillaries (Shakib et al., 1968), and that the previous theory that retinal capillaries develop from veins (Michaelson, 1948) is wrong.

The more mature parts of the vascular bed are characterized in this way by the formation of blood vessels which differ in function and in luminal width. The capillary network, too, becomes less dense and assumes a less uniform appearance. The most striking changes occur in the capillary network in the immediate vicinity of vessels which have been transformed into arterioles. On either side of these arterial vessels, zones develop in which capillaries disappear. These capillary-free zones are not primarily present, as used to be assumed, but develop due to retraction of capillaries and reduced lateral budding from arterial vessels (Engerman and Meyer, 1965).

The primordium of the capillary network initially forms in the layer of nerve fibres and ganglion cells, from which blood vessels subsequently invade deeper layers of the retina to form a second plexus of capillaries in the inner nuclear layer. Studying rats, Engerman and Meyer (1965) observed degeneration of many capillaries in the inner layer of the blood vessels during the development of the outer layer of capillaries.

The network of the retinal vasculature shows steady centrifugal expansion based on the formation of new vessels in the zone of transition between the vascularized retina and the avascular periphery. Human retinal vessels reach the ora serrata on the nasal side by about the 7th—8th month, whereas in the temporal portion of the fundus the retina is vascularized only about as far as the equator at this time (Cogan, 1963). The delay in vascularization of the temporal as compared with the nasal half of the retina has been confirmed by several histological and clinical observations in premature infants.

At indirect ophthalmoscopy the non-vascularized part of the retinal periphery manifests itself as a pale zone in premature infants. The presence of such a zone therefore signifies that the retinal vascularization is not yet completed. On the basis of this ophthalmologically visible criterion, Fletcher (1955) found that neonates with a body weight of 2000 g as a rule had an entirely vascularized retina. Roth (1970) determined the gestational age of mostly prematurely born babies on the basis of various neurological and physical findings, and ophthalmoscopically found vascular maturation for the first time at 31 weeks. Vascularization was found to be complete in all infants with a gestational age of 38 weeks and over.

The vascularization of the peripheral retina in the eyes of immature and premature babies has also been studied histologically (Foos and Kopelow, 1973; Saga and Uemura, 1977). Foos and Kopelow (1973) found a fully vascularized retina in 10% of the eyes of infants with a gestational age of 28 weeks, and 70% of the eyes at a gestational age of 36 weeks. These authors found a completely vascularized retina in all full-term infants.

The above shows that the gestational age at which the retinal periphery is fully vascularized, can vary widely. Other histological studies have confirmed this (Kushner et al., 1977). Distinct differences in the rate of retinal vascularization between the two eyes in the same individual have been observed but are rare (Foos and Kopelow, 1973).

In eyes with a not yet fully vascularized retina, the peripheral zone of advancing vasculature proved to show a fimbriated pattern. The peripheral avascular zone was always at its widest in the temporal and superior part of the fundus. In several of these eyes, the boundary between the vascular and the avascular retina curved abruptly back in central direction near the horizontal meridians, thus producing a V-shaped notch. A notch of this kind was found in 12% of the eyes with immature vascularization (Foos and Kopelow, 1973). It indicates incomplete or retarded fusion of the superior and inferior vascular complexes near the horizontal meridians, these authors maintain.

Histologically, the avascular part of the normal foetal retina shows cystic defects between the processes of Müller cells in the nerve fibre layer. These cysts are visible at low magnification, not only in flat-mount preparations but also in cross-sections (Figure 2). Some authors have reported the remarkable observation that such cystic changes are not found in eyes with the features of retrolental fibroplasia (Kushner et al., 1977).

The above studies show that the human retina is as a rule fully vascularized by the time of birth, and sometimes even before this. This does not mean that the retinal vasculature shows an adult pattern at this time, and particularly not the peripheral retina, which matures last. According to Cogan (1963), the immature configuration at the end of the intrauterine period is clearly visible especially in flat-mount preparations of the retina. It is not until about the 5th month after birth that the retinal vasculature shows its adult configuration with meshes of varying shape and size, and only about that time are mural cells discernible in the vascular walls (Cogan, 1963).

## 1.5 Anatomy of the vasculature of the peripheral retina

The blood vessels of the peripheral retina form a network which is much less dense and extends much more in a single plane than is the case in the posterior pole. The peripheral retina is considerably thinner than the posterior retina. A marked decrease in thickness is particularly noticeable between equator and ora serrata; in fact the neuroretina near the ora serrata is only half as thick as near the equator (Daicker, 1972). A true three-dimensional configuration of the vascular network, as present in the posterior pole, does not exist in the

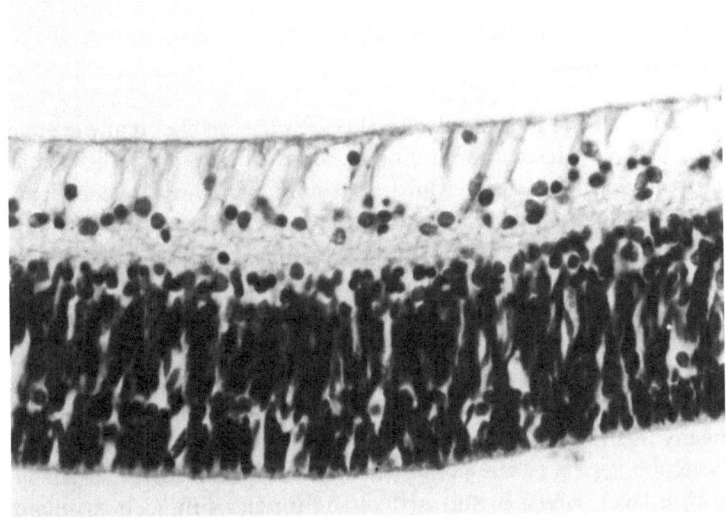

Figure 2. Cross-section through the neuroretina in the region of the equator, in the same eye as in Figure 1. The nerve fibre layer shows cystic spaces between the processes of Müller cells. No development of blood vessels is discernible as yet (× 50).

peripheral retina (Toussaint et al., 1961). The density of the capillary bed, expressed in the total length of capillaries per retinal surface area unit, markedly diminishes from the posterior pole to the periphery, and at the equator is about a quarter of the density near the optic disc (Toussaint and Danis, 1970). Measured at the same distance from the optic disc, the density of the capillary bed in the temporal sector proved to exceed that in the nasal sector; and somewhat lower density was found in the superior and inferior sectors of the fundus (Toussaint and Danis, 1970).

The outer boundary of the peripheral vascular bed near the ora serrata is formed by capillaries, and at some sites by venules, which drain blood from a few slightly more centrally localized capillaries. Such venules, which constitute the most peripheral parts of the retinal vascular bed and curve in central direction to drain the blood in larger venous branches, are described by some German-speaking authors as "Wurzelvenen" (root veins) (Zollinger, 1944; Daicker, 1972). Sometimes these vessels extend over a longer distance more or less parallel to the ora serrata before curving in central direction. In that case they are sometimes referred to as arcade vessels (German: "Arkadenvenen"). Arcade vessels of great length are rare in human subjects (Daicker, 1972), but are regularly found in some mammals such as dogs (Mutlu and Leopold, 1964).

The capillary-free zone around the arteries, already observed in the previous century by His (1980), increases in width towards the periphery of the fundus, where it attains a width of about 0.12 mm (Michaelson, 1954).

### 1.6 Structure of the retinal vessels and the vitreoretinal juncture of the peripheral fundus

The structure of the individual retinal vessels in the region of the equator, as observed at light microscopy in cross-sections of the retina, differs hardly (if at all) from that of the vessels in the posterior pole. Spitznas and Bornfield (1977) maintain that the capillaries in the extreme periphery of the retina have an abnormally wide lumen, but Daicker (1972) observed this only in the abovementioned "Wurzelvenen" and arcade vessels.

A histological peculiarity of the retinal vessels in the extreme periphery of the fundus is the presence of a perivascular halo which consists of delicate collagen fibrils, basal lamina material, dense bodies, vesicles and parts of macrophages (Spitznas and Bornfield, 1977). Luciano et al. (1977) histochemically identified glycoproteins in this halo, which can vary in thickness.

The blood vessels of the peripheral retina are localized superficially in the nerve fibre layer, which in this part of the fundus is thin. As in the posterior retina, the blood vessels are surrounded by a continuous envelope of glia cells which separates blood vessels from nerve cells.

The close anatomical relation between the retinal vessels, particularly in the peripheral fundus, and the vitreoretinal juncture is of significance in the mechanism by which this juncture, and even the cortical vitreous, develop changes in response to vascular disturbances. At light-microscopic examination the vitreoretinal juncture is distinguishable as a homogenous membrane on the inner surface of the retina; this membrane averages $2-3\mu$ in thickness and is described as inner limiting membrane. At electron-microscopic examination this membrane proves to consist of two layers: a basal lamina and a thicker layer of vitreous fibrils which, on the vitreous side, are connected with the basal lamina (Gärtner, 1966). The basal lamina is separated from the plasma membrane of the glia cells of the retina by a narrow electron-lucent space (Foos, 1972).

The vitreoretinal juncture shows considerable structural differences in different portions of the fundus: it is very thin in the region of the ora serrata at the site of the vitreous base, and in central direction becomes thicker and thicker until it attains 6 times its initial thickness in the posterior pole (Foos, 1972).

Aother difference concerns the so-called attachment plaques by which the Müller cells are connected with the basal lamina. These plaques are observed only in the peripheral retina but are absent in the posterior pole (Foos, 1972).

The vitreoretinal juncture is usually separated from the retinal blood vessels by a glial layer which consists of processes of the Müller cells. This layer can be absent in blood vessels localized very superficially in the neuroretina, as they often are in the periphery of the fundus. In that case there is often a direct connection between the vascular wall and the vitreoretinal juncture. Such connections can be found in normal eyes, and are therefore also known as physiological vitreovascular adhesions (Gärtner, 1962b).

At the level of superficially localized vessels the vitreoretinal juncture sometimes shows defects (Foos, 1977) through which processes of glia cells can invade the cortex of the vitreous and form local vitreoretinal adhesions (Daicker et al., 1977). Similar defects of the basal lamina in the vitreoretinal juncture, with local growth of glial tissue to the vitreous space, can also be present without any direct relation to retinal blood vessels. They have been observed in foetal as well as in adult eyes (Daicker et al., 1977).

Gärtner (1962b) demonstrated light-microscopically that normal retinal blood vessels can in some cases even leave the stroma of the neuroretina and, over some distance, take an epiretinal course through the vitreous space.

CHAPTER 2

# CLINICAL EXAMINATION OF PERIPHERAL RETINAL BLOOD VESSELS AND CIRCULATION

A limited number of methods are available for clinical examination of the vasculature and circulation of the peripheral retina. This chapter discusses the principal techniques and aids used in this context, with emphasis on the practical possibilities and limitations of the various methods.

One difficulty in this respect is that the normal peripheral retina shows many interindividual variations. It is consequently not always possible to establish with certainty whether a slight anomaly should be regarded as a variant of the normal or as a minimal expression of an (hereditary) affection. This uncertainty prevails in particular in the study of families with DEVR.

It is therefore of importance to determine which vascular phenomena observed in contact lens studies and fluorescein angiography cannot be interpreted as normal.

## 2.1 Indirect ophthalmoscopy

Indirect ophthalmoscopy, using either a monocular or binocular instrument, is a valuable and widely used method for examination of the peripheral fundus. For examination of patients with only slight vascular abnormalities in the peripheral retina, however, indirect ophthalmoscopy has two disadvantages if compared with contact lens biomicroscopy, which is subsequently discussed: the magnification of the fundus features is insufficient for adequate visualization of the vascular ramifications peripheral to the equator. Magnification can be somewhat enhanced by using a weaker condensing lens or positive adapter lenses in the ophthalmoscope, but these measures have their limitations. The second disadvantage of indirect ophthalmoscopy is the difficulty of assessing the (preretinal) vitreous.

Since vascular affections of the retina manifest themselves in the inner retinal layers and the preretinal vitreous may be involved, it is important to use a method which permits adequate examination of the posterior and peripheral vitreous.

For these two reasons I have preferred to examine my patients and their relatives by slit-lamp biomicroscopy, which ensures better visualization of details in the fundus and the preretinal vitreous space than does indirect ophthalmoscopy. Whenever possible, I have performed the examination bilaterally in complete mydriasis. Indirect ophthalmoscopy yielded no sup-plemental findings and consequently was omitted in most cases. It was per-formed only in cases in which contact lens examination was not feasible.

## 2.2 Three-mirror contact lens examination

The technique of slit-lamp biomicroscopy with the aid of a three-mirror contact lens has been described in detail in other publications (Busacca et al., 1957; Eisner, 1973; Tolentino et al., 1976). The method is superior for a study of the peripheral retinal vasculature and the preretinal vitreous.

For observations on the peripheral fundus, the three-mirror contact lens has the great advantage that it eliminates optical aberrations which result from the angle of incidence of the beam at the corneal surface. Not only does this enhance the definition of the fundus features but it also reduces the rec-tangular distortion of these features (Niesel, 1975). According to Lotmar (1971), astigmatism increases very markedly outside the 80° area even with a contact lens. Since indentation reduces the angle of observation for the peri-pheral fundus, this method is of importance for reduction of astigmatism.

The definition of details in the peripheral fundus shows considerable dif-ferences in different eyes. This is due to differences in optical aberrations due to the slant of the beam and media turbidities, especially in the peripheral vitreous. As a result, the definition of features can differ even in different sec-tors of the same eye.

### 2.2.a *The biomicroscopic features of the normal vasculature of the peripheral retina*

In the normal fundus, the peripheral ramifications of the central retinal artery and vein show an even distribution over the various retinal sectors. The lumi-nal width of the ramifications steadily diminishes towards the periphery. Bio-microscopically, it is usually no longer possible to decide whether the vessels in the region of the equator are arterial or venous vessels. This can be achieved only by following these vessels as far as the posterior fundus.

Peripheral ramifications of retinal vessels can usually be followed as far as the ora serrata region. In the clinical diagnosis of mild cases of DEVR it is im-portant to establish the presence of small retinal branches in the peripheral portion of the equator region and the central portion of the ora serrata region. Since the primary lesions of the condition are based on a developmental dis-order of the retinal vasculature, which becomes manifest in the temporal sec-tor of the peripheral retina, demonstration of avascularity in this area is an important contribution to diagnostic certainty.

Optimal illumination is of great importance for observation of the most peripheral ramifications of the retinal vasculature. The intensity of illumination of the slit-lamp should be much higher than that used in examining the posterior fundus. The contrast of small retinal vessels against the background of the choroid can be enhanced by the use of a green or green-yellow filter, but this should not absorb too much light! Indentation makes it possible to observe the most peripheral portion of the retina as far as the ora serrata. For visualization of the small vascular branches in the peripheral retina, indentation is of limited value because the blood in these branches is pushed away, and this does not exactly enhance their visibility.

This is why I have made but little use of an indentation funnel in my study. Before completion of the contact lens examination, indentation of the sclera in the temporal sector was effected in most cases by exerting mild pressure with the radial part of the tip of the middle finger, meanwhile ensuring fixation of the three-mirror contact lens between thumb and index finger of the same hand. This method can only be used for temporal indentation, which for my purpose was usually sufficient.

Since the capillary bed of the retina cannot be visualized biomicroscopically, the vascularity of the peripheral retina has to be determined (in this examination) on the basis of observations on the smaller peripheral arteries and venous branches. A suitable method is to identify a relatively large vascular branch posterior to the temporal equator, and to follow its ramifications as close to the ora serrata as possible. In normal eyes this is usually possible as far as about 1–2 disc diameters central to the ora serrata.

It is not always possible to distinguish retinal vessels as far as the ora serrata region in normal eyes. As already pointed out, optical aberrations or delicate turbidities of the media can impede detailed observations.

In eyes with peripheral retinal degenerative changes – e.g. snailtracks and diffuse chorioretinal degeneration, with or without myopia – retinal vessels are often biomicroscopically indistinguishable in the affected areas. And in fluorescein angiography these areas often show diminished or absent perfusion.

Although the vasculature of the normal peripheral retina is highly variable, abrupt termination of the vascular bed in the equatorial region of the fundus (as found in DEVR) is an unmistakable indication of pathology. This finding is in fact the principal criterion in differentiating between the affected and unaffected members of a family (see Chapter 4).

## 2.3 Photography and fluorescein angiography of the peripheral fundus

There are several methods of making photographs of the peripheral fundus. Depending on the method, the following equipment can be used:
– slit lamp camera and contact lens
– fundus camera with (wide angle) contact lens objective
– hand-held fundus camera with interposed condensing lens (indirect

method)
— normal fundus camera without further aids.

For slit-lamp photography, a mirror contact lens can be used (Klein et al., 1974). This ensures relatively high magnification but entails a narrow image angle. Transscleral illumination of the fundus is possible (Slezak and Kenyeres, 1975).

Pomerantzeff (1975) designed a fundus camera with a contact lens objective to ensure direct contact with the cornea of the eye examined. This camera makes it possible to depict the entire fundus as far as the equator at a single exposure, but of course at low magnification.

The technique of fundus photography with a hand-held fundus camera and an interposed condensing lens is optically comparable with indirect ophthalmoscopy. This technique is especially suitable for young children examined under anaesthesia (Nagata and Tsuruoka, 1972).

Photography of the peripheral fundus with a normal fundus camera without further aids requires camera adjustment at an angle with the optical axis of the eye. An advantage is that no separate technical adjustments are required. Another advantage, particularly important for depiction of smaller details, is the relatively high magnification. Disadvantages of this technique are the relatively narrow angle and the difficult manoeuvres required for proper camera adjustment. A prerequisite with this technique is good cooperation on the part of the patient, who is required to train his eyes in extreme directions of gaze without executing interfering movements of the eyes or head. To photograph the temporal periphery, the camera has to be pivoted in nasal direction, and the anatomy of the patient's nose may in some cases impair this manoeuvre.

All photographs of the peripheral fundus of patients mentioned in this study were obtained by the lastmentioned method. Like all other known techniques of photography of the peripheral fundus, it entails considerable astigmatism, which increases as the angle between the optical axis of the camera objective and the optical axis of the eye examined widens.

Some fundus cameras have a corrective device to reduce astigmatism (Aan de Kerk, 1973). Although a considerable degree of correction can be achieved in this way (Busse and Mittelman, 1976), it is impossible to neutralize all the optical aberrations due to the slant of the light rays passing through the refracting media of the eye examined. These optical aberrations manifest themselves on photographs of the peripheral fundus, even in normal eyes; and, particularly on flurorescein angiograms, they can be confused with perfusion disorders.

The purpose of flurorescein-angiographic examination of the peripheral fundus as performed in the persons described in this thesis, was to demonstrate developmental disorders of the peripheral retinal vasculature. Some of the problems encountered in this context were far from small. Apart from the abovementioned optical aberrations and technical problems of access to the equatorial region in some cases, diagnosis was impeded in other cases by the extremely peripheral localization of the lesions. The next subsection lists several characteristics of the fluorescein angiogram of the normal peripheral fundus, and discusses features which should be interpreted as pathological. Mention will also be made of some possible artefacts, produced by the abovementioned optical aberrations.

## 2.3.a The fluorescein angiogram of the normal peripheral fundus

The characteristics and artefacts to be discussed here were encountered in fluorescein angiography performed by the technique we used. Several features of the normal fluorescein angiogram of the peripheral fundus obtained by similar techniques, have been discussed by Sata (1972), Asdourian and Goldberg (1979) and Miyakubo and Numaga (1980).

With the technique used it was usually impossible to depict retinal vessels localized peripheral to the midline between equator and ora serrata.

The fluorescein angiogram of the equatorial region of the normal fundus shows the following characteristics:

*Choroid*

-   The first filling of the choroidal arteries with fluorescein as a rule precedes the filling of the retinal arteries by a few seconds. This finding contradicts a report by Archer et al. (1970), who observed approximately simultaneous filling. Their angiograms, however, mainly covered the area slightly central to the equator, where the difference in time between choroidal and retinal filling is less marked, or even absent.
-   The flush of the choriocapillaris is less intensive in the periphery than in the posterior pole. Particularly anterior to the equator, the fluorescence of the choriocapillaris is substantially less marked than posterior to the equator. This phenomenon probably results in part from the less intensive circulation in the periphery. It has been established anatomically that the structure of the peripheral choriocapillaris is less dense and coarser than that in the posterior pole, and that a larger area is supplied from a single arteriole (Shimizu and Ujiie, 1976).

The phenomenon of hypofluorescence of the choriocapillaris anterior to the equator is probably accentuated by optical factors. Even in complete mydriasis it is usually inevitable that part of the incident light from the fundus camera fails to enter through the pupil of the eye. Partly because of this, the illumination of the most peripheral portion of the fundus is weaker than that of the region posterior to the equator, and consequently the peripheral choriocapillaris is depicted as relatively hypofluorescent. With a few modern cameras it is possible to adapt the shape of the illumination pupil optically to the requirements of peripheral fundus photography.

We were unable to confirm the report that the peripheral choriocapillaris is entirely invisible on the fluorescein angiogram (Bec et al., 1980).

*Retina*

— The blood flow in all vessels of the equatorial retina is significantly slower than that in the posterior fundus. This has its consequences for fluorescein angiography. The interval between exposures can be longer than in angiography of the posterior pole, but the series of exposures should be continued longer. Not infrequently, filling of small peripheral vascular branches is still observed even after a full minute. When late exposures are omitted, it may be erroneously concluded that a perfusion disorder of the peripheral retina is involved.
— On the fluorescein angiogram, the peripheral vascular bed is less dense than that in the posterior pole; and the periarterial capillary-free zones are wider.
— As a result of the abovementioned optical aberrations, the photograph is usually only partly in sharp definition. That part of the photograph that depicts the most peripheral part of the fundus usually shows the least definition and the least contrast. This phenomenon can produce the erroneous impression that the peripheral retina is poorly perfused, or not at all.

The visibility of peripheral retinal vessels on the angiogram can vary widely in normal eyes. These differences are in part caused by variations in the background fluorescence of the choroid. The darker the latter appears, the more readily can the retinal vascular bed be distinguished.

On the fluorescein angiogram of the peripheral fundus, the following features should be regarded as abnormal:
— Any leakage from retinal vessels.
— Non-perfusion of the peripheral retina.

PART II

DISTURBED DEVELOPMENT OF THE PERIPHERAL RETINAL
VESSELS

CHAPTER 3

# CLINICAL STUDIES OF FAMILIES WITH DOMINANT EXUDATIVE VITREORETINOPATHY

## 3.1 Materials and methods

The probands of seven of the nine families with DEVR had been referred to our department in view of their eye abnormalities. In none of them had the diagnosis DEVR been established prior to the investigation at our institute. The probands of two families (the F family and the I family) were not patients of our department. All the members of the various families examined were of Dutch nationality. The majority were living in the eastern part of The Netherlands.

The ophthalmological examinations mentioned in this thesis were performed by the methods and with the aid of the equipment specified below.

*Slit-lamp examination*

In most cases this examination was made using the Rodenstock type RD 2000 slit lamp. Contact lens examinations were made with a Haag Streit three-mirror contact lens according to Goldman. Like the photographic and fluorescein-angiographic examinations, this examination was performed in maximal mydriasis. The mydriatics used were usually 0.5% tropicamide and 5% phenylephrine, administered several times in combination.

*Fundus photography and fluorescein angiography*

For photographic and fluorescein-angiographic examination of the fundus we used a Kowa fundus camera type RC-W and a Zeiss fundus camera. For fluorescein angiography the Kowa camera was equipped with Spectrotech filters type SE-40 and SB-50, and the Zeiss camera with Zeiss filters type 500 and 520. Some exposures were made with the Canon CF60Z fundus camera.

Nearly all steroscopic photographs were obtained by making two or more exposures in succession and, in the intervals, slightly shifting the camera in the horizontal plane. Stereo-pairs were later selected from the available exposures. Photographs of the peripheral fundus were obtained by slanting the fundus camera without use of a mirror contact lens or other optical aids. For fluorescein angiography generally about 5 ml of a 20% solution of sodium fluorescein was rapidly injected into a vein of the forearm.

Colour photographs were made on Kodachrome 64 ASA film, with a green filter interposed in many instances. Kodak tri X film was used for fluorescein angiography. The latter film was developed in Promicrol with the aid of a Mafi rotary processor.

### Measurement of visual fields

The visual fields were examined with the aid of a photometrically standardized Goldmann perimeter (V-4 test object: 1000 asb; eyeball illumination: 31.5 asb). We used only the kinetic method.

### Electroretinography and electro-oculography

A photoscopic and a scotopic electroretinogram (ERG) was obtained in several cases; electro-oculography (EOG) was usually performed in the same cases. Apparatus and set-up for this procedure have been described by Thijssen et al. (1974).

### Dark adaptation

Dark adaptation was examined in some cases, using the Goldmann-Weekers adaptometer. In all cases dark adaptation of both eyes was examined simultaneously in mydriasis. The examination was continued for 25 minutes.

### Colour vision

Colour vision tests used were the Tokyo Medical College test (TMC), the American Optical Hardy Rand Rittler test (AOHRR), the Ishihara test (1970 version), the New colour test, Panel D-15, desaturated Panel D-15, the Farnsworth 100 HUE test, and the test with Nagel's anomaloscope (type 11). The source of illumination consisted of six Philips fluorescent tubes, colour 57, colour rendering index 96, providing 1750 lux at the level of the desk.

### Ultrasonography

Ultrasonographic examination of the eyeball was performed in a few instances, mostly involving eyes whose fundus could not be visually examined due to media turbidities. Some eyes with clear media, moreover, were biometrically examined. Ultrasonography was carried out with the Kretz unit type 7200 MA (A-scan) and the Bronson-Turner unit (B-scan).

## 3.2 The A family

*Introduction*

This was the first family in The Netherlands in which DEVR was diagnosed. A family study was performed at the Nijmegen University Department of Ophthalmology by Nijhuis, who described some fluorescein-angiographic findings obtained in this family (Nijhuis et al., 1979).

In 1979 and 1980, virtually all affected family members known at that time were re-examined by me, along with a number of those in whom no or only dubious changes had been found. Ophthalmological examinations were also made of a number of persons not previously examined. In this way the pedigree was extended.

*Proband V-25 (16-06-56)*

*History*

At age 3, this female patient was referred to our Department by the family doctor, who suspected a divergent eye position. The child's general health was good. There was no history of prematurity or neonatal oxygen administration.

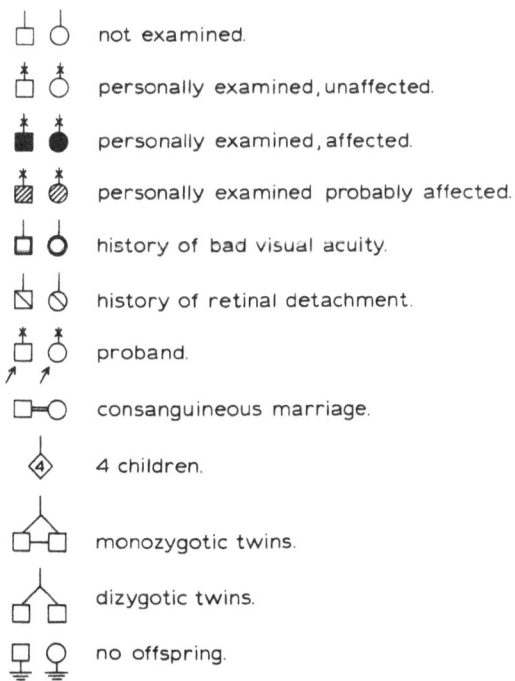

Figure 3. Explanation of symbols used in the pedigrees of the families with DEVR (A through I).

24

Pregnancy and parturition had been normal.

Several persons in the family reportedly had eye anomalies: both parents had strabismus and reportedly poor visual acuity in one eye. Similar anomalies were believed to be present in a number of aunts and paternal cousins of this patient.

*Ophthalmological examination (age 3)*

Visual acuity      Not accurately determinable.

Eye position       Straight. Conspicuously wide positive kappa
                   angle.

Media              ODS: Clear.

Fundi              ODS: In both posterior poles abnormal configur-
                   ation of the retinal vessels with temporal ectopia
                   of the macula. No retinal detachment.

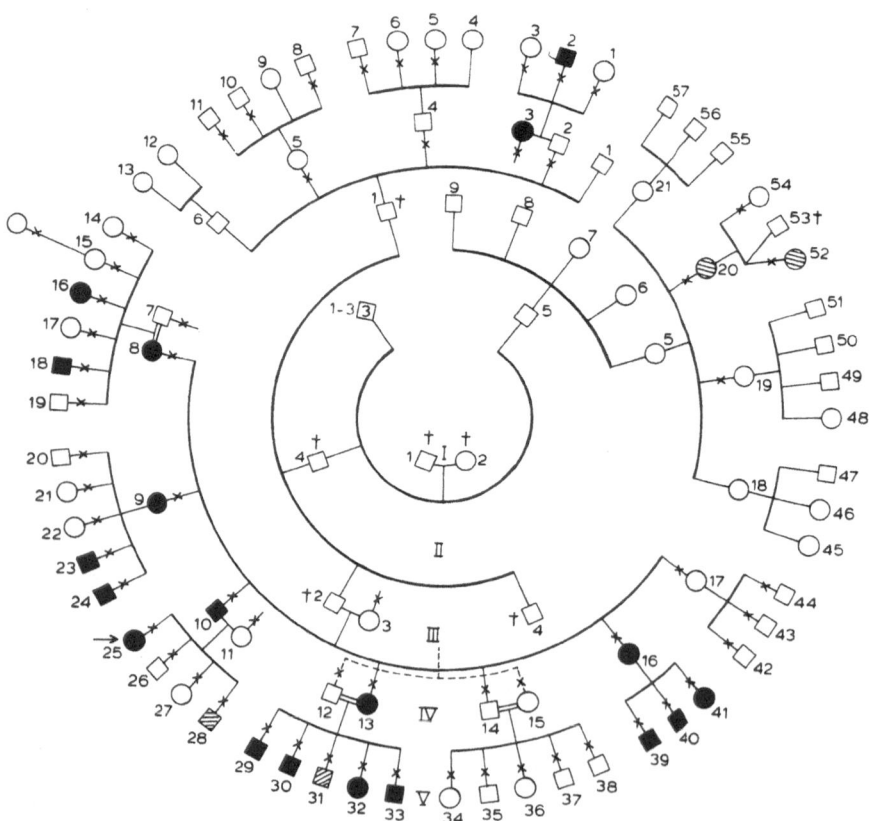

Figure 4. Pedigree of the A family.

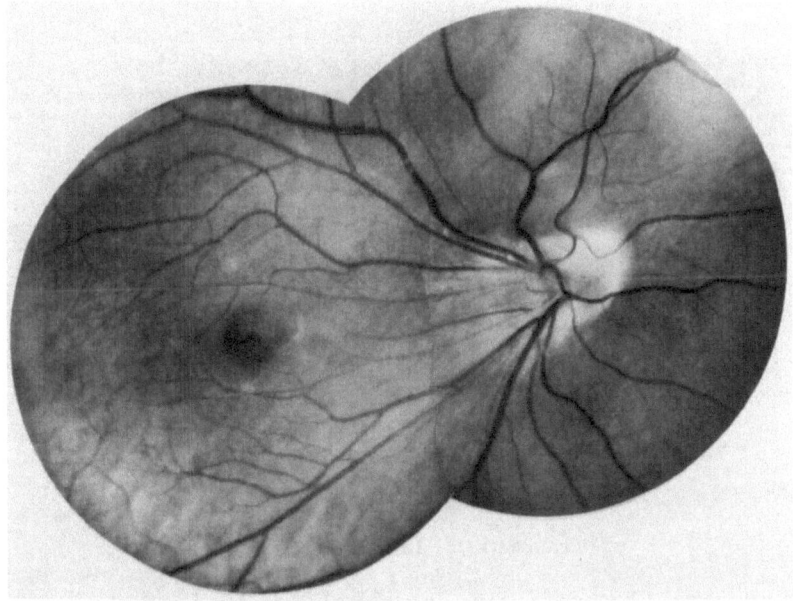

Figure 5 (V-25). Right eye. Stretched course of the retinal vessels and temporal ectopia of the macula.

*Ophthalmological examination (age 8)*

| | |
|---|---|
| Visual acuity | VOD: cyl. − 2.5 axis 0° 0.6. |
| | VOS: cyl. − 3.0 axis 0° 0.6. |

*Ophthalmological examination (age 10)*

| | |
|---|---|
| Visual acuity | VODS: As before. |
| Binocular vision | Present. |
| Media | Vitreous turbidities, especially anterior to the peripheral fundus OS. |
| Fundi | ODS: Abnormally stretched course of the retinal vessels from the disc to the inferior temporal sector, with ectopia of both maculae in the same direction (Figure 5). In the left posterior pole the vascular deformation is more marked than in the right, and the features of so-called dragged disc have developed (Figure 6). Cicatrices and some retinoschisis in the temporal periphery of both fundi. |

*Ophthalmological examination (age 18)*

Patient had again been referred by her own ophthalmologist, who had found severely reduced visual acuity OS due to retinal detachment.

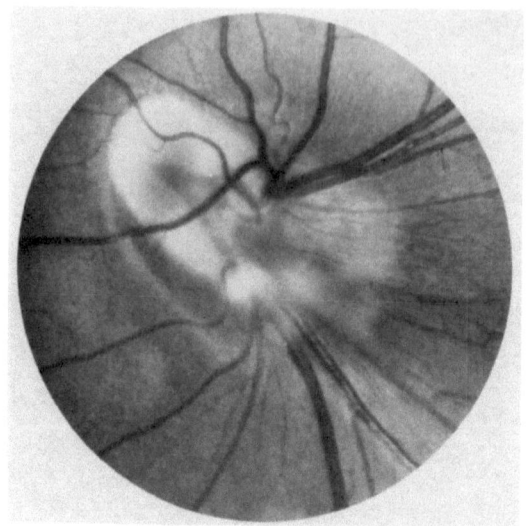

Figure 6 (V-25). Left eye. Dragged disc.

| | |
|---|---|
| Visual acuity | VOD: S + 0.5/Cyl. − 3.5 axis 5° 0.8. |
| | VOS: Cyl. − 2.5 axis 170° 1/60. |
| Anterior segments | OD: Normal. |
| | OS: Some cortical posterior cataract. |
| Fundi | OD: Unchanged. |
| | OS: Retina detached around the centre of the posterior pole, but partly in situ slightly inferior to the centre of the posterior pole. This part is surrounded by a circular fold of detached retina which protrudes in the vitreous (Figure 7). |
| Therapy | Operative treatment of OS does not seem feasible. The temporal periphery of the fundus OD is treated by Argon laser coagulation in the region anterior to the equator, in several sessions. The superior nasal sector is likewise coagulated. No complications. |

*Ophthalmological examination (age 20)*

| | |
|---|---|
| Visual acuity | VOD: Cyl. − 2.5 axis 5° 0.5. |
| | VOS: 1/60. |
| Fluorescein angiogram | OD: Deformation of the retinal vessels in the posterior pole due to traction from the temporal periphery and ectopia of the macula, which is likewise deformed. Fairly marked diffuse leakage from all retinal vessels in and around the posterior |

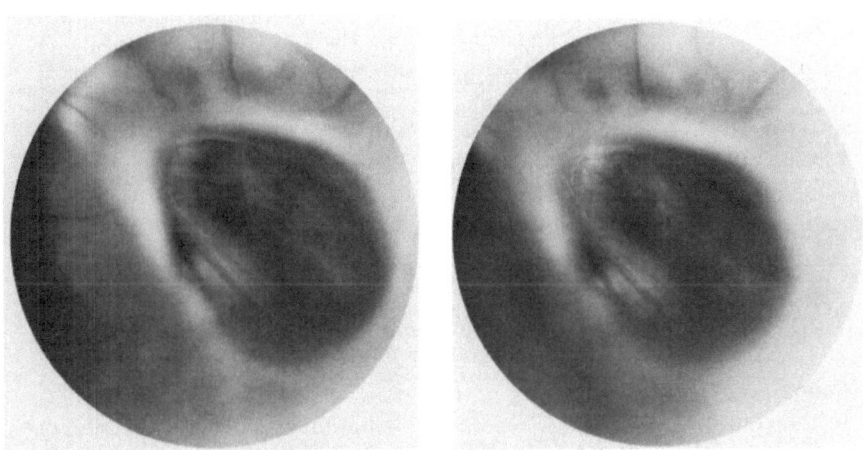

Figure 7 (V-25). Stereo-photograph. Left eye, 8 years later. The retina around the centre of the posterior pole is elevated in a circular fold.

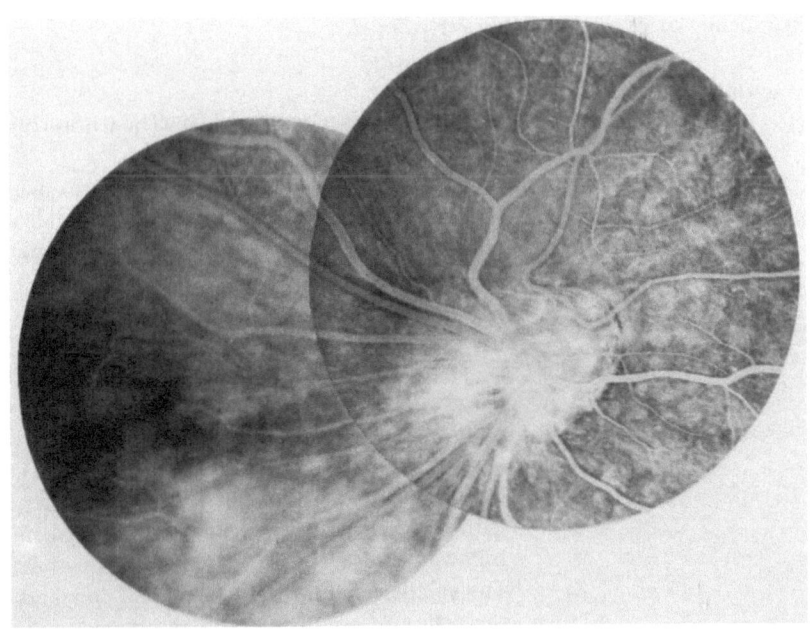

Figure 8 (V-25). Right eye. Fluorescein angiogram. Diffuse leakage in the posterior pole in the late phase.

pole (Figure 8). Many coagulation scars are visible anterior to the equator. No visible neovascularization.

| | |
|---|---|
| ERG | OD: Scot. b-wave $180\,\mu V$; OS: $30\,\mu V$. |
| EOG | OD: Lp/Dt: 307; Dt: $163\,\mu V$. |
| | OS: Lp/Dt: 79; Dt: $63\,\mu V$. |
| Dark adaptation | Binocular: Slightly disturbed cone adaptation. |
| Colour vision | OD: Slightly disturbed: too many errors in the 100 Hue test; the Nagel anomaloscope reveals a shift to red. |
| | OS: Not determinable. |

*Course*

In the course of 1977 and 1978, signs of irritation are found in both anterior segments, without many subjective complaints. A positive flare is found bilaterally, and some cells are found in the aqueous humour. Intraocular pressure is not increased. The symptoms are treated with eye drops (1% dexamethasone phosphate and 1% atropine sulphate).

*Ophthalmological examination in January 1980 (age 23)*

| | |
|---|---|
| Visual acuity | VOD: S − 0.5/Cyl. − 2.75 axis 175° 0.5. |
| | VOS: No light perception |
| Intraocular pressure | OD: 12 mm Hg. |
| | OS: 8 mm Hg. |
| Anterior segments | OD: Normal. |
| | OS: Many posterior synechiae. The lens is totally cataractous and shows calcifications. |
| Vitreous | OD: Filamentous retrolental structure, behind which a large optically empty space is visible as a result of detachment of a large part of the posterior vitreous membrane. |
| | OS: Not assessable due to the cataract. |
| Fundi | OD: The vascular pattern of the posterior pole is as previously described, and seems unchanged (Figure 5). The attachment of the posterior vitreous membrane to the retina is clearly visible near the nasal equator. Abnormally stretched configuration of the postequatorial retinal vessels with a radial course. The retinal vessels can be followed as far as the extreme nasal periphery. The vascularization of the temporal periphery of the retina is not readily assessable due to many coagulation scars. No visible neovascularizations, retinal defects or exudates. |

| | |
|---|---|
| Fluorescein angiogram | OD: Features unchanged since October 1976. |
| Ultrasonography | OD: Axis length 21 mm (A-scan) |
| | OS: Axis length 20 mm. Echoes throughout the vitreous space. The sclera gives high reflexes suggestive of calcifications. |
| Therapy | For cosmetic reasons the strabismus OS is corrected by retroposition of the external rectus muscle (10 mm) and resection of the internal recturs muscle (5 mm). Subsequently the white, cataractous lens is excised. The cosmetic result is satisfactory. |

*General examination*

No general complaints other than periodical headaches. In view of the eye abnormalities the patient was paediatrically examined at age 8; no abnormalities were found. The patient is of rather gracile habitus; the maxilla is rather high. General physical examination reveals no other abnormalities.

*Internal and haematological examination (1979)*

| | |
|---|---|
| Radiological findings | Normal chest X-ray. |
| Laboratory findings | ESR 6 mm in one hour. |
| | Hb 9.2 mmol/l. |
| | WBC 6.5 × $10^9$/l; normal differentation. |
| | Platelets 266 × $10^9$/l. |
| Enzymes | SGOT 16 U/l. |
| | SGPT 14 U/l. |
| | LDH normal. |
| | Alkaline phosphatase normal. |
| Electrolytes | Na 138 mmol/l. |
| | K 3.6 mmol/l. |
| | Cl 105 mmol/l. |
| | $HCO_3$ 25.0 mmol/l. |
| Other serum values | Urea 3.3 mmol/l. |
| | Creatinine 68 μmol/l. |
| | Glucose 4.2 mmol/l. |
| | Protein spectrum normal. |
| Coagulation | The bleeding time was increased on two occasions and normal on one occasion. Otherwise normal. |
| Serology | Toxoplasmosis: negative complement fixation test and immunofluorescence. |
| Oxygen dissociation | Normal oxygen affinity of haemoglobin. |

## Summary and conclusion

A female patient with marked bilateral vitreoretinal changes which at the age of about 15 led to traction detachment in the left eye, with subsequent total vitreous organization and cataract. Although the primary vascular lesions can no longer be accurately assessed due to previous treatments and media turbidities, they are consistent with a diagnosis of severe dominant exudative vitreoretinopathy.

## Subject IV-10 (28-04-23)

### History

The proband's father had reportedly suffered from poor vision in the left eye since early childhood. This eye had shown strabismus, for which corrective surgery had been performed at an early age. There was no history of premature birth.

### Ophthalmological examination

| | |
|---|---|
| Visual acuity | VOD: S − 2.0 0.6. |
| | VOS: 1/60, good light projection. |
| Cycloplegic refraction | OD: S − 4.0. |
| | OS: S + 3.0. |
| Intraocular pressure | OD: 18 mm Hg. |
| | OS: 14 mm Hg. |
| Eye position | Divergent strabismus OS, about 10°. |
| Anterior segments | ODS: No abnormalities other than slight cortical opacities in the lens of OD. |
| Vitreous | OD: Normal structure; Delicate white particles. |
| | OS: Syneresis. Delicate white particles. Preretinal vitreous membrane. |
| Fundi | OD: Abnormal stretching of a few small vascular branches which extend from the disc in temporal direction immediately above and below the macula. Many vascular branches terminate abruptly just anterior to the temporal equator. The nonperfused retinal periphery shows slight white without pressure. No defects, exudates or neovascularizations. |
| | OS: The vascular configuration of the posterior pole is virtually the same as that in OD. An irregular zone of atrophy of pigment epithelium and choriocapillaris is seen temporal to the disc. Temporal to the posterior pole, the preretinal vitreous contains a membrane which shows some defects and, central to the equator, attaches to the |

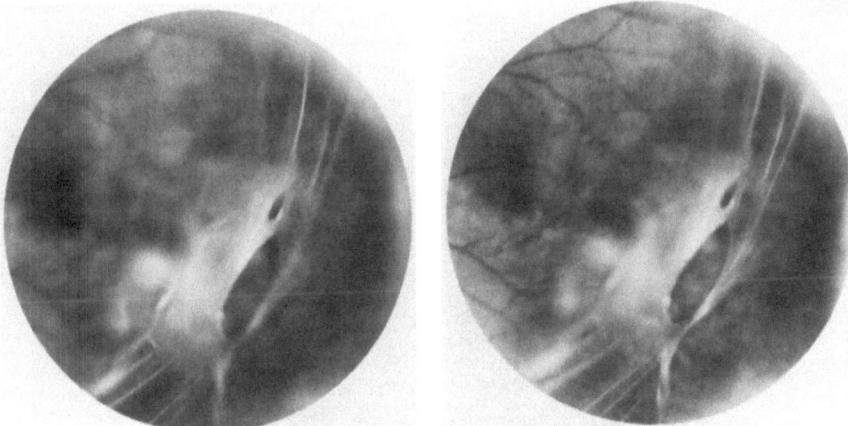

Figure 9 (IV-10). Stereo-photograph. Left eye. Attachment of vitreous membrane to the retina temporal to the posterior pole.

retina (Figure 9). In this area the retina contains numerous vascular branches, some of which are tortuous. These terminate in a slightly meandering liminal zone. The retina peripheral to this zone is avascular. No retinal defects, exudates or neovascularizations.

Fluorescein angiogram    ODS: Significant leakage from the retinal vascular branches in the temporal equator region.

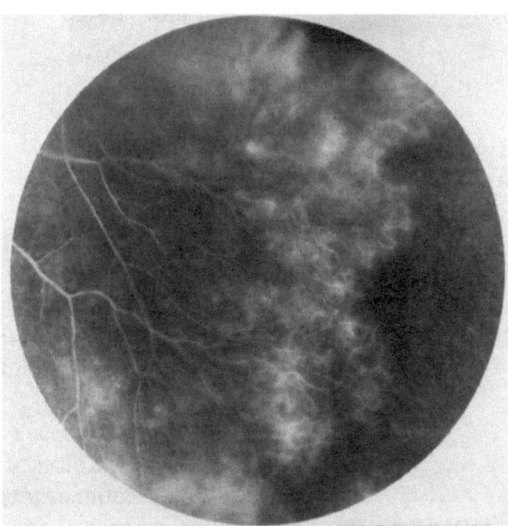

Figure 10 (IV-10). Left eye. Late phase of the angiogram shows non-perfusion of the peripheral retina and fluorescein leakage from numerous vascular branches in the equatorial retina.

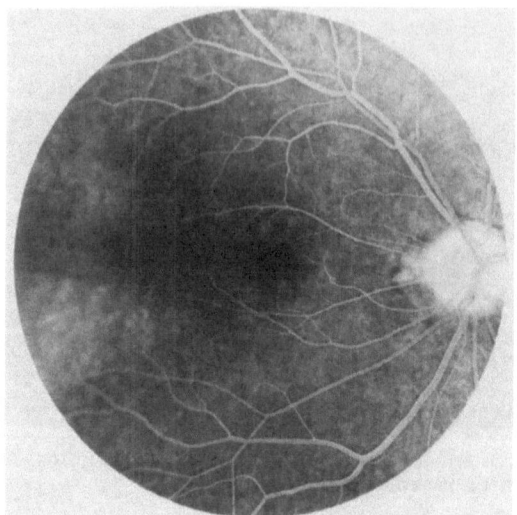

Figure 11 (IV-10). Right eye. Late phase of the angiogram shows some slight leakage from macular capillaies and hyperfluorescence of the disc.

Non-perfusion of the temporal retinal periphery (Figure 10). The late exposures show slight leakage from capillaries in both posterior poles, especially around the macula, and striking hyperfluorescence of both discs (Figure 11).

ERG  
Scotopic b-wave OD: 210 $\mu$V.  
Scotopic b-wave OS: 185 $\mu$V.  
Photopic b-wave OD: 60 $\mu$V.  
Photopic b-wave OS: 50 $\mu$V.

EOG  
OD: Lp/Dt 233; DT 338 $\mu$V.  
OS: Lp/Dt 153; Dt 450 $\mu$V.

Dark adaptation  
Binocular: Subnormal.

Colour vision  
OD: Normal.  
OS: Disturbed: red-green defect HRR.

Ultrasonography  
Axis length OD: 21.5–23 mm.  
Axis length OS: 21.5–23 mm.

A-scan  
In both eyes, the eye axis length varies slightly when measured at different sites of the posterior pole.

B-scan  
OD: In vertical section the sclera of the posterior pole proves to show a strikingly marked curvature. The horizontal section reveals an insufficient curvature on the temporal, and a more or less normal curvature on the nasal side of the posterior pole.

OS: In the vertical plane the curvature of the posterior pole is excessive, and in the horizontal section the curvature of the sclera is more marked on the temporal than on the nasal side.

## Follow-up

Repetition of the ophthalmological examination and fluorescein angiography 36 months after the first examination, failed to reveal any significant changes.

## Conclusion

The vascular changes of both fundi are entirely consistent with a diagnosis of DEVR.

## Subject IV-11

Ophthalmological examination of the mother of V-25 revealed amblyopia of the left eye as a result of anisometropia. Both fundi were normal.

## Conclusion

No manifestations of DEVR.

## Subject V-28 (17-07-64)

## History

Sustained severe perforation of the left eyeball when falling in glass at the age of 1 year. The eye has since become totally atrophic and blind. No history of premature birth or neonatal oxygen administration.

## Ophthalmological examination

| Visual acuity | VOD: 1.25 uncorrected. |
| | VOS: No light perception. |
| Anterior segments | OD: Normal. |
| | OS: Dish prosthesis. |
| Vitreous | OD: Nothing unusual apart from a few delicate white particles. |
| Fundi | OD: The posterior pole presents an entirely normal appearance. A few tortuous venous branches are visible in the temporal equator region. However, the vascularization of the equator region seems complete, and no circumscribed transition to a non-vascularized retinal periphery is visible. A small peripheral retinal defect is visible near 7 o'clock. No other changes are observed. |
| Fluorescein angiogram | OD: Slightly tortuous vascular branches in the temporal sector of the equator; fluorescein leak- |

age from small venous branches occurs at some sites near 8 o'clock and 9 o'clock (Figure 12). No demonstrable disorder of peripheral retinal perfusion. The late exposures show no leakage from perimacular capillaries, but the disc is slightly hyperfluorescent.

| | |
|---|---|
| EGR | OD: Scotopic b-wave 205 $\mu$V. |
| | Photopic b-wave 50 $\mu$V. |
| EOG | OD: Lp/Dt 219; Dt 400 $\mu$V. |
| Dark adaptation | OD: Normal. |
| Colour vision | OD: Normal. |

*Follow-up*

At ophthalmological examination 36 months after the first examination, visual acuity, media and fundus of the right eye were unchanged. The fluorescein angiogram was likewise identical.

*Conclusion*

In this 14-year-old boy, whose left eye had been destroyed in an accident, the periphery of the fundus OD showed minimal ophthalmoscopic and angiographic lesions which may have resulted from a very slight manifestation of DEVR. However, the diagnosis cannot be established with certainty.

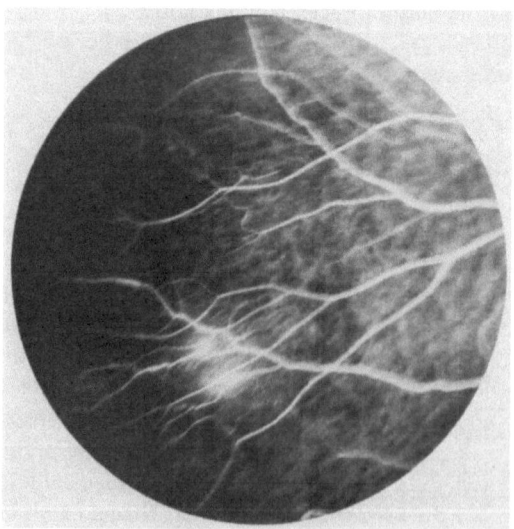

Figure 12 (V-28). Right eye. Fluorescein leakage from a few equatorial retinal vessels in the late phase.

*Subject IV-8 (10-06-19)*

*History*
No visual complaints. Good general health. No history of premature birth.
This subject is the female partner in a consanguineous marriage.

*Ophthalmological examination*

| | |
|---|---|
| Visual acuity | VOD: S + 1.9/Cyl. − 2.25 axis 90° 1.0. |
| | VOS: S + 1.75/Cyl. − 1.75 axis 85° 1.0. |
| Intraocular pressure | ODS: 12 mm Hg. |
| Eye position | Straight. |
| Anterior segments | ODS: Both corneae are somewhat hazy due to minimal light scatter in the endothelium. No evidence of cornea guttata. |
| Vitreous | ODS: Normal structure. |
| Fundi | ODS: From the disc, the retinal vessels take a slightly stretched course to the inferior temporal sector, with minimal ectopia of both maculae in the same direction. The temporal retinal vessels terminate in numerous small ramifications near the equator, and peripheral to this the retina is slightly whitish and entirely avascular (Figure 13). |
| Fluorescein angiogram | ODS: Significant leakage from the small vessels near the temporal equator (Figure 14). Non-perfusion of the retina, at least on the temporal side. |

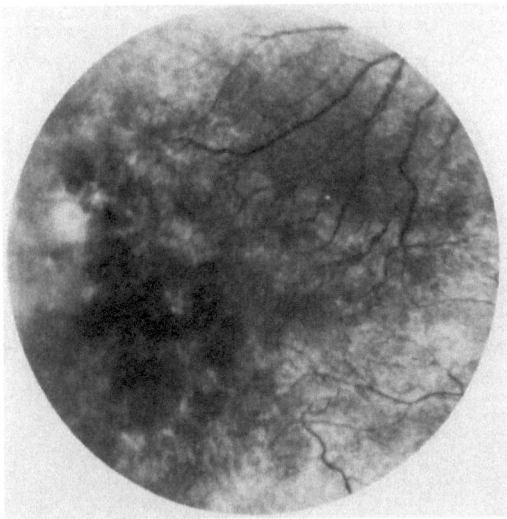

Figure 13 (IV-8). Right eye. Numerous retinal vessels localized in the temporal equatorial zone.

The avascular zone of the retina extends in central direction near the horizontal meridian and thus forms a wedge-shaped notch between the smallest branches of the superior and inferior temporal vessels (Figures 14 and 15). No neovascularization. The early exposures of both posterior poles reveal minimal dilations of the perimacular capillaries; late exposures show unmistakable leakage from these vessels. Some fluorescein leakage is visible also at the discs.

| | |
|---|---|
| Visual fields (Goldmann) | Slight absolute limitation of the visual field in the superior nasal quadrant ODS. |
| ERG | OD: Scotopic b-wave: $170\,\mu V$. |
| | OS: Scotopic b-wave: $230\,\mu V$. |
| | OD: Photopic b-wave: $50\,\mu V$. |
| | OS: Photopic b-wave: $50\,\mu V$. |
| EOG | OD: Lp/Dt 168; Dt $350\,\mu V$. |
| | OS: Lp/Dt 148; Dt $725\,\mu V$. |
| Dark adaptation | Binocular: Slightly subnormal. |
| Colour vision | ODS: Virtually normal; a few non-specific errors in the Panel D-15 test. |

*Follow-up*

Examinations of visual acuity, media and fundi, and fluorescein angiography of posterior poles and temporal peripheral fundi were repeated after 36 months. The results were unchanged.

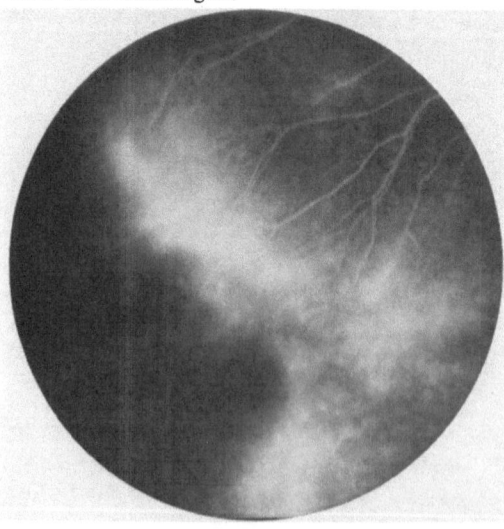

Figure 14 (IV-8). Fluorescein angiogram of the same region as in Figure 13. Fluorescein leakage from the branches in the zone adjacent to the avascular retina.

*Conclusion*
Bilateral changes of the retinal vasculature, consistent with a diagnosis of DEVR.

*Subject V-16 (09-10-53)*

*History*
Visual acuity in the right eye has always been poor. During the school years, some time was devoted to treatment by occulsion of the left eye. Strabismus operations were performed at age 10 and age 12. The right eye became totally blind by about age 20. No history of premature birth or neonatal oxygen administration.

*Ophthalmological examination*

| | |
|---|---|
| Visual acuity | VOD: No light perception. |
| | VOS: S − 1.25/Cyl. − 2.0 axis 20° 0.6. |
| Intraocular pressure | ODS: 12 mm Hg. |
| Eye position | OD: Convergent strabismus. |
| Anterior segments | OD: The iris shows posterior synaechiae. The aqueous shows a positive flare and contains cells. The lens shows subcapsular posterior and cortical cataract. |
| | OS: Normal. |

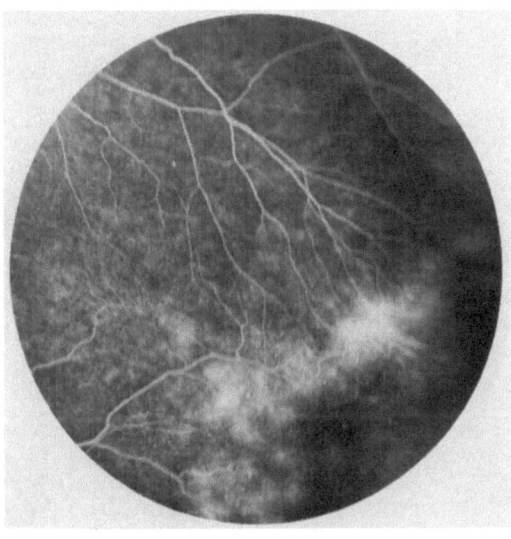

Figure 15 (IV-8). Left eye. Fluorescein angiogram shows the same features as in the right eye.

Vitreous

OD: Many turbidities and membranes throughout the vitreous space.

OS: Normal retrolental vitreous structure. Posterior vitreous detachment with condensations in the posterior vitreous membrane.

Fundi

OD: Large intraretinal and subretinal exudates scattered in the fundus. Particularly in the temporal periphery the retina seems to be lifted (Figure 16). Further fundus details obscured by media turbidities.

OS: The temporal vascular branches of the retina in the posterior pole are slightly stretched. Numerous small ramifications of these vessels are localized central to the temporal equator. Anterior to the equator, they terminate in a rather meandering liminal zone which demarcates the non-vascularized retinal periphery. At the level of this juncture, a small exudate is visible near 3 o'clock. No neovascularizations or retinal defects.

Fluorescein angiogram

OS: Unmistakable leakage from the small retinal vessels localized immediately central to the juncture with the avascular temporal retinal periphery (Figure 17). Fluorescein leakage also occurs in a few more posteriorly localized zones parallel to

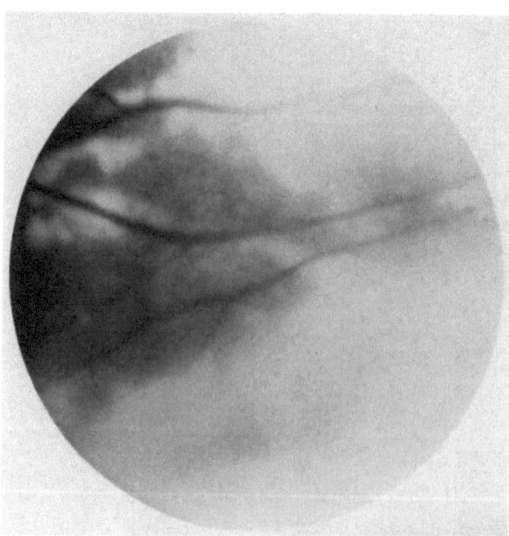

Figure 16 (V-16). Right eye. Large subretinal exudates in the temporal fundus.

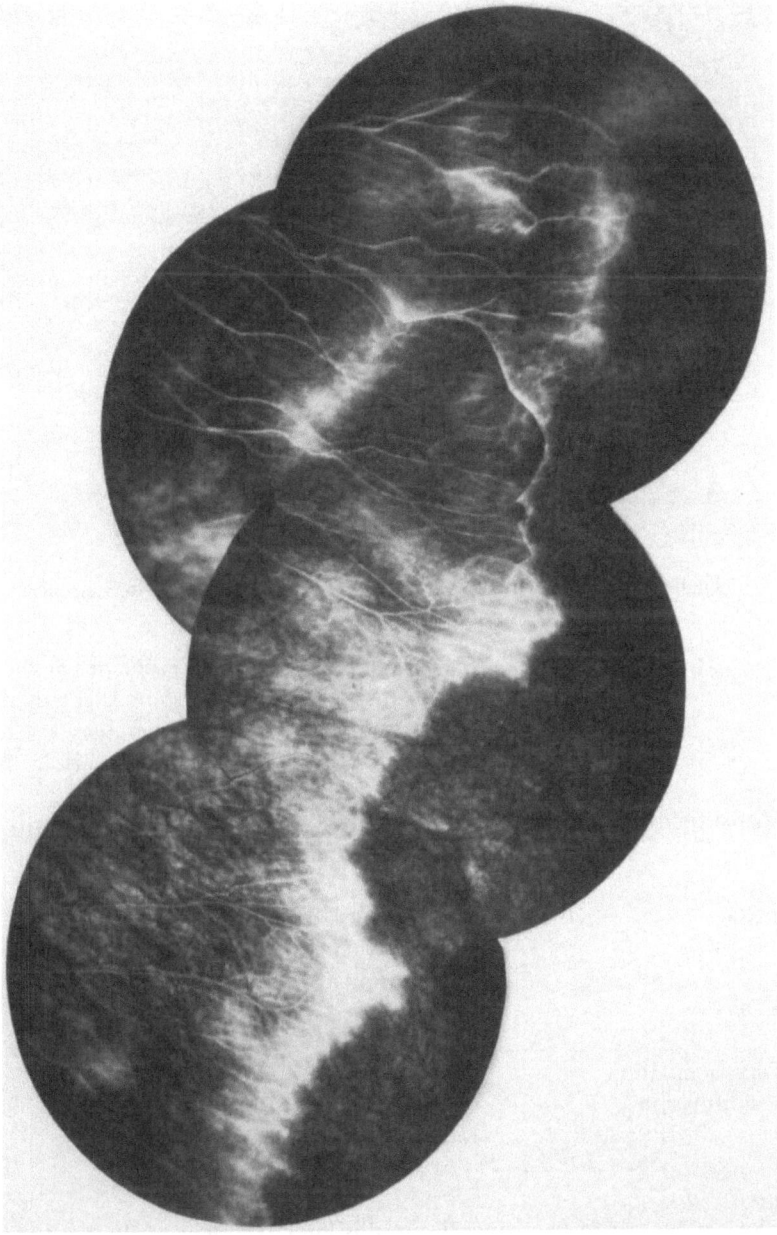

Figure 17 (V-16). Left eye. Late phase of the angiogram shows non-perfusion of the peripheral retina.

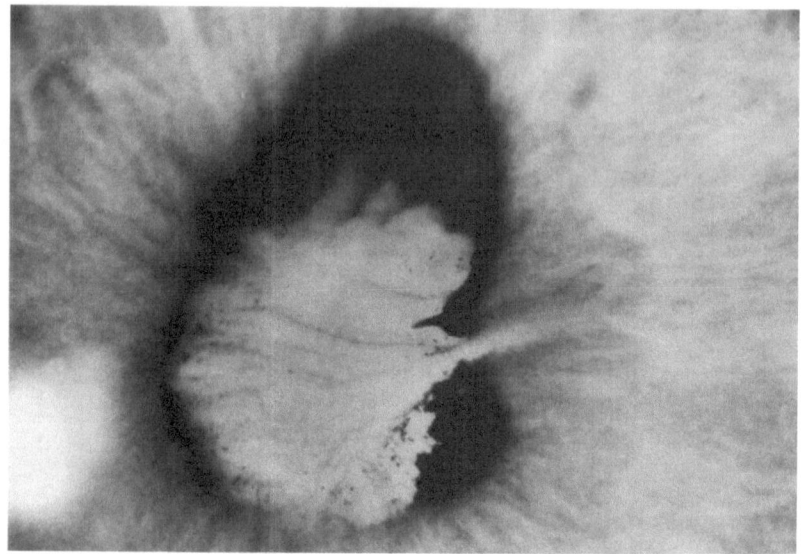

Figure 18 (V-16). Right eye. Complicated cataract with posterior synechiae.

the juncture. Some retinal capillaries at the centre of the posterior pole show slight dilations. Slight fluorescein leakage from these vessels is visible in the late phase, when the disc is hyperfluorescent.

| | |
|---|---|
| Visual fields (Goldmann) | OS: Distinctly diminished central sensitivity, and slight limitation of the III-4 isopter in the nasal visual field. |
| ERG | OD: Not recordable. |
| | OS: Scotopic b-wave: $300\,\mu V$. |
| | Photopic b-wave: $90\,\mu V$. |
| EOG | OD: Reversed polarity; |
| | OS: Lp/Dt 232; Dt $700\,\mu V$. |
| Dark adaptation | OS: Normal. |
| Colour vision | OS: Slightly disturbed. Slight shift to red on Nagels anomaloscope. |

*Follow-up*

The patient was re-examined 36 months later. The lens of the right eye had meanwhile become totally cataractous, showing a shrunken anterior lens capsule connected with the iris via synechiae (Figure 18). The fundus could no longer be examined. Visual acuity, media and fundus of the left eye were unchanged, as was the fluorescein angiogram.

*Conclusion*

Bilateral fundus changes with loss of light perception in the right eye as a result of exudative and tractional retinal detachment. The findings are entirely consistent with a diagnosis of severe DEVR.

*Subject V-18 (07-08-57)*

*History*

I did not personally examine this family member, because he was on active service as a sailor. In December 1975 he was examined by Nijhuis, who supplied me with the fundus photographs. There were no visual complaints. No history of premature birth or neonatal oxygen administration.

*Ophthalmological examination*

| | |
|---|---|
| Visual acuity | VOD: 1.0 uncorrected. |
| | VOS: 1.0 uncorrected. |
| Eye position | Unknown |
| Anterior segments | ODS: Normal. |
| Vitreous | ODS: No distinct abnormalities. |
| Fundi | ODS: The temporal ramifications of the retinal vessels take a slightly stretched course in temporal direction. Particularly the temporal sector of the peripheral fundus shows extensive white without pressure, and some snailtracks in the area anterior |

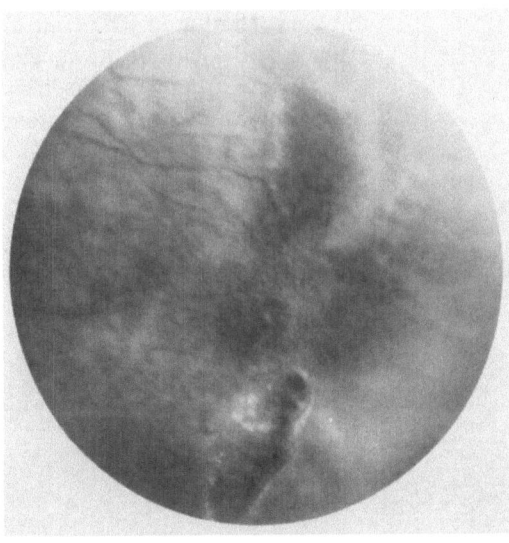

Figure 19 (V-18). Left eye. The avascular retinal periphery shows white without pressure and snailtrack-like lesions.

to the equator. Central to these seemingly avascular areas, the retinal vessels terminate in numerous ramifications (Figure 19).

*Conclusion*

The vascular changes in both fundi are consistent with a diagnosis of DEVR.

*Subject IV-9 (29-09-21)*

*History*

No visual complaints. The birth weight is unknown, but there is no record of premature birth.

*Ophthalmological examination*

| | |
|---|---|
| Visual acuity | VOD: S − 1.75/Cyl. − 1.0 axis 125° 0.6. |
| | VOS: S − 1.0/Cyl. − 1.0 axis 30° 0.8. |
| Intraocular pressure | ODS: 16 mm Hg. |
| Anterior segments | Normal |
| Vitreous | Normal structure, no cells. |
| Fundi | ODS: Slightly stretched course of the retinal vessels in both posterior poles, and probably some ectopia of the maculae in temporal direction. The retinal vessels terminate in small ramifications peripheral to the equator of both fundi, and the extreme periphery of the retina is not perfused in this area. The fundus OD contains a small white exudate at the level of the equator near 8 o'clock. Areas with atrophy of the pigment epithelium and choriocapillaries are scattered in the periphery of both fundi. No retinal defects or neovascularizations. |

*Follow-up*

At examination 36 months later, visual acuity and the features of both fundi were unchanged.

*Conclusion*

Vascular lesions of the retina in both fundi, consistent with a diagnosis of DEVR.

*Subject V-23 (17-07-57)*

*History*

VODS was reportedly slightly diminished from early childhood on. There are complaints of muscae volitantes. No record of premature birth or neonatal oxygen administration.

*Ophthalmological examination*

| | |
|---|---|
| Visual acuity | VOD: S − 4.25 0.5. |
| | VOS: S − 2.75 0.5. |
| Eye position | Straight. |
| Anterior segments | ODS: Normal. |
| Vitreous | ODS: Slight syneresis. |
| Fundi | ODS: Abnormally stretched vessels in both posterior poles with some temporal ectopia of the maculae. In the temporal equator region the retinal vasculature terminates in irregular ramifications. Some of the terminal ramifications are visible as white dendrite-like structures near 9 o'clock in the right fundus (Figure 20). Non-vascularized retinal periphery of the temporal fundus ODS. No exudates or neovascularizations. In the left fundus, the extreme periphery of the retina in the nasal upper quadrant is likewise avascular. |
| Fluorescein angiogram | ODS: Aberrant configuration of the retinal vasculature in both fundi and non-perfusion of the temporal retinal periphery anterior to the equa- |

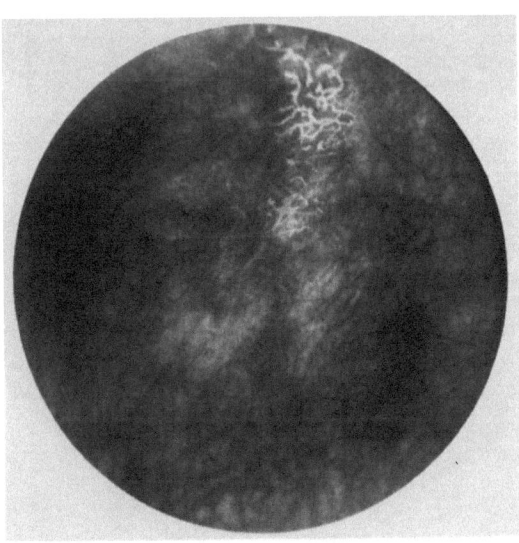

Figure 20 (V-23). Right eye. The terminal ramifications of the retinal vessels are visible as white dendrite-like structures.

44

tor. Near the 9 o'clock meridian OD, the zone of aberrant terminal ramifications deviates slightly in central direction. The white dendrite-like structures in this area are clearly recognizable as the extreme ramifications of the retinal vessels, which evidently have not occluded completely (Figure 21). At one site in the avascular retinal zone, delicate vessels arise from the capillaries of the liminal zone. Late exposures of the posterior pole show hyperfluorescence of both discs but no leakage from the macula.

*Follow-up*
Fundi, visual acuity and media remained unchanged throughout a period of 40 months.

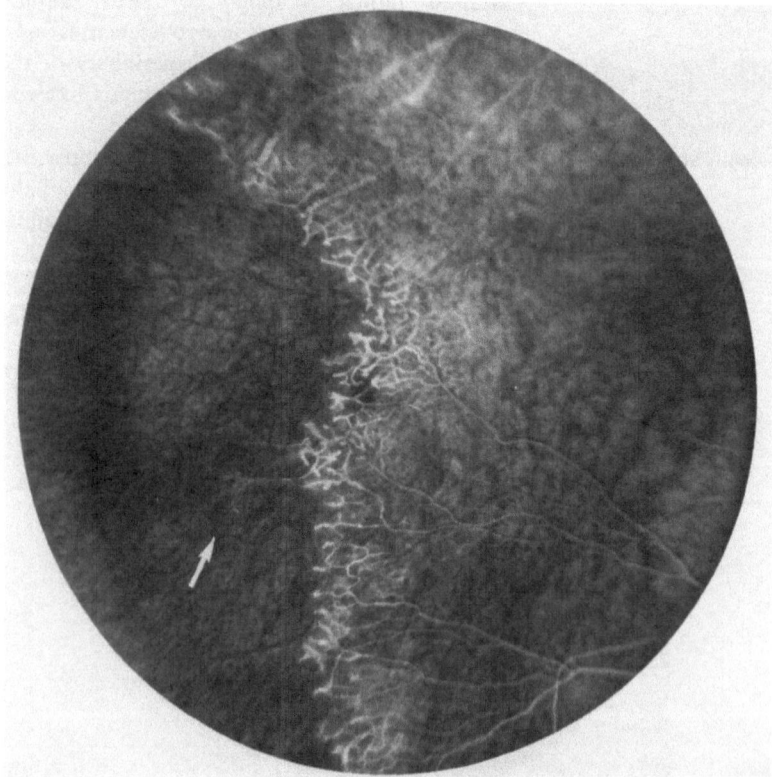

Figure 21 (V-23). Fluorescein angiogram of the same region as in Figure 20. The sclerosed ramifications are partly perfused. At one site, very slender blood vessels enter the avascular retina (arrow).

*Conclusion*
Bilateral vascular lesions of the peripheral retina, consistent with a diagnosis of DEVR.

*Subject V-24 (18-02-62)*

*History*
The left eye has had poor visual acuity and shown divergent strabismus from the start. As a child, this patient sustained a small lesion of the right eye caused by a glass splinter. The birth weight was 3100 g. There is no record of premature birth or neonatal oxygen administration.

*Ophthalmological examination*

| | |
|---|---|
| Visual acuity | VOD: S − 2.0/Cyl. − 1.0 axis 0° 0.8. |
| | VOS: 1/60. |
| Eye position | The left eye, which is hardly capable of any fixation, shows about 15° divergent strabismus. The right eye has an increased positive kappa angle. |
| Anterior segments | OD: Small corneal scar near the inferior temporal limbus. |
| | OS: Normal. |
| Vitreous | OD: Normal. |
| | OS: The central vitreous is of normal structure but contains delicate white particles. Membranes extending in the temporal preretinal vitreous space attach to a white tissue mass localized in the extreme inferior temporal retinal periphery and the pars plana. This mass is connected with the posterior lens capsule near the equator. |
| Fundi | OD: Slight inferior temporal ectopia of the macula. Temporal to the posterior pole the configuration of the retinal vasculature is aberrant: this area comprises numerous ramifying vessels, some of which are tortuous. Their smallest ramifications terminate abruptly near the equator. The avascular retinal periphery shows evidence of degeneration. No exudates or neovascularizations. |
| | OS: This fundus shows the classical features of a falciform retinal fold. The vessels on the disc are distorted in inferior temporal direction. From the disc, a raised radial fold of the retina extends through the centre of the posterior pole to the extreme fundus periphery (Figure 22), where the |

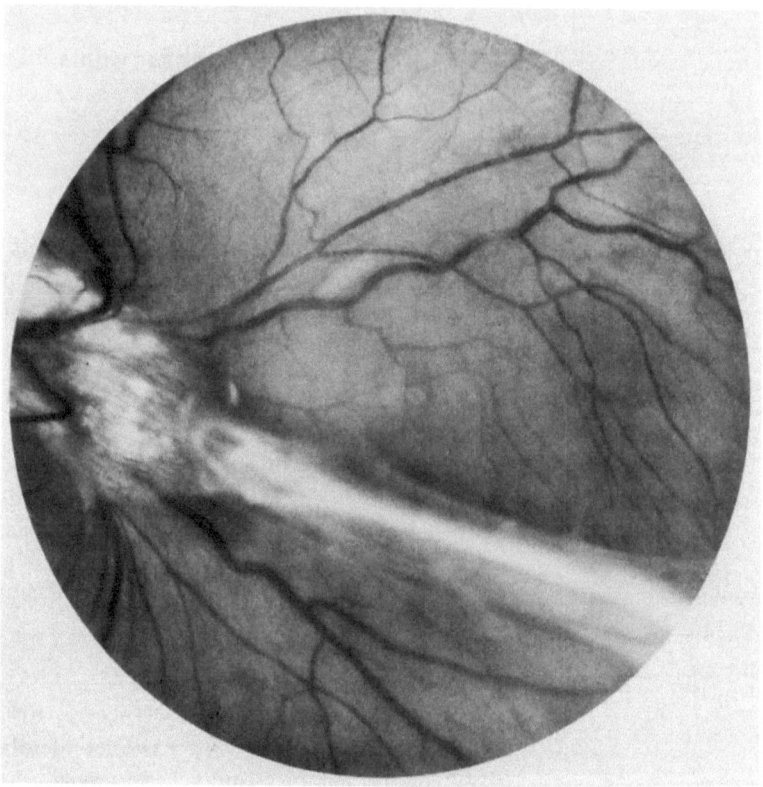

Figure 22 (V-24). Left eye. Falciform retinal fold.

duplicature ends in a white tissue mass which is connected with the lens equator and the pars plana near 4 o'clock. The anterior rim of the retinal fold presents a glittering white appearance, but no remnants of hyaloid vessels are visible. Several retinal vascular branches form a fold in the inferior temporal sector of the posterior pole. In this area a vitreous membrane containing a defect attaches to the apex of the retinal fold (Figure 23).

Fluorescein angiogram

OD: Exposures of the temporal equator region clearly reveal the abrupt terminations of the retinal vasculature and non-perfusion of the peripheral retina. Between the extreme ramifications of the superior and inferior temporal retinal vessels, a V-shaped avascular retinal area extends in central direction (Figure 24). Slightly later ex-

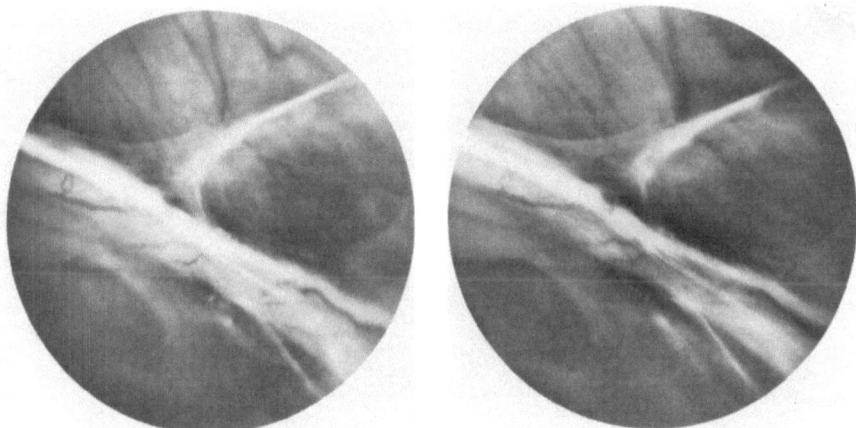

Figure 23 (V-24). Stereo-photograph. Left eye. Attachment of membrane to apex of falciform fold. Several retinal vessels localized in the fold.

posures clearly show leakage from the most peripheral vessels in this region. The disc is hyperfluorescent in the late exposures.

OS: Evident non-perfusion of the peripheral retina in the temporal equator region immediately superior to the falciform fold. The white tissue mass connected with the distal part of the falciform fold shows marked fluorescein leakage (Figure 25).

| | |
|---|---|
| ERG | OD: Scotopic b-wave: $315\,\mu V$. |
| | Photopic b-wave: $100\,\mu V$. |
| | OS: Scotopic b-wave: $310\,\mu V$. |
| | Photopic b-wave: $70\,\mu V$. |
| EOG | OD: Lp/Dt 241; Dt $425\,\mu V$. |
| | OS: Lp/Dt 171; Dt $300\,\mu V$. |
| Dark adaptation | Binocular: Normal. |
| Colour vision | OD: Normal. |
| | OS: Not testable due to poor fixation. |

*General physical examination*

General health has always been good. General physical examination reveals nothing abnormal apart from a slightly elevated palate and some atrophy of the ball of both thumbs.

*Radiological examination*

X-rays of the skull and hands reveal no abnormalities.

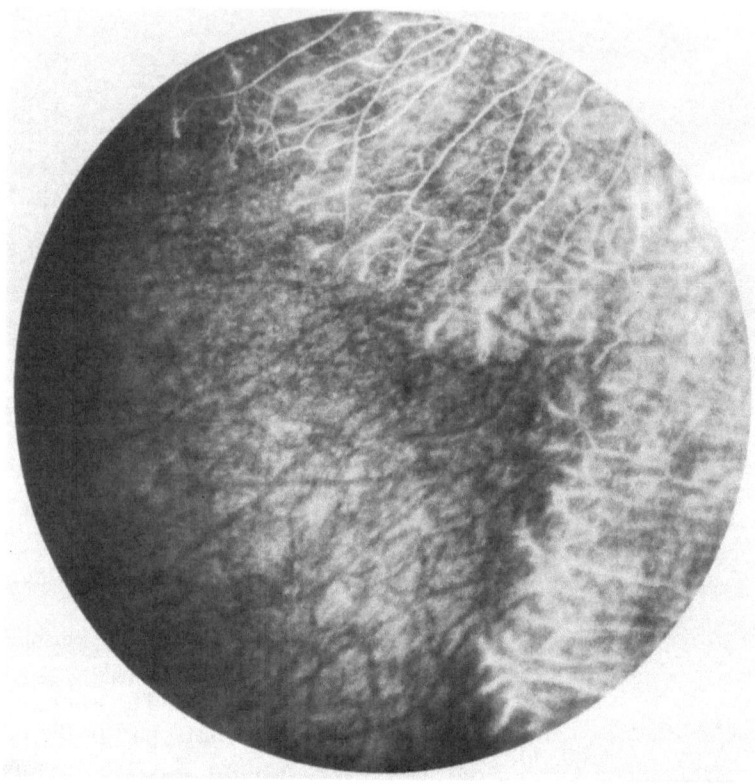

Figure 24 (V-24). Right eye. Fluorescein angiogram. The retinal vasculature terminates in the equatorial zone in small aberrant ramifications. Note the wedge-shaped configuration of the avascular zone.

*Laboratory studies*

| | |
|---|---|
| Blood | Electrolytes, blood gases, liver enzymes, total protein pattern and protein, creatinine, cholesterol and triglyceride values are normal. |
| Urine | Protein and reduction: negative. Sediment: normal. Amino acids: normal. |
| Immunological studies | Lipoproteins, haptoglobin and foetoprotein are normal. IgG and IgA are normal. IgM slightly increased. |
| Haematological studies | ESR, Hb and blood count: Normal values. Foetal haemoglobin: 1% (normal). |
| Blood coagulation studies: | Slightly prolonged Quick and cephalin time at first examination. Slightly increased fibrin breakdown products. Subsequently, however, no distinct abnormalities are found. |

*Follow-up*

The patient was re-examined 38 months after the initial examination. The divergence of the right eye had been cosmetically corrected by a strabismus operation performed elsewhere. There was no evidence of progression of the ophthalmological abnormalities.

*Conclusion*

Bilateral abnormalities of the retinal vasculature consistent with a diagnosis of DEVR, and complicated by falciform retinal detachment in the left eye.

*Subject IV-13 (02-11-24)*

*History*

No visual complaints. A history of premature birth (birth weight about 1500 g). Reportedly no neonatal oxygen administration.

*Ophthalmological examination*

| | |
|---|---|
| Visual acuity | VOD: 1.0, uncorrected. |
| | VOS: 1.0, uncorrected. |
| Eye position | Straight |
| Anterior segments | ODS: Some slight opacities in the anterior and the posterior cortex of both lenses. |
| Vitreous | ODS: Slight syneresis, no cells. |

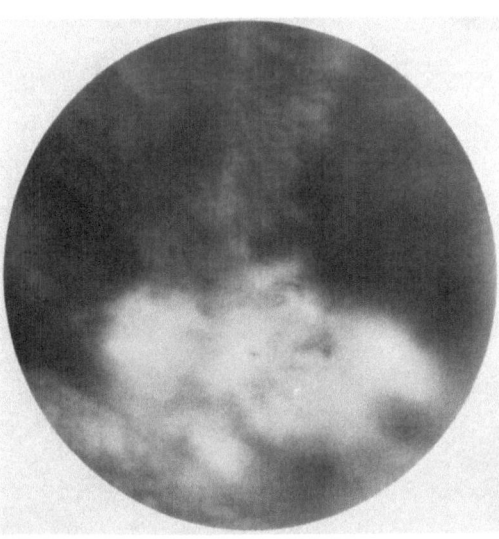

Figure 25 (V-24). Left eye. Fluorescein leakage from the peripheral tissue mass in the late phase of the angiogram. Non-perfusion of the peripheral retina (top right).

| | |
|---|---|
| Fundi | ODS: Virtually normal configuration of the retinal vessels in both posterior poles. Some tortuosity of the small vessels in the midperiphery of both fundi. The temporal fundus periphery in both eyes shows no distinct retinal vessels but there are no visible defects, exudates or degenerative changes. |
| Fluorescein angiogram | OS: Early exposures show minor dilatations of the retinal capillaries in the macular region (Figure 27). The disc is hyperfluorescent and in fact shows slight fluorescein leakage in the immediate vicinity. |
| | OD: The late exposures of the temporal equator region and posterior pole show the same changes as the fundus OS. No neovascularizations. |

*Follow-up*

Re-examination (including fluorescein angiography) after 36 months revealed no progression of the changes.

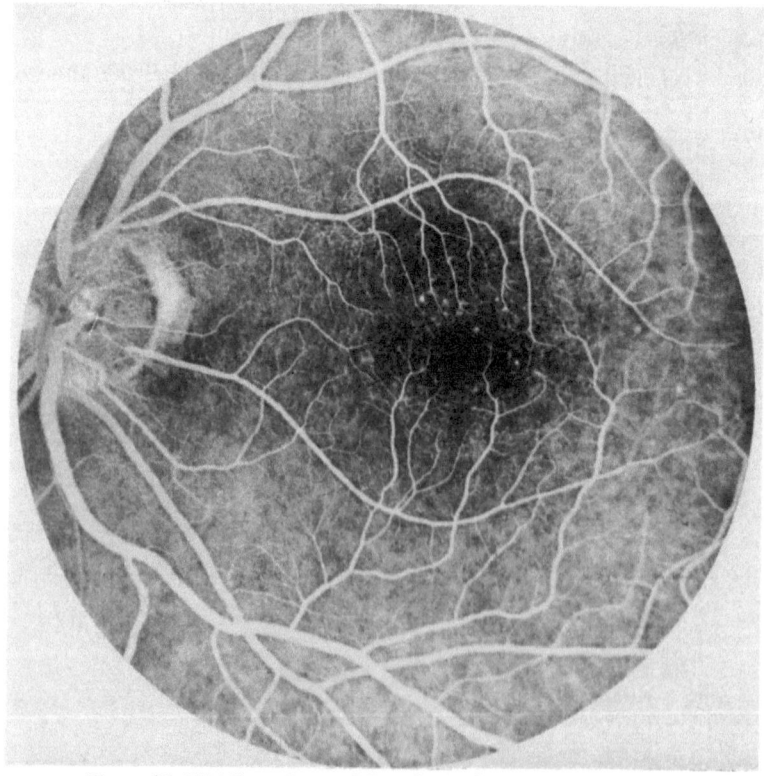

Figure 26 (IV-13). Left eye. Dilatations of macular capillaries.

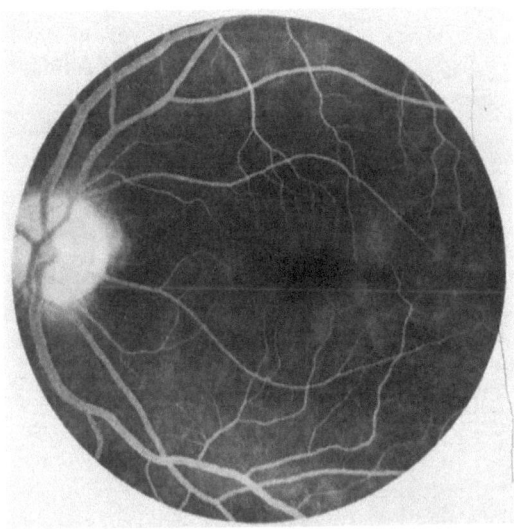

Figure 27 (IV-13). Left eye. Late phase of the angiogram showing leakage from capillaries in the macular region and on the disc.

## Conclusion
Bilateral retinal vascular lesions consistent with a diagnosis of DEVR.

## Subject IV-12 (16-06-23)

### History
The husband of IV-13 is remotely related to her. There are no visual complaints. The birth weight was 4000 g. A genealogical study could not demonstrate a family relationship between the spouses, but excluded any relationship closer than the 8th degree.

### Ophthalmological examination

| | |
|---|---|
| Visual acuity | VOD: S + 0.75 1.0. |
| | VOS: S + 1.5/Cyl. − 0.5 axis 90° 1.0. |
| Media | ODS: Normal. |
| Fundi | OD: Slight venous stasis retinopathy with some scattered minor retinal haemorrhages. Both fundi show moderate sclerotic changes of the arterial retinal vasculature. |
| Fluorescein angiogram | OD: Slightly increased circulation time. Some minor leakage of fluorescein from the larger venous branches in the posterior pole and in the macular region. |
| | OS: No abnormalities in the posterior pole. The |

temporal equator region in both eyes shows normal perfusion of the retina.

*General internal examination*
No changes other than slight hypertension and some obesity.

*Conclusion*
Slight venous stasis retinopathy of the right eye and signs of vascular sclerosis in both fundi. No symptoms of DEVR.

*Subject V-29 (26-07-53)*

*History*
The left eye is reportedly lazy and has never had good visual acuity. No amblyopia treatment has been given. General health has always been good. Birth weight was low (2300 g) but reportedly there was no neonatal oxygen administration.

*Ophthalmological examination*

| | |
|---|---|
| Visual acuity | VOD: 1.25, uncorrected. |
| | VOS: 0.16, uncorrected. |
| Eye position | Straight. |
| Anterior segments | ODS: Normal. |
| Vitreous | ODS: Normal structure, no cells. |
| Fundi | ODS: Slightly stretched course of the retinal vessels in both posterior poles, and possibly some inferior temporal ectopia of the maculae. Very delicate radial folds in the macular region OS. In both fundi the temporal retinal vessels terminate in multiple ramifications in the equator region. Peripheral to this the avascular retina shows a whitish colour (white without pressure). |
| Fluorescein angiogram | OS: The early phase clearly reveals that the retinal vasculature in the temporal equator region terminates in a zone of aberrant, slightly dilated terminal branches from which unmistakable leakage is visible in the later exposures. Near the 4 o'clock meridian, this zone deviates slightly in central direction. One site shows very intensive local leakage immediately peripheral to the ex- |

treme zone of capillaries (Figure 28). The early phase shows slightly irregular and dilated capillaries in the macular region, from which unmistakable leakage is visible after some time. The late phase shows hyperfluorescence of the disc.

OD: Late exposures of the right fundus likewise show non-perfusion of the temporal retinal periphery, leakage from capillaries central to this area, and leakage in the macular region as well as hyperfluorescence of the disc.

Visual fields (Goldmann)    OD: Slight absolute limitation of the nasal visual field.

OS: The superior nasal quadrant shows a marked absolute limitation of the visual field which extends to just within the $20°$ area.

*Follow-up*

Re-examination of visual acuity, media and fundi (including fluorescein angiography) after 38 months revealed no signs of progression.

*Conclusion*

Bilateral retinal vascular changes consistent with a diagnosis of DEVR.

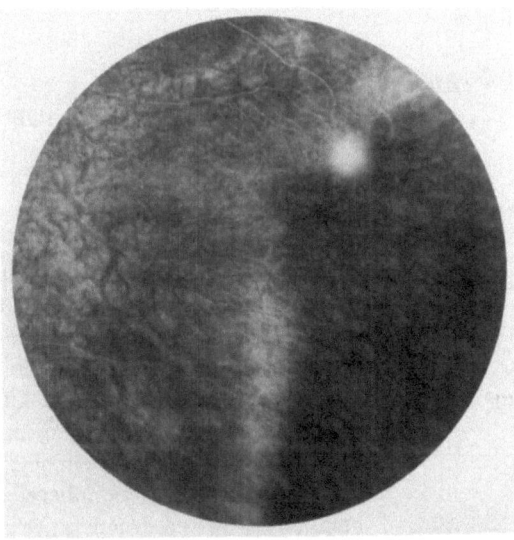

Figure 28 (V-29). Left eye. Leakage in the liminal zone from peripheral ramifications and from one small neovascularization. Note the wedge-shaped configuration of the avascular retinal zone.

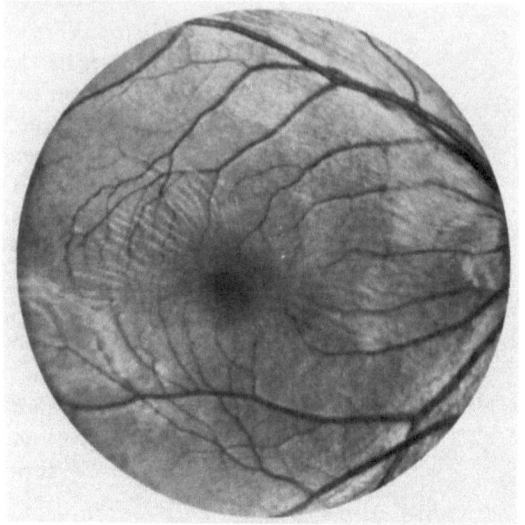

Figure 29 (V-30). Right eye. Delicate perimacular radial folds.

*Subject V-30 (07-08-54)*

*History*

No visual complaints. Birth weight 2800 g. No neonatal oxygen administration. Good general health.

*Ophthalmological examination*

| | |
|---|---|
| Visual acuity | VOD: S + 3.0/Cyl. − 1.0 axis 140° 0.6. |
| | VOS: S + 3.5/Cyl. − 0.75 axis 20° 0.8. |
| Eye position | Straight |
| Anterior segments | ODS: Normal. |
| Vitreous | ODS: Normal structure, no cells. |
| Fundi | ODS: In the retina, delicate radial folds are visible around the foveola in the centre of both posterior poles (Figure 29). The vessels take a slightly stretched course in temporal direction, and there seems to be minimal ectopia of both maculae in the same direction. Some tortuous small vessels are visible in the mid-periphery of both fundi. The temporal retinal periphery seems to be avascular but shows no degenerative changes. |
| Fluorescein angiogram | ODS: Non-perfusion of the temporal periphery. The zone of retinal vessels along the central margin of the avascular zone shows fluorescein leak- |

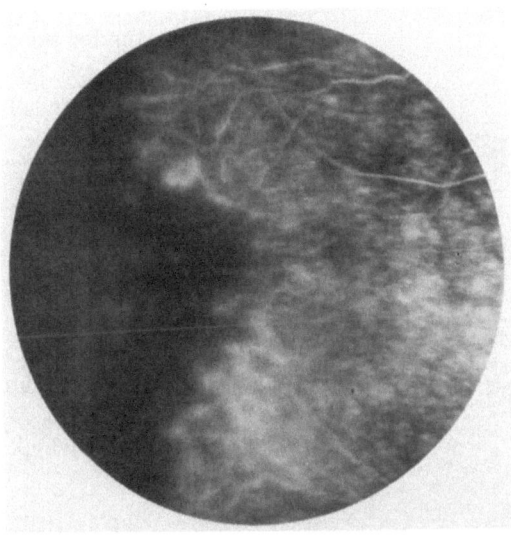

Figure 30 (V-30). Right eye. Non-perfusion of the peripheral retina on the fluorescein angiogram.

age (Figure 30). Slight dilatation of a few macular capillaries, from which unmistakable fluorescein leakage is visible in the late phase. Leakage is visible also at the level of the discs and their immediate vicinity.

*Conclusion*
Bilateral retinal vascular changes consistent with a diagnosis of DEVR.

*Subject V-31 (02-09-58)*

*History*
No visual symptoms. Birth reportedly premature (birth weight 1500 g). Kept in the incubator for some time after birth, but no record of the duration of incubator management or oxygen administration.

*Ophthalmological examination*

| | |
|---|---|
| Visual acuity | VOD: S − 4.5 1.0. |
| | VOS: S − 4.0 1.0. |
| Eye position | Straight. |
| Anterior segments | ODS: Normal. |
| Vitreous | ODS: Normal. |
| Fundi | ODS: Normal pattern of retinal vessels in the posterior pole in both eyes. The temporal peri- |

phery of the right fundus shows no distinct abnormalities, but in the left fundus the retina in this region presents a whitish appearance anterior to the equator and is avascular.

Fluorescein angiogram — The posterior poles are normal. The temporal equator region OD shows no distinct changes other than a defect in the pigmented layer, but the angiogram of this area is not entirely in sharp definition. The same region in the left fundus does show changes: posterior to the equator a fair number of more or less parallel vascular branches seem to terminate abruptly. Nowhere, however, is fluorescein leakage visible. In the late phase both discs are slightly hyperfluorescent.

*Conclusion*

Slight abnormalities in the fluorescein angiogram of the left eye, suggestive of incomplete vascularization of the temporal retinal periphery. A diagnosis of DEVR is uncertain in this case because the changes can also be a manifestation of slight retrolental fibroplasia.

*Subject V-32 (06-12-61)*

*History*

Esotropia was reportedly discovered in infancy and treated by operative correction at age 5. No amblyopia treatment mentioned. VODS has always been good.

*Ophthalmological examination*

Visual acuity — VOD: S + 0.5 1.0.
VOS: S + 0.5 1.0.

Eye position — Convergent strabismus OS, about $10°$.

Anterior segments — ODS: Normal.

Vitreous — ODS: Bilaterally, the retrolental vitreous is of normal structure and contains no cells. In the left eye the preretinal periphery of the vitreous space contains some delicate turbidities.

Fundi — ODS: Normal configuration of the retinal vasculature in both posterior poles. Superior and temporal to the macula of the left eye, a pigment epithelium area the size of one disc diameter shows atrophy. In both fundi the periphery shows various tortuous retinal vessels but no other retinal vascular changes.

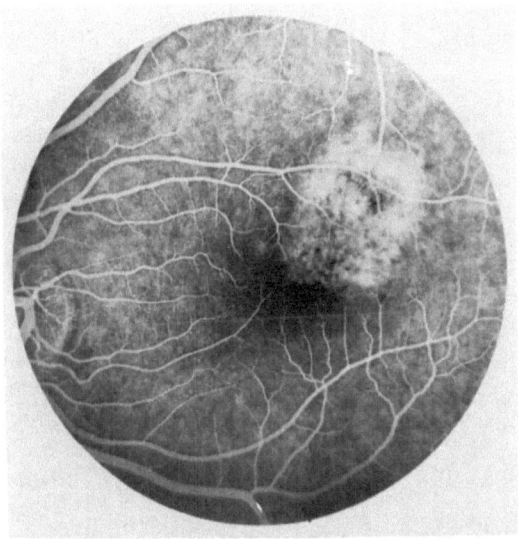

Figure 31 (V-32). Left eye. Fluorescein angiogram. Hyperfluorescent zone due to atrophy of the retinal pigment epithelium.

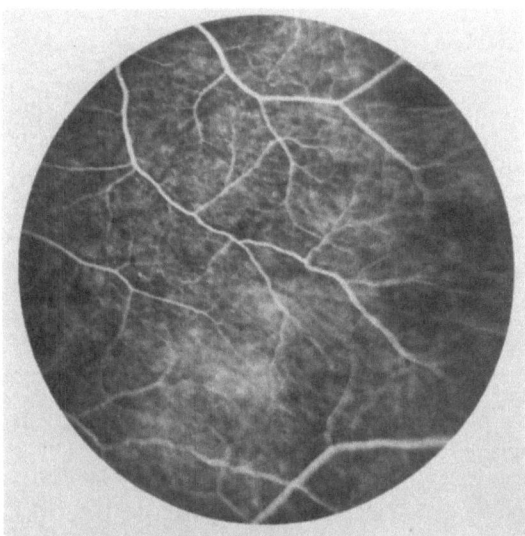

Figure 32 (V-32). Left eye. Slight fluorescein leakage in the late phase of fluorescein angiography.

| | |
|---|---|
| Fluorescein angiogram | OS: The early phase of the posterior pole clearly reveals the atrophic area of the pigment epithelium as hyperfluorescent area (Figure 31). Late exposures of the temporal fundus reveal tortuous vessels with some fluorescein leakage (Figure 32). No abrupt transition to a non-perfused retinal periphery is fluorographically visible. The late phase shows unmistakable hyperfluorescence of the disc. |
| | OD: The late exposures of the posterior pole show a hyperfluorescent disc but no leakage in the macular region. The region central to the equator shows no changes other than a few tortuous retinal vessels. There are no exposures of the equatorial zone of sufficiently sharp definition. |
| Visual fields (Goldmann) | ODS: No distinct abnormalities. |

*Follow-up*

No evidence of progression was found at re-examination after 39 months.

*Conclusion*

Slight bilateral vascular changes in the retinal periphery with fluorescein leakage in the left eye, based on a mild manifestation of DEVR.

*Subject V-33 (03-01-66)*

*History*

Convergence of the right eye reportedly present since early infancy, with poor visual acuity. Strabismus correction at age 4. No amblyopia treatment on record. The birth weight was 2500 g. Nutritional problems necessitated hospitalization for a few days after birth. No record of neonatal oxygen administration.

*Ophthalmological examination*

| | |
|---|---|
| Visual acuity | VOD: 1/60, uncorrected. |
| | VOS: Cyl. − 0.5 axis 0° 1.0. |
| Eye position | OD: Convergent strabismus, about 7°. |
| Anterior segments | ODS: Normal. |
| Vitreous | ODS: Normal structure, no cells. |
| Fundi | ODS: In both posterior poles the retinal vessels take a slightly stretched course in temporal direction but there is no distinct ectopia of the maculae. The pattern of the retinal vasculature in the |

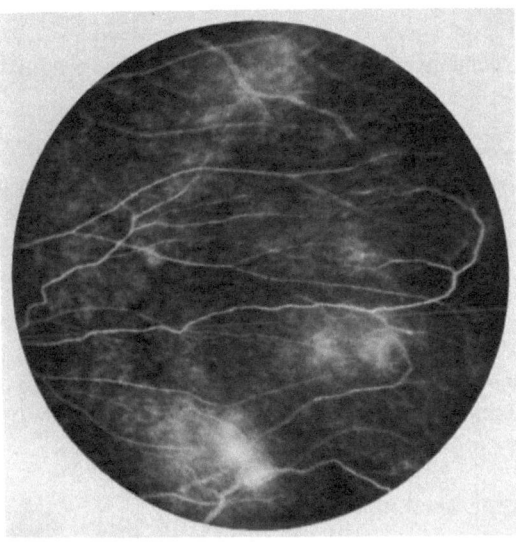

Figure 33 (V-33). Left eye. Abnormal configuration of retinal vessels in the temporal equatorial zone and slight fluorescein leakage in the retina.

temporal sector of both posterior poles is slightly aberrant: relatively many vessels with a fairly parallel course are localized in this part of the two fundi. Some of these vessels are markedly tortuous. No retinal defects, exudates or neovascularizations.

Fluorescein angiogram OD: The early exposures of the posterior pole show no changes apart from a slightly peculiar configuration of the retinal vessels; specifically, there are no capillary dilatations in the macular region. The retinal circulation time is normal. The equatorial zone near 9 o'clock shows a fairly large number of retinal vessels whose venous branches are abnormally tortuous. Some of these branches curve near the equator, and several show some fluorescein leakage. Avascularity of the peripheral retina is not demonstrable fluorographically. The late exposures of the posterior pole show no leakage in the macula but the disc is hyperfluorescent.

OS: Late exposures of the temporal equator region show fluorescein leakage from slightly aberrant vascular branches. Avascularity of the peripheral retina is not demonstrable (Figure 33).

*Follow-up*
Visual acuity, media and fundi were unchanged at re-examination 36 months later.

*Conclusion*
Bilateral peripheral retinal vascular changes, suggestive of a mild manifestation of DEVR.

*Subject IV-16 (13-10-29)*

*History*
Visual acuity OD has always been poor. Cataract examination OD at age 27, probably for cosmetic reasons. The right eye has been totally blind for some years. No history of premature birth.

*Ophthalmological examination*

| | |
|---|---|
| Visual acuity | VOD: No light perception. |
| | VOS: S − 0.5/Cyl. − 2.5 axis 65°. |
| Intraocular pressure | OD: 21 mm Hg. |
| | OS: 20 mm Hg. |
| Eye position | Divergent strabismus, 20°. |
| Anterior segments | OD: Clear cornea. The anterior chamber is of virtually normal depth. The iris is atrophic and, in part, connected via synechiae with a totally opaque white tissue mass which occludes the entire pupillary aperture. |
| | OS: Normal. |
| Vitreous | OD: Not assessable. |
| | OS: Normal structure of the retrolental vitreous. Anterior to the temporal fundus periphery the vitreous shows some delicate condensations. |
| Fundi: | OS: Disc, macula and vessels in the posterior pole present a normal appearance. Central to the temporal equator the retina comprises a slightly increased number of vessels of more or less parallel arrangement. The antero-equatorial retina shows white without pressure. Retinal vessels are not visible in this area. Anterior to the equator, two small retinal defects are visible near the 12 o'clock position. |
| Fluorescein angiogram | OS: Near 4 o'clock, the retinal vasculature terminates anterior to the equator in small irregular ramifications from which fluorescein leaks (Figure 34). The retina peripheral to this is not per- |

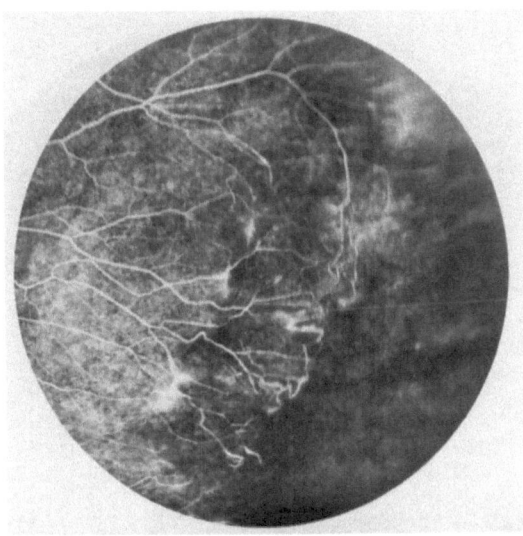

Figure 34 (IV-16). Left eye. Fluorescein angiogram. Tortuous branches in the inferior temporal sector of the fundus and non-perfusion of the peripheral retina.

|  |  |
|---|---|
|  | fused. A few small capillary telangiectases in the macular region show slight fluorescein leakage. In the late phase, the disc is hyperfluorescent. |
| ERG | OD: Not recordable. |
|  | OS: Scotopic b-wave: $190\,\mu V$. |
|  | Photopic b-wave: $30\,\mu V$. |
|  | Flicker fusion frequency: 50 Hz. |
| EOG | OD: Flat type 1. |
|  | OS: Lp/Dt 176; Dt $637\,\mu V$. |
| Dark adaptation | OS: Normal. |
| Colour vision | OS: A slight protan defect is found both with the anomaloscope and in the Farnsworth 100 Hue test. |

*Therapy*
Both retinal defects in the periphery of the fundus OS were treated by laser coagulation, without subsequent complications.

*Follow-up*
Re-examination after 37 months revealed no signs of progression. The fluorescein angiogram showed no abnormalities other than a few scars caused by the Argon laser treatment.

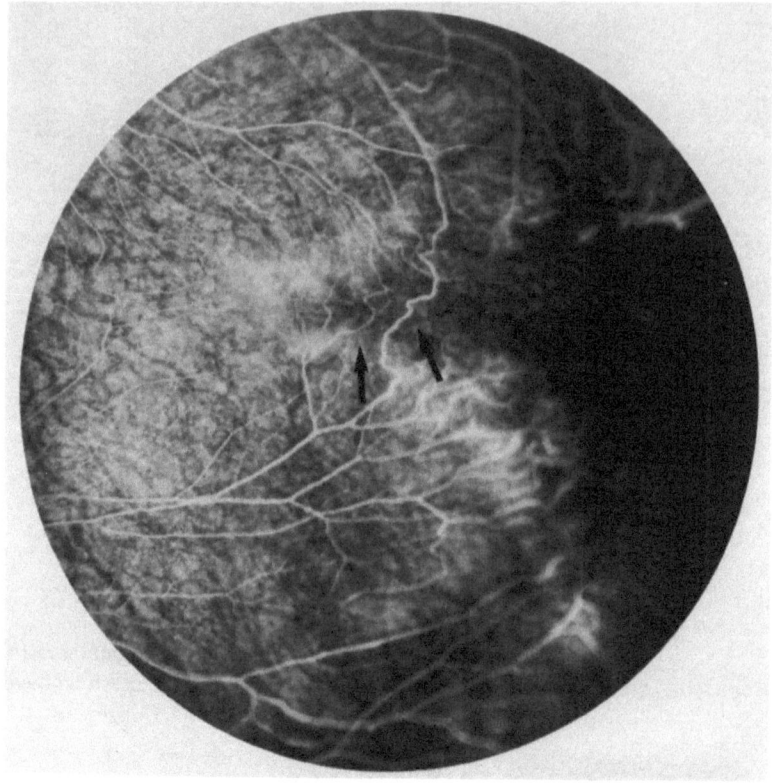

Figure 35 (V-39). Left eye. Fluorescein angiogram of equatorial zone near 3 o'clock. Tortuous shunt vessels between superior and inferior temporal retinal vessels (arrows).

*Conclusion*

Total vitreous organization and retinal detachment OD; vascular lesions of the temporal retinal periphery OS with a few retinal defects. The findings are consistent with a diagnosis of DEVR.

*Subject V-39 (17-02-55)*

*History*

No visual complaints. Good general health. No record of premature birth or neonatal oxygen administration.

*Ophthalmological examination*

| Visual acuity | VOD: C − 0.5 axis 170° 1.25. |
| | VOS: S + 0.75/ Cyl. − 1.5 axis 70° 1.25. |
| Eye position | Straight |
| Anterior segments | ODS: Normal. |

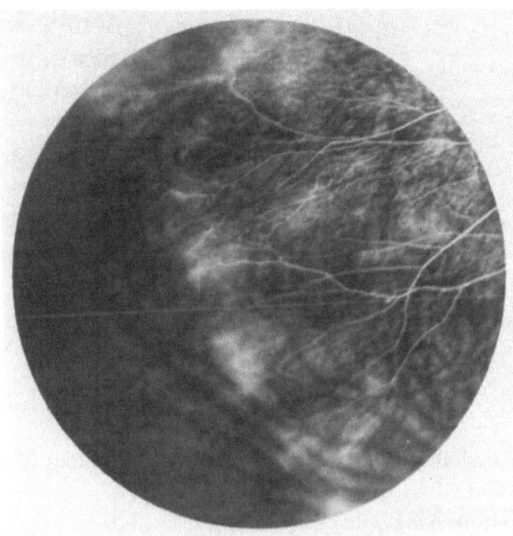

Figure 36 (V-39). Right eye. Numerous vessels terminate abruptly near the temporal equator.

| | |
|---|---|
| Vitreous | ODS: Normal. |
| Fundi | ODS: Both posterior poles are of normal appearance. The temporal mid-periphery shows an abundance of retinal vascular branches, some of which are tortuous. Peripheral to this, the retina seems avascular, but this part shows no degenerative changes. |
| Fluorescein angiogram | OS: The early phase shows no lesions of the posterior pole. In the temporal equator region the retinal vessels terminate in multiple ramifications from which fluorescein leaks. The peripheral retina is avascular. A few tortuous shunts between peripheral branches of the superior and the inferior temporal retinal vessels are near 3 o' clock (Figure 35). The disc is hyperfluorescent in the late phase. No leakage in the macular region. |
| | OD: In the temporal equator region the retinal vasculature terminates in aberrant, leaking ramifications (Figure 36). Late exposures of the posterior pole show slight leakage in the macular region and disc hyperfluorescence. |
| Visual fields (Goldmann) | OD: No distinct limitations. |
| | OS: Slight limitation of the nasal visual field. |

| ERG | OD: Scotopic b-wave: $310\,\mu$V. |
|---|---|
| | Photopic b-wave: $60\,\mu$V. |
| | OS: Scotopic b-wave: $210\,\mu$V. |
| | Photopic b-wave: $45\,\mu$V. |
| EOG | OD: Lp/Dt 213; Dt $300\,\mu$V. |
| | OS: Lp/Dt 217; Dt $288\,\mu$V. |
| Colour vision | ODS: Tendency to a blue-yellow defect. |

*Follow-up*

Re-examination after 34 months revealed no signs of progression. The fluorescein angiogram was unchanged.

*Conclusion*

Bilateral retinal vascular lesions consistent with a diagnosis of DEVR.

*Subject V-40 (01-03-58)*

*History*

No visual complaints other than slightly diminished visual acuity OS. Good general health. No record of premature birth or neonatal oxygen administration.

*Ophthalmological examination*

| Visual acuity | VOD: S + 0.5. 0.8. |
|---|---|
| | VOS: S + 1.5/Cyl. − 1.5 axis 0° 0.6. |
| Eye position | Straight. |
| Anterior segments | ODS: Normal. |
| Vitreous | ODS: Normal. |
| Fundi | ODS: Vascular configuration in both posterior poles slightly stretched in temporal direction with slight ectopia of the maculae in the same direction. On the temporal side of both posterior poles, the retina contains numerous vascular branches which do not seem to continue to the extreme periphery. The retinal periphery shows no exudates, defects or pigmentations. |
| Fluorescein angiogram | OS: The early phase of the posterior pole shows no capillary dilatations. The equatorial zone near 3 o'clock contains an abnormally large number of vascular branches which terminate abruptly immediately anterior to the equator: local non-perfusion of the peripheral retina. Leakage of fluorescein from these vessels. The late phase |

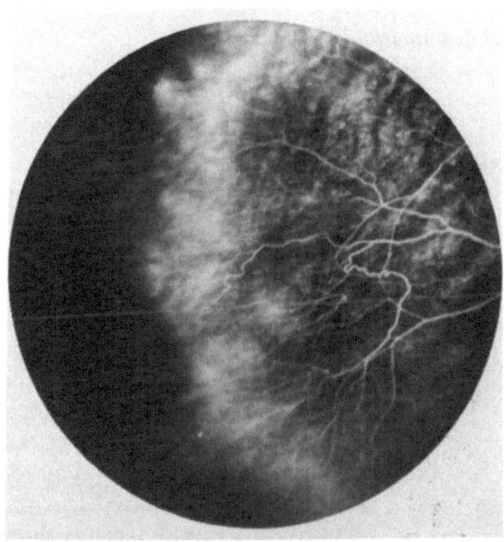

Figure 37 (V-40). Right eye. Fluorescein angiogram shows tortuous venous branches and leakage in the zone adjacent to the avascular retina.

shows a hyperfluorescent disc but no leakage in the macular region.

OD: The late phase of the posterior pole and the temporal equatorial zone shows the same changes as those observed in the fundus OS (Figure 37). No signs of neovascularizations.

| | |
|---|---|
| ERG | OD: Scotopic v-wave: $330 \mu V$. |
| | Photopic h-wave: $70 \mu V$. |
| | OS: Scotopic b-wave: $370 \mu V$. |
| | Photopic b-wave: $55 \mu V$. |
| EOG | OD: Lp/Dt 250; Dt $300 \mu V$. |
| | OS: Lp/Dt 204; Dt $300 \mu V$. |
| Dark adaptation | Binocular: Normal. |
| Colour vision | ODS: Normal. |

*Conclusion*

Bilateral vascular changes of the retinal periphery, consistent with a diagnosis of DEVR.

*Subject V-41 (23-10-61)*

*History*

Patient has been wearing spectacles since age 3. VODS reported to have always been subnormal. No record of premature birth or neonatal oxygen administration.

*Ophthalmological examination*

| | |
|---|---|
| Visual acuity | VOD: S $-$ 1.25/Cyl. $-$ 1.5 axis 20° 0.6. |
| | VOS: S $-$ 3.0/Cyl. $-$ 0.25 axis 25° 0.4. |
| Eye position | Straight. |
| Anterior segments | ODS: Normal. |
| Vitreous | ODS: Retrolental vitreous of normal structure, without cells. The preretinal vitreous in the temporal fundus periphery shows slight turbidities. |
| Fundi | ODS: In the posterior poles, the small vessels inferior and superior to the macula show no perimacular curvature but take an abnormally stretched course in temporal direction. Both maculae show slight ectopia in the same direction. Temporal to both posterior poles, numerous vascular branches are closely packed in the retina. Some are very tortuous. These vessels terminate abruptly in a whitish zone near the equator. Peripheral to this zone, which is particularly distinct in the right fundus, no vessels are visible in the retina. In both fundi this avascular retinal portion shows small circular defects. A minor retinal haemorrhage is visible in the left fundus near the equator at the level of the 4 o'clock meridian (Figure 38). No exudates. |

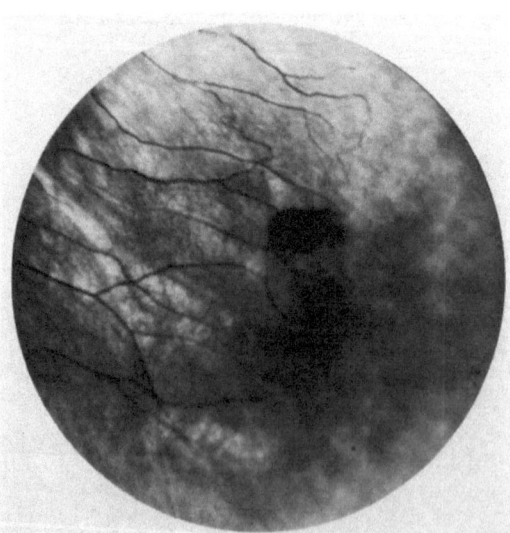

Figure 38 (V-41). Left eye. Minor retinal haemorrhage at the level of the most peripheral ramifications.

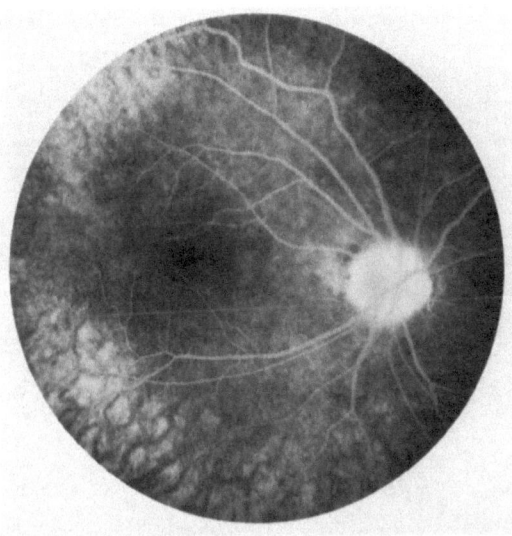

Figure 39 (V-41). Right eye. Hyperfluorescence of the disc in the late phase of fluorescein angiography.

| | |
|---|---|
| Fluorescein angiogram | OD: The retinal vasculature terminates temporally in aberrant ramifications which leak fluorescein. The peripheral retina outside the equator is avascular. Near the 9 o'clock meridian the avascular zone even extends locally in central direction to a level posterior to the equator. At one site, intensive fluorescein leakage is seen from a small neovascularization just outside the zone of the terminal ramifications of the retinal vasculature. No leakage in the macular region, but the disc is hyperfluorescent in the late phase (Figure 39). |
| | OS: Late exposures of the temporal periphery show changes similar to those found in the right fundus. Here, too, a large portion of the peripheral retina is non-perfused, and locally the avascular zone even extends to slightly central to the equator (Figure 40). No neovascularizations. In the late phase the disc is hyperfluorescent. |
| ERG | OD: Scotopic b-wave: $230\,\mu V$. |
| | Photopic b-wave: $30\,\mu V$. |
| | OS: Scotopic b-wave: $310\,\mu V$. |
| | Photopic b-wave: $50\,\mu V$. |
| EOG | OD: Lp/Dt 190; Dt $400\,\mu V$. |
| | OS: Lp/Dt 212; Dt $400\,\mu V$. |

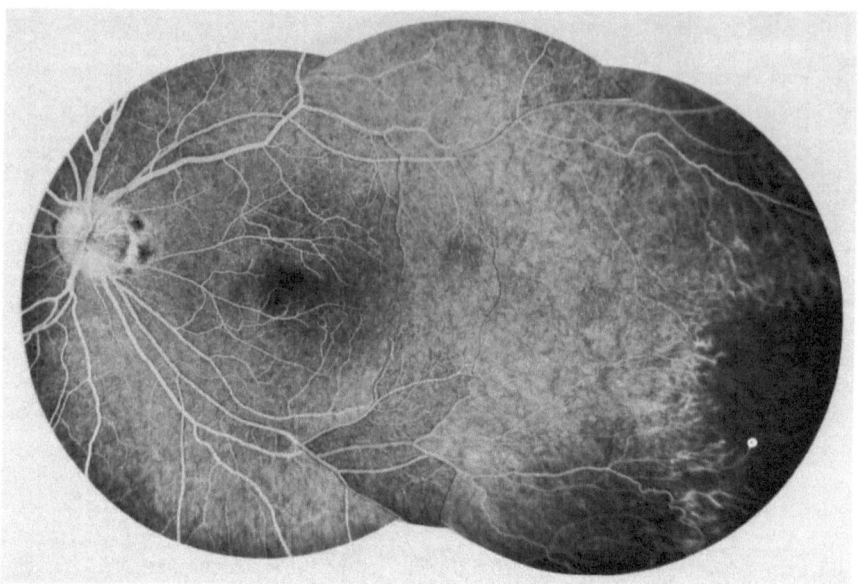

Figure 40 (V-41). Left eye. Near 3 o'clock, the avascular retinal periphery extends central to the equator.

Dark adaptation          Binocular: Normal.
Colour vision            ODS: Normal.

*Follow-up*
Visual acuity, media and fundi were unchanged at re-examination after 37 months. The fluorescein angiogram was likewise unchanged.

*Conclusion*
Bilateral retinal vascular changes consistent with a diagnosis of DEVR.

*Subject V-52 (05-09-57)*

*History*
Since 1972 our department has known this young woman to be suffering from severe bilateral proliferative retinopathy of uncertain aetiology. Convergent strabismus OD was diagnosed at age 6; one year later VOD proved to be 0.3, and extensive fundus changes were found in this eye. General health was good. The patient had been prematurely born as one of a pair of twins. The twin brother died within a few weeks of birth. The exact duration of the pregnancy is not known. The patient's birth weight was 2500 g. After birth she was placed in an incubator for a total of six weeks. Her condition during this period is reported not always to have been good, and it seems likely that

a relatively large amount of oxygen was administered (which concentrations and during which periods?). The frequency of blood analyses is unknown, as are the values found. The patient's relationship to the previously described persons was not discovered until the family study was virtually completed.

*Ophthalmological examination (1972)*

| | |
|---|---|
| Visual acuity | VOD: 0.5/60. |
| | VOS: S + 2.5 1.0. |
| Eye position | Convergent strabismus OD. |
| Intraocular pressure | OD: 8/7.5 |
| | OS: 8/7.5 (Schiøtz tonometer). |
| Anterior segments | OD: The aqueous humour shows an unmistakable positive flare and some cells. Some subcapsular cataract formation. |
| | OS: Normal. |
| Vitreous | OD: Strands and membranes. Many cells. |
| | OS: Normal. |
| Fundi | OD: In the posterior pole there are gross scars in the retina, which is partly detached. Haemorrhages and fibrovascular proliferations in the temporal periphery. |
| | OS: The posterior pole presents a normal appearance. Some preretinal haemorrhages are visible in the inferior temporal sector. |

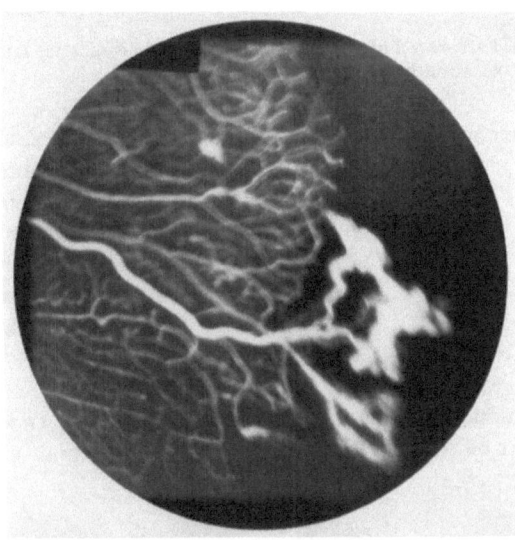

Figure 41 (V-52). Left eye. Fluorescein angiogram. The arteriovenous phase shows non-perfusion of the retina anterior to the temporal equator and a neovascularization of fair size, supplied by an artery with a wide lumen.

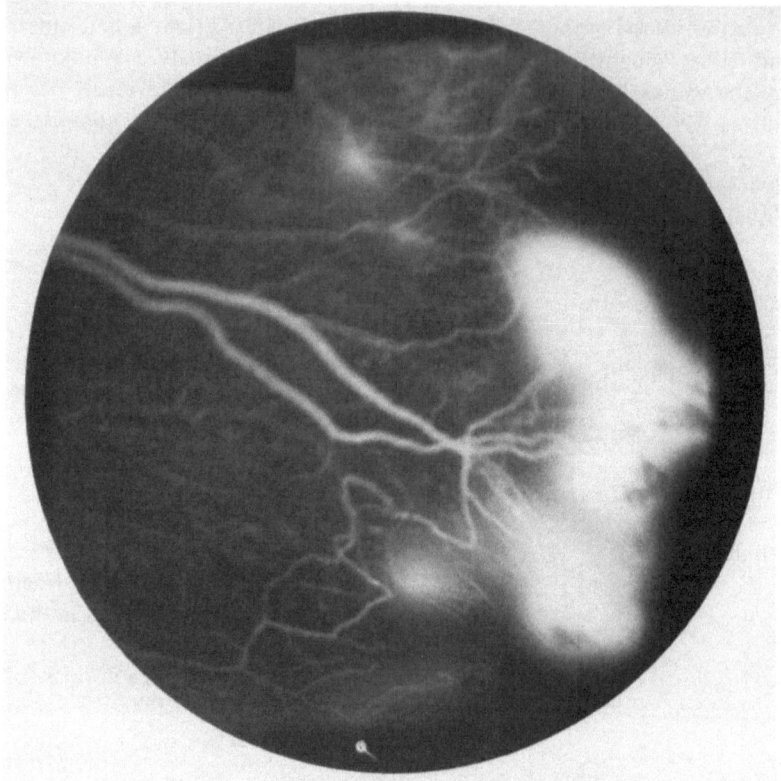

Figure 42 (V-52). Left eye. Fluorescein angiogram. A few seconds later than in Figure 41, intensive leakage from the neovascularization is visible.

Fluorescein angiogram      OS: In the early phase, the retinal vasculature near 4 o'clock terminates in small, blind-ending ramifications near the equator. Immediately peripheral to this a preretinal vascular proliferation is supplied by an arteriole of fair size (Figure 41). Intensive fluorescein leakage from the neovascularization within a few seconds (Figure 42).

*Therapy*
Intensive coagulation of the equatorial zone between 2 and 5 o'clock and direct treatment of the neovascularization with the Xenon arc coagulator. No complications.

Fluorescein angiogram      OS: The coagulations have almost totally des-
(1975)      troyed the neovascularizations. The vascular bed of the retina is of reduced density central to the

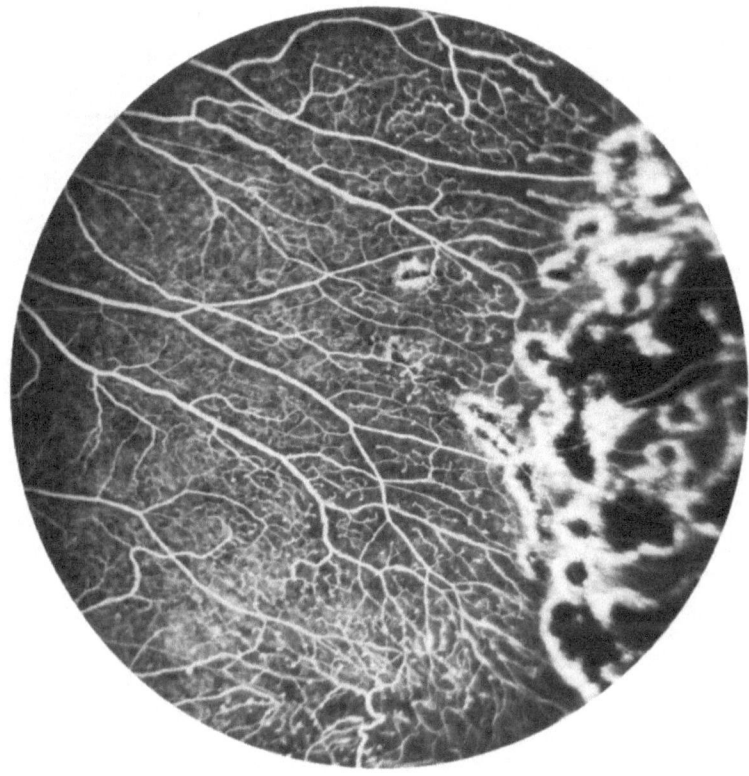

Figure 43 (V-52). Left eye. Coagulation has totally destroyed the neovascularization. The capillary bed of the retina central to the scars is of abnormal structure and shows blind-ending vascular buds.

coagulation scars. Several capillaries end blindly in saccular dilatations or small vascular loops (Figure 43). The posterior pole is intact and shows no fluorescein leakage in the late phase.

*Further course (until 1980)*
The condition of the retina OS remains good. VOS remains 1.0. Up to 1974 the right eye has gradually developed total retinal detachment as a result of traction and subretinal exudation. There is no longer any light perception.

*General and internal examination.*
An extensive clinical examination was made. General physical examination revealed nothing abnormal. Routine haematological and coagulation studies yielded entirely normal findings.

72

## Conclusion

The fluorescein angiogram of the left fundus suggests a disorder of the peripheral retinal vascularization, complicated by secondary vascular proliferations. In the right eye the latter have led to total retinal detachment. The vascular lesions may be due to neonatal oxygen administration or result from DEVR. It is also possible that both have played a role in the pathogenesis.

### Subject IV-20 (20-01-29)

#### History
No visual complaints and no record of premature birth or neonatal oxygen administration.

#### Ophthalmological examination

| | |
|---|---|
| Visual acuity | VOD: S + 0.75/Cyl. − 0.25 axis 30° 0.8. |
| | VOS: S + 1.0 1.0. |
| Eye position | Straight |
| Intraocular pressure | ODS: 15 mm Hg. |
| Anterior segments | ODS: Normal. |
| Vitreous | ODS: Normal structure. no cells. |
| Fundi | ODS: Normal posterior pole. No distinct changes at indirect ophthalmoscopy of the periphery of both fundi. |

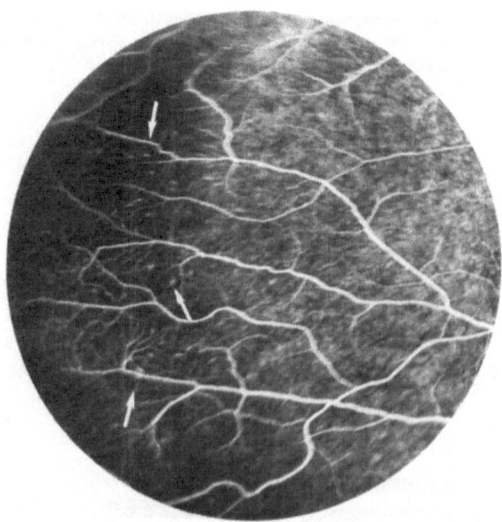

Figure 44 (IV-20). Right eye. Slight leakage in the temporal sector of the retina shortly after the arteriovenous phase of the angiogram (arrows).

73

Fluorescein angiogram      OD: Early exposures of the temporal equatorial zone near 9 o'clock show slight dilatations of several capillaries. The capillary network in this region is of fairly low density. Soon, there is some slight fluorescein leakage from a few capillaries and from a segment of a small venous branch near the equator (Figure 44). No evidence of an avascular zone in the peripheral retina.
OS: The peripheral exposures are of insufficient quality for proper evaluation. As in OD, the disc shows some hyperfluorescence in the late phase, and there is no leakage in the macular region.

*Conclusion*
Slightly subnormal visual acuity and slight vascular changes of the peripheral retina of the right eye. It is possible (but not certain) that the changes represent a mild manifestation of DEVR.

### 3.3 The B family

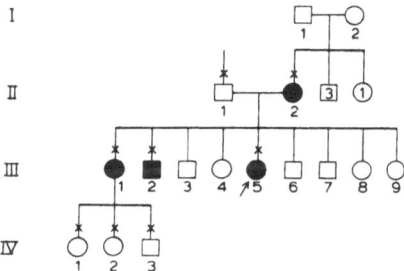

Figure 45. Pedigree of the B family.

*Introduction*

In October 1978 the proband of this family was referred to the University of Nijmegen Department of Ophthalmology in view of bilateral total retinal detachment with a very poor prognosis. The fundi of this 14-year-old girl showed such distinct abnormalities that we decided to submit the other family members to ophthalmological examination. In the proband's mother and her older brother and sister, this examination disclosed unmistakable changes which confirmed a diagnosis of DEVR. Unfortunately, we failed to convince the parents of the importance of examining the remaining children.

*Proband III-5 (11-07-64)*

*History*

This 14-year-old girl was transferred to our department from another university hospital, for operative treatment of bilateral retinal detachment. She was reported to have had visual complaints since no more than a month. Previously, the parents had never noticed anything out of the ordinary so far as her eyes or eyesight were concerned. The eldest brother reportedly had one blind eye, but no other eye abnormalities were said to exist in the family. During an interview with the parents, they were found to show a marked tendency to dissimulate ailments. The history was consequently regarded as unreliable. The girl's general health was believed to be good, apart from complaints about headaches. There was no record of premature birth or neonatal oxygen administration. Apart from medication with prednisone (40 mg every other day) and amoxicillin (3 x 375 mg/day), the girl had received no medication or operative ophthalmological therapy prior to admission to our department.

*Ophthalmological examination*

| | |
|---|---|
| Visual acuity | VOD: Light perception |
| | VOS: 1/60. |
| Intraocular pressure | OD: 7 mm Hg. |
| | OS: 10 mm Hg. |
| Eye position | Divergent strabismus OD; no nystagmus. |
| Anterior segments | ODS: The corneae are clear. The vitreous contains cells and shows a flare (Tyndall phenomenon). The lenses are clear and show no luxation. |
| Vitreous | ODS: The vitreous contains many pigment particles and cells. Many membranes are visible throughout the vitreous space, but especially in the preretinal part. |
| Fundi | OD: Total detachment of the retina, which protrudes into the central part of the vitreous space. Between 11 and 1 o'clock, the retina shows a very large rupture from the extreme fundus periphery to immediately superior to the posterior pole. The central boundary of this rupture is a thick ridge of curled-up retina (Figure 46). Particularly in the inferior quadrant, the retina shows whitish structures and is thickened, probably as a result of glia proliferations. The vascular pattern temporal and inferior to the posterior pole is abnormal: there are stikingly numerous tortuous retinal vessels with a more or less parallel course (Figure 47). It is difficult to observe the |

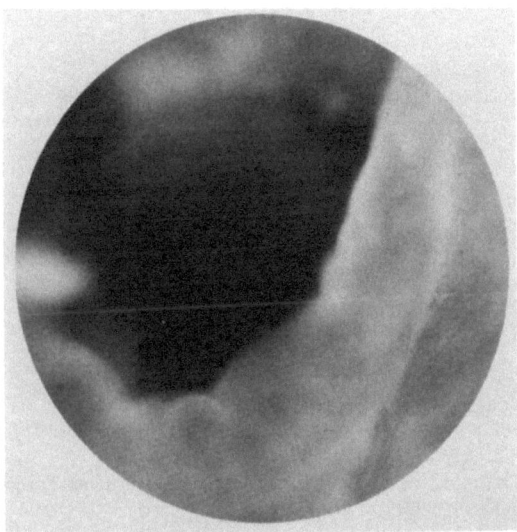

Figure 46 (III-5). OD. Large retinal rupture in the superior quadrants.

retinal vessels in the temporal fundus periphery, due to preretinal vitreous membranes in this region. No distinct exudates of vascular proliferations are visible.

OS: Like OD, this eye shows total detachment of the retina, which protrudes into the vitreous space superior and inferior to the posterior pole. The centre of the retina shows a fairly flat detachment. Around the posterior pole the posterior vitreous seems detached. Along the boundary of this detachment there is pronounced traction due to fibrous organization of the posterior vitreous membrane. The temporal retinal periphery shows striking vascular lesions: numerous vascular branches terminate abruptly slightly central to the equator. From this site arise large, sea fanlike vascular proliferations localized anterior to the peripheral retina. Some of these have caused minor haemorrhages (Figure 48). In some areas these neovascularizations show distinct fibrotic organization. The temporal retinal periphery, so far as visible, is avascular. Large subneuroretinal exudates are visible in the temporal and superior nasal areas (Figure 49). No distinct retinal defects are visible.

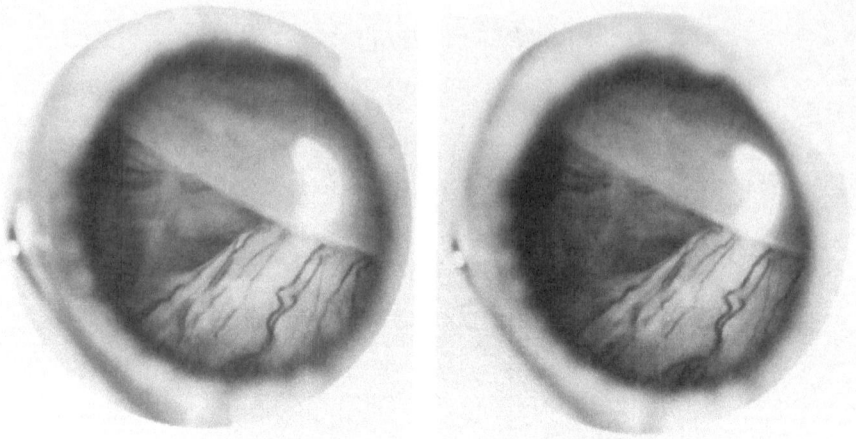

Figure 47 (III-5). Stereo-photograph OD. Total retinal detachment. The course of the retinal vessels is strikingly parallel.

| | |
|---|---|
| ERG | As expected in total retinal detachment, responses are hardly recordable. Only from the left eye can minimal potentials be derived. |
| EOG | OD: Lp/Dt 116. |
| | OS: Lp/Dt 108. |
| Ultrascanography | A-scan and B-scan confirm total retinal detachment with extensive vitreous membranes. |

*General physical examination*
History                    No complaints apart from intermittent headaches.

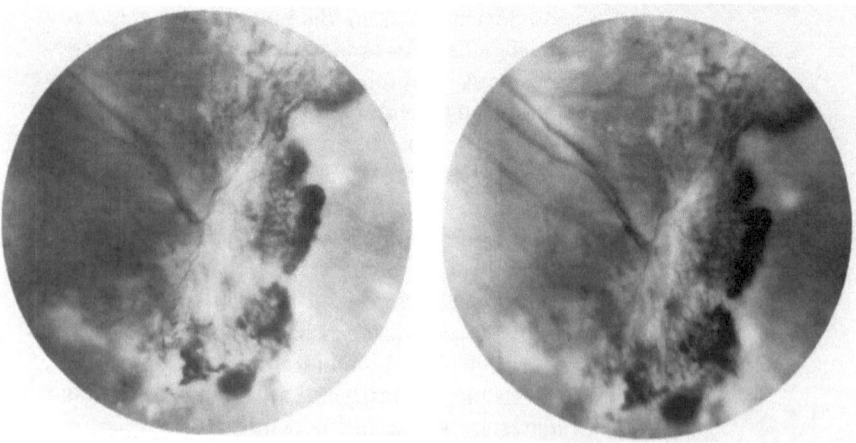

Figure 48 (III-5). Stereo-photograph OS. Large neovascularizations arise from the central boundary of the avascular retina. The vessels extend anterior to the retina.

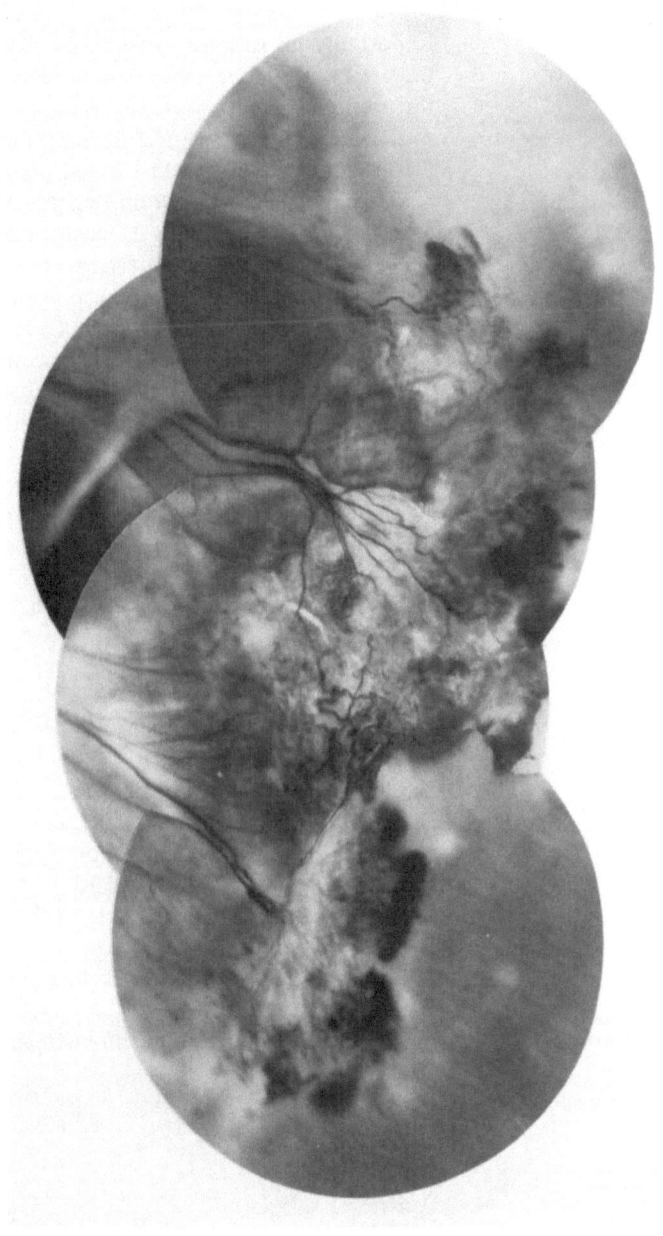

Figure 49 (III-5). OS. Composition of the vascular changes in the inferior temporal quadrant. Large subretinal exudates are partly visible (top).

| | |
|---|---|
| | Reportedly no serious illness in the patient's history. Family: Hypertension reportedly exists in the mother's family. |
| Examination | A slender, rather slight girl without conspicuous features in general habitus. Blood pressure 140/85 (RR); pulse rate 80/min, regular. Head and neck: Small congenital haemangioma of the lower lip on the right side. The teeth are carious despite dental care during the previous stay in hospital. A few teeth have been extracted. Chest: Apart from a soft systolic souffle which seems functional, no cardiac or pulmonary changes. Abdomen: Normal. Spine: Lumbar scoliosis. Extremities: Normal. |
| Radiology | Chest X-ray: Normal. Dentition: No changes of mandibular or maxillary dentition other than absence of a few teeth. Paranasal sinuses: Normal. Orbits: Normal. |
| ECG | No distinct changes other than a slightly shortened R-S time. |
| Laboratory findings | Leucocyte count $7000/mm^3$<br>ESR 3 mm in the first hour.<br>Hb 9.2 mmol/l.<br>Haematocrit 0.44<br>Platelets $228\,000/mm^3$.<br>Differentation: neutrophils 57, eosinophils 2, basophils 1, lymphocytes 39, monocytes 1. |
| Plasma electrolytes | Na 140. K 4.38. Cl 102. $HCO_3$ 30. |
| Serum levels | Glucose (fasting) 4.4 mmol/l. Urea 5.15 mmol/l. Creatinine 57 mmol/l. |
| Enzymes | CPK 2 U/l. LDH 161 U/l. Alkaline phosphatase 108 U/l. |
| Hb electrophoresis | No abnormal haemoglobin demonstrable. |
| Total protein | 69 g/l. |
| Serum protein spectrum | Normal. |
| AST | 300 U. |
| Rose test | Negative. |
| Latex | Negative. |
| ANF | Negative. |
| Toxoplasma | Immunofluorescene negative. Complement fixation test negative. |
| Toxocara | Complement fixation test negative. |
| Ascaris | Complement fixation test negative. |
| Mantoux test | Negative. |

| Urine | Glucose negative. Acetone negative. |
| 24-hour urine | Creatinine 6.7 mmol/l. Homocystine negative. Hydroxyproline 494 μmol/l. |
| Coagulation studies | Bleeding time (Ivy): 2 min 1 sec − 3 min 55 sec − 2 min 58 sec. |
| | Coagulation time (Lee-White): 6 min 25 sec − 6 min 35 sec − 7 min 6 sec. |
| | Thromboplastin time (Quick): 13 sec − 13 sec. |
| | Thrombotest (Owren): more than 100%. |
| | Cephalin-kaolin time (Langdell-Margolis): 30 sec − 29 sec. |
| | Fibrinogen content (Clauss-Vermijlen): 3555 mg/l. |
| | Thrombin time: 24 sec − 23 sec. |

*Therapy*

An operation was performed on the right eye 10 days after admission. Via the pars plana, a vitrectomy was performed at which the many tough vitreous strands were removed. Again via the pars plana, silicon oil was then introduced into the vitreous space. At the same time, subretinal fluid was drained off via a puncture in the equatorial sclera near the 9 o'clock position. During this procedure, silicon oil leaked through the large retinal defect, and unfortunately this subretinal oil could not be properly removed. The subretinal silicon oil caused persistence of virtually total retinal detachment after the operation. In view of the poor prognosis of a second operation, this was not performed. An operation on the left eye was contemplated but, after discussion of the chances with the parents, not performed. Shortly after discharge from our hospital, the patient was transferred to a home for visually handicapped children.

*Subject III-2 (30-03-55)*

*History*

This 23-year-old eldest brother of the proband reportedly had had poor visual acuity in the left eye from the start. By about age 7, the left eye was reported to have become totally blind. As long as the patient can remember, VOD has never been adequate and may have further diminished in the past few years. In the course of childhood an ophthalmologist prescribed correcting spectacles. No ophthalmological treatment of any kind has been given. The previously established diagnosis is unknown. Birth weight is unknown but there is no record of premature birth or neonatal oxygen administration. At age 17 the patient was hospitalized, reportedly for meningitis. Moderate hyper-

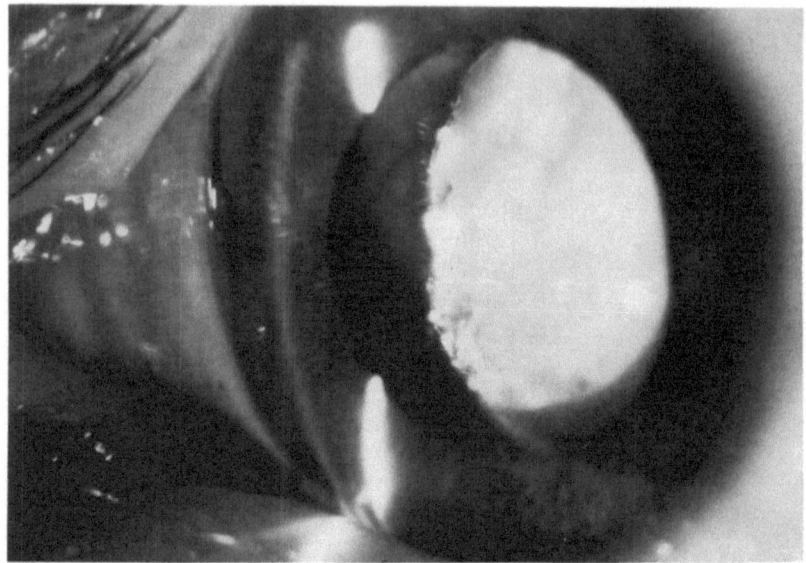

Figure 50 (III-2). OS. Totally cataractous, atrophic lens.

tension was diagnosed a few years before we saw this patient, and for this reason he was using Moduretic and Temesta tablets.

*Ophthalmological examination*

| | |
|---|---|
| Visual acuity | VOD: S − 6.5 0.5. |
| | VOS: no light perception. |
| Intraocular pressure | ODS: 12 mm Hg. |
| Eye position | Divergent strabismus OS. No nystagmus. |
| Anterior segments | OD: Normal. |

OS: Incipient band keratopathy near the corneal limbus. The aqueous humour shows no flare and contains no cells. The pupil shows no direct response to light. There is some atrophy of the pigmented layer of the iris, but no synechiae are visible. The lens is totally cataractous, and shows atrophy of the anterior lens capsule and calcifications (Figure 50). As a result of this atrophy, it is possible to look past the superior nasal side of the lens into the vitreous space.

Vitreous      OD: there is a rather ropey structure with some liquefaction. The posterior vitreous membrane is detached from the retina and shows delicate circular opacities.

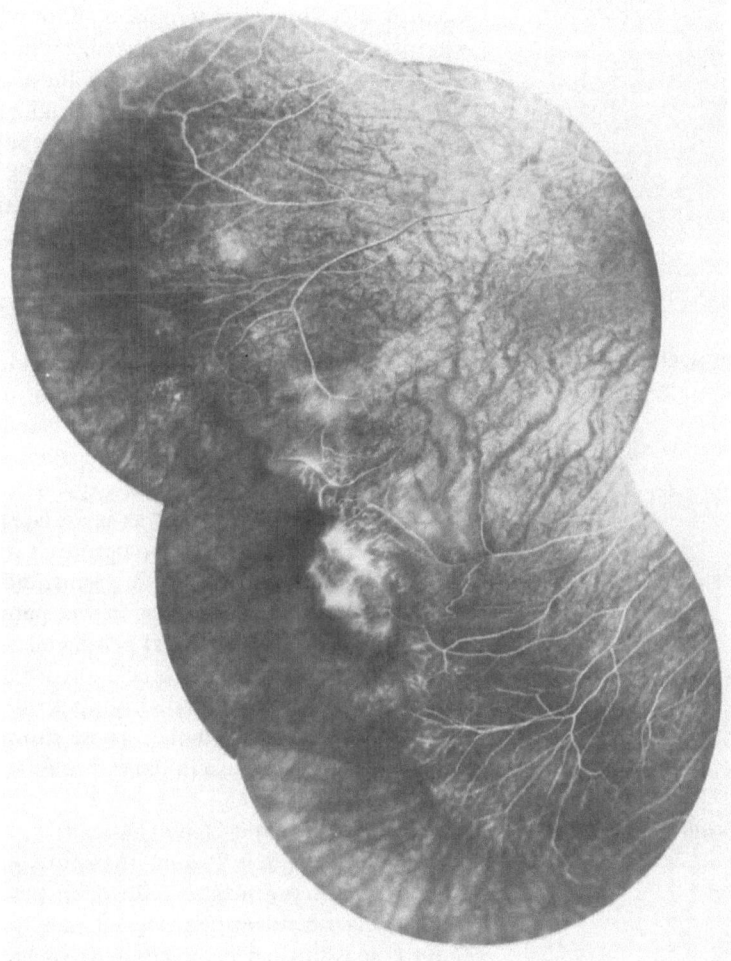

Figure 51 (III-2). OD. Fluorescein angiogram. Composition of the temporal equatorial zone shows numerous vascular ramifications ending abruptly. Fluorescein leakage from a small neovascularization.

Fundi

OS: Only the superior nasal part of the anterior vitreous space can be observed. Here, the vitreous shows cells and a thick fibrovascular tissue mass.

OD: The choroid shows an atrophic area on the temporal side of the disc. The temporal vascular branches take a strikingly stretched course from the disc, radiating to the fundus periphery. The macula shows slight ectopia in the inferior temporal sector, numerous closely packed branches of retina vessels are visible. At the level of the equator these branches terminate abruptly (non-vascularization of the peripheral retina). The boundary between the vascular and the avascular part of the retina meanders slightly and roughly follows the course of the equator. In the superior and in the inferior part of the fundus, this boundary gradually extends in the direction of the extreme periphery, where it disappears from view. There are no defects or exudates.

OS: This fundus is not adequately visible due to the media opacities.

Fluorescein angiogram    OD: The above described abnormal vascular pattern in the inferior temporal quadrant of the retina is readily visible (Figure 51). The vasculature terminates abruptly in delicate irregular ramifications showing dilation of some capillaries, from which fluorescein is seen to leak in the late phase. The peripheral retina shows no perfusion whatsoever in the area photographed. Pigmented layer and choroid show no changes in the peripheral fundus. Just outside the most peripheral zone of the retinal vessels there is a small network of neovascularization from which fairly marked fluorescein leakage is seen. The late phase shows very slight fluorescein leakage in the centre of the posterior pole.

Ultrasonography    OD: The axis length is 28 mm (A-scan).

OS: The axis length is 20 mm. The entire vitreous space contains organizations in which the retina can no longer be identified. The sclera of the posterior pole is thickened and contains calcium.

## General condition

A few months prior to the last ophthalmological examination the patient was admitted to a department of internal medicine with acute arthritic symptoms and fever. An exhaustive examination failed to elicit the cause of the acute polyarthritis. This examination disclosed no congenital abnormalities or any other changes possibly related to his eye condition.

## Therapy

At the hospital in his place of residence the patient was treated on several occasions by Argon laser coagulation in the temporal periphery of the right fundus. No complications developed.

*Course*

We saw this patient again about two years after our first examination. Visual acuity was unchanged. In the temporal fundus periphery the avascular part of the retina contained several coagulation scars. The small neovascularization was no longer visible. The fundus features were otherwise unchanged. We discussed the possibility of a cosmetic lens extraction, with anterior vitrectomy if necessary, and correction of the strabismus OS.

*Conclusion*

Dominant exudative vitreoretinopathy. Severe proliferative vitreous organizations with total retinal detachment OS

*Subject III-1 (27-03-54),*

*History*

No visual complaints. No record of ophthalmological examination. Birth weight unknown. No history of premature birth or neonatal oxygen administration. Good general health.

*Ophthalmological examination*

| | |
|---|---|
| Visual acuity | VOD: C − 0.25 axis 0° 0.8. |
| | VOS: C − 0.5 axis 0° 0.8. |
| Eye position | Straight. |
| Anterior segments | ODS: Normal. |
| Vitreous | ODS: Normal structure of the retrolental vitreous, although it contains some cells. Slight vitreous opacities immediately preretinal in the temporal periphery of both fundi. |
| Fundi | ODS: Slightly abnormal configuration of, in particular, the temporal branches of the retinal vessels in the posterior pole: the normal curvature round the posterior pole is slightly diminished, and the maculae show some ectopia in temporal direction. The temporal retinal periphery shows no retinal vasculature. No exudates or retinal defects. |
| Fluorescein angiogram | OD: In the temporal equatorial zone, the retinal vasculature terminates in short aberrant ramifications from which some fluorescein leaks. No abnormalities of the pigmented layer and choroid. No leakage in the macular region, but the disc shows marked hyperfluorescence in the late phase (Figure 52).<br>OS: The temporal retina is perfused only as far as |

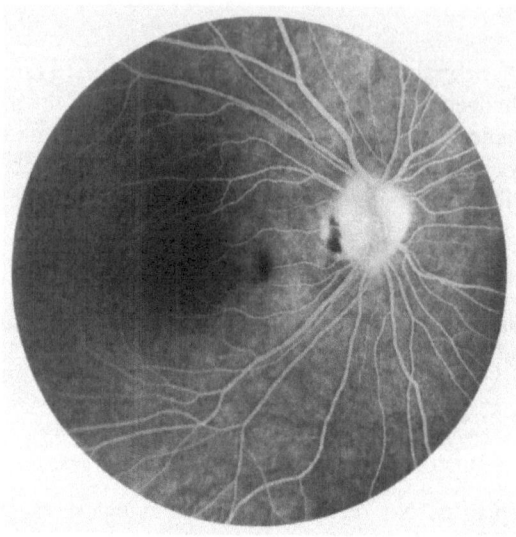

Figure 52 (III-1). OD. Late phase of the angiogram shows hyperfluorescence of the disc. The retinal vasculature is slightly deformed.

the equator. The most peripheral zone of the vasculature consists of aberrant vascular loops and blind-ending small vessels which are often slightly dilatated and leak fluorescein (Figure 53).Outside this area the avascular retina shows a small cicatrix of the pigmented layer, but no other changes of RPE and choroid are visible. The disc shows marked hyperfluorescence in the late phase, but there is no leakage in the macular region.

| | |
|---|---|
| Visual fields (Goldmann) | ODS: Slight limitation of the III-4 isopter in the inferior nasal quadrant. No other changes. |
| Ultrasonography | ODS: Axis length of both eyeballs 23 mm (A-scan). Normal curvature of the posterior pole. |

*Conclusion*
Unmistakable symptoms of DEVR in the fundus periphery ODS. No complications.

*Subject II-2 (27-05-34)*

*History*
This 44-year-old mother of the proband had no history of visual complaints; there was no record of previous ophthalmological examination.

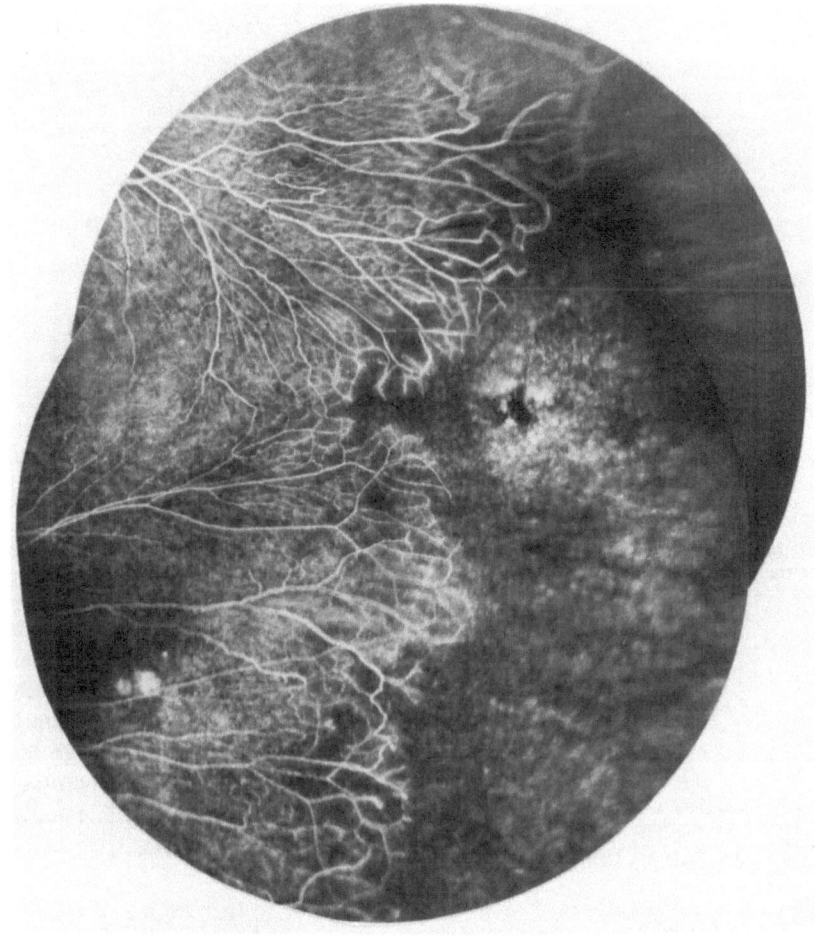

Figure 53 (III-1). OS. The angiogram shows aberrant ramifications of retinal vessels central to the zone of non-perfusion.


*Ophthalmological examination*
Unfortunately, a complete ophthalmological examination could not be made. The examination was limited to indirect ophthalmoscopy of the fundus. Colour photographs of the fundi were also made. On the basis of the findings thus obtained, however, DEVR could be diagnosed with certainty.

Fundi                     In the posterior poles of both fundi the temporal branches of the central retinal artery and vein show an abnormally stretched course in temporal direction. Both maculae show some ectopia in inferior temporal direction (Figure 54). The disc

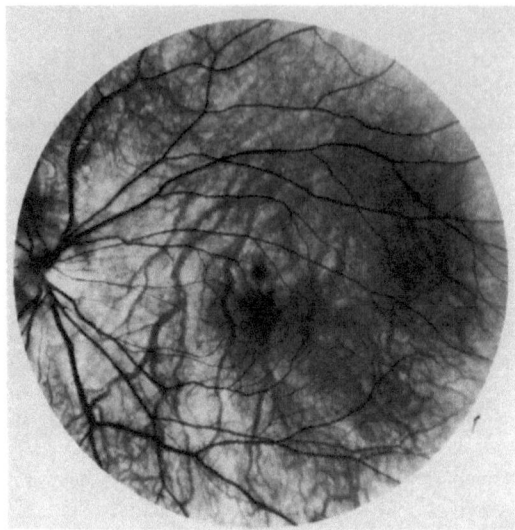

Figure 54 (II-2). OS. Stretched vessels in the posterior pole of the retina and slight ectopia of the macula. (The dark spot above the macula is a photographic artefact.)

OD shows a temporal cone. The peripheral retina ODS is not completely vascularized on the temporal side. The avascular part contains delicate pigmentations. Central to the equator, the inferior temporal vascular retina shows a fair sized tear. At the site of this defect, the retina is lightly elevated by traction (Figure 55). No visible neovascularizations or subretinal exudates.

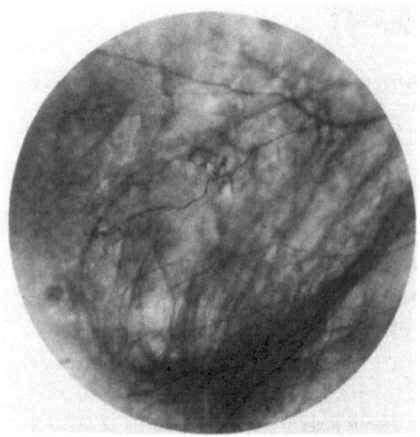 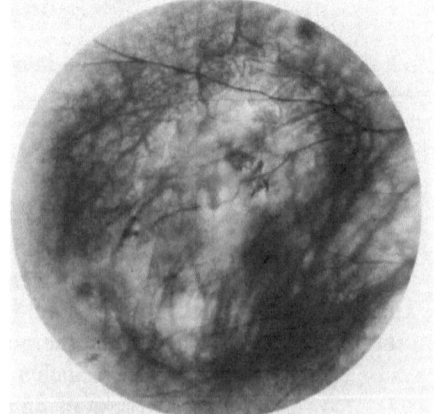

Figure 55 (II-2). Stereo-photograph OD. Retinal tear central to the equator in inferior temporal quadrant.

*Course*

Further examination or treatment was impossible due to lack of motivation on the part of the patient.

*Conclusion*

Unmistakable bilateral retinal vascular changes consistent with a diagnosis of DEVR. Horseshoe tear in the retina OD.

## 3.4 The C family

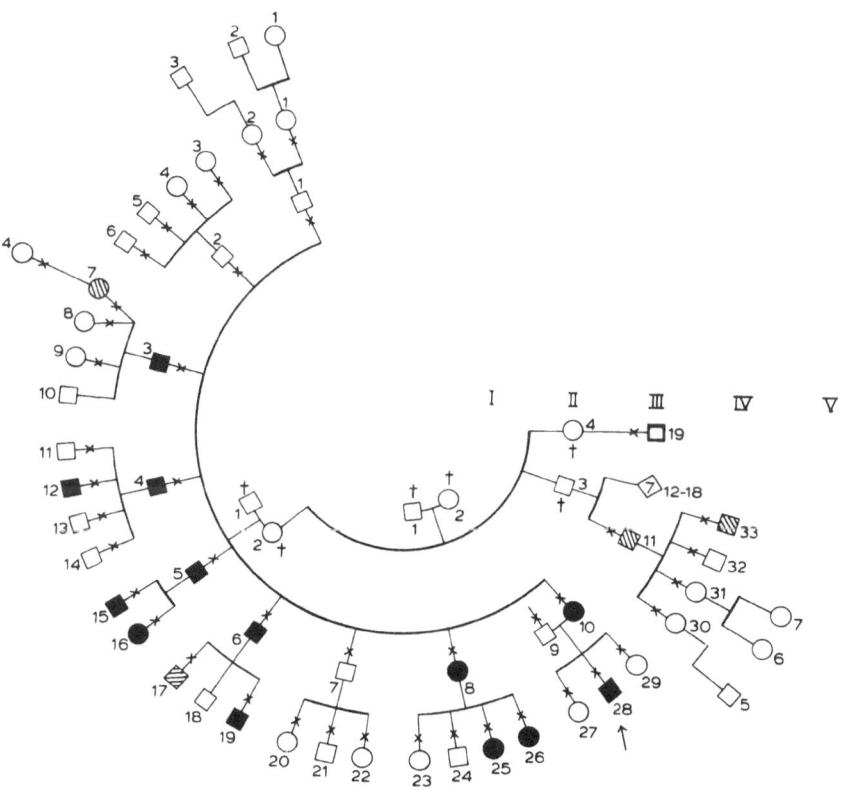

Figure 56. Pedigree of the C family.

*Introduction*

The proband of this family was identified by chance during the study of the A family. The proband's father (IV-2 in the pedigree of the A family) showed no distinct symptoms of DEVR, but the proband's mother was found to show unmistakable symptoms of DEVR in both eyes. A relationship between the proband's mother and the A family was not demonstrable through three preceding generations. This is why a separate pedigree was composed. Consequently the code of the proband of the C family and his mother's code differ from their respective codes in the pedigree of the A family (vide infra). It is quite possible that the A family and the C family are related via ancestors: both families come from the same region in The Netherlands, which until recently has been rather isolated. No exhaustive genealogical study of the two families has so far been performed.

*Proband IV-28 (18-04-56) – Code in the A family: V-2*

*History*
No visual complaints. Ophthalmological examination was performed in view of a blood relationship to the A family via the father, No record of premature birth or neonatal oxygen administration.

*Ophthalmological examination*

| | |
|---|---|
| Visual acuity | VOD: S + 0.5. 1.25 |
| | VOS: S + 0.5. 1.25 |
| Eye position | Straight. Positive kappa angle. |
| Anterior segments | ODS: Normal. |
| Vitreous | ODS: Hyaloid canal clearly visible due to delicate condensations. Vitreous structure otherwise normal. No signs of a persistent hyaloid artery. |
| Fundi | ODS: Disc and macula present a normal appearance. The configuration of the retinal vessels in the posterior pole is normal. Both maculae are localized slightly superior to the horizontal meridian through the disc centre, but there is no distinct ectopia. Numerous ramifications of retinal vessels are localized in the area central to the temporal equator. The arterioles in this area show a decidedly stretched course, and several venules are abnormally tortuous. These vessels terminate abruptly anterior to the equator, leaving the peripheral retina avascular at this site. The nasal periphery of the retina shows an intact vasculature. No exudates, neovascularizations or defects of the retina. |
| Fluorescein angiogram | OD: The early phase reveals no changes in the posterior pole. The temporal retinal periphery is not perfused. An arteriovenous anastomosis extends over a short distance along the boundary |

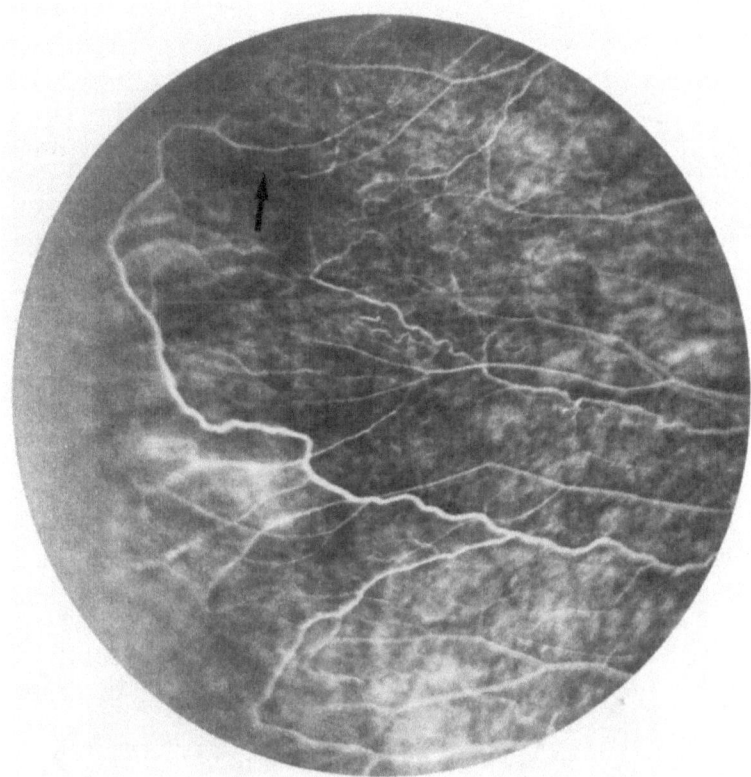

Figure 57 (IV-28). OD. Some fluorescein leakage in the late phase of the angiogram from a few arterioles central to the equator. Some tortuous venous branches. Note the arterio-venous anastomosis (arrow).

between the avascular and the vascular retina (Figure 57). Fluorescein leakage in the liminal zone is slight. The disc is hyperfluorescent in the late phase.

OS: The abnormal configuration of retinal vessels and the tortuous course of some venules are clearly visible (Figure 58). The slightly more peripheral exposures show the termination of the retinal vessels anterior to the equator, and fluorescein leakage from these vessels. The disc is very hyperfluorescent in the late phase, and there is even some fluorescein leakage in the surrounding retina (Figure 59).

## Conclusion

Unmistakable vascular changes in the temporal retinal periphery ODS, consistent with a diagnosis of DEVR.

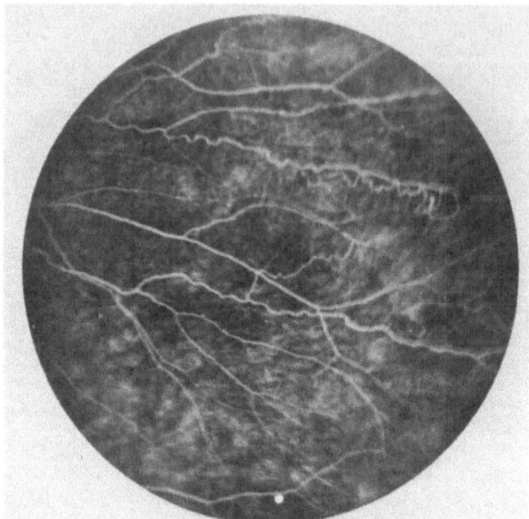

Figure 58 (IV-28). OS. Fluorescein angiogram reveals tortuous venous branches.

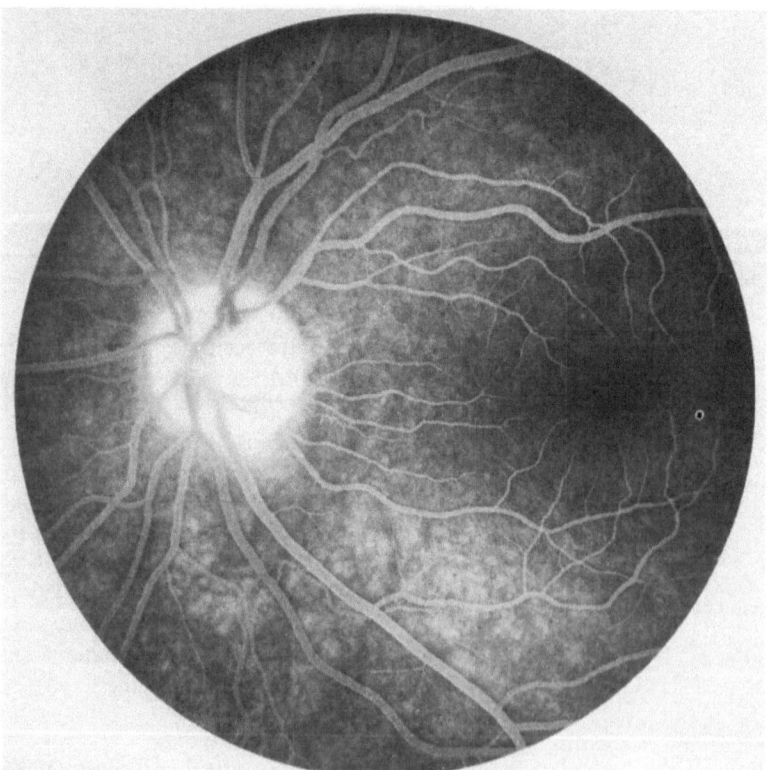

Figure 59 (IV-28). OS. Marked hyperfluorescence of the disc in the late phase of the angiogram.

*Subject III-10 (27-06-27) – Code in the A family: IV-3*

*History*

No visual complaints. Strabismus corrected in childhood (preoperative eye position and type of operation unknown). Birth weight unknown, but no record of premature birth or neonatal oxygen administration.

*Ophthalmological examination*

| | |
|---|---|
| Visual acuity | VOD: S + 5.0/Cyl. − 2.0 axis 15° 0.6. |
| | VOS: S + 4.5 0.8. |
| Eye position | Straight. Wide positive kappa angle. |
| Anterior segments | ODS: Normal. |
| Vitreous | ODS: Normal structure, no cells. |
| Fundi | ODS: In the posterior poles the temporal vascular branches take an abnormally stretched course in temporal direction. Both maculae show some ectopia in temporal direction. The retina between the posterior pole and the temporal equator contains an abnormally large number of vessels with a strikingly parallel course. Several venules in this area are abnormally tortuous. Slightly peripheral to the temporal equator, the retinal vessels terminate in aberrant ramifications, which form a circumscribed zone adjacent to the avascular part of the retina localized peripheral to them. The avascular retina shows some white without pressure. In OS, the inferior temporal sector of this part of the retina shows a few small exudates, immediately peripheral to the terminal ramifications. There are no retinal defects or neovascularizations. |

*Conclusion*

Unmistakable bilateral peripheral retinal vascular changes consistent with a diagnosis of DEVR.

*Subject III-3 (24-09-19)*

*History*

No visual complaints. Birth weight unknown. No record of premature birth.

*Ophthalmological examination*

| | |
|---|---|
| Visual acuity | VOD: 1.0, uncorrected. |
| | VOS: 1.0 with correction (refraction unknown). |

| | |
|---|---|
| Eye position | Straight. |
| Anterior segments | ODS: Normal. |
| Vitreous | ODS: Normal. |
| Fundi | OD: Normal posterior pole. In the temporal equatorial zone between 8 and 10 o'clock there are numerous small retinal vessels, taking a more or less parallel course in radial direction. The small venous branches in this area are very slightly tortuous. Anterior to the equator, the vessels in this area cannot be followed entirely. There are no exudates or defects in the retina. |
| | OS: Normal posterior pole. Posterior to the temporal equator, between 2 and 4 o'clock, abnormally numerous small retinal vessels take a radial course. The small venous branches in this area are abnormally tortuous. The retinal vessels terminate abruptly peripheral to the equator. At 3 o' clock the boundary between the vascular and the avascular part of the retina shows a wedge-shaped notch, where the latter part extends farther in posterior direction. Many delicate superficial pigmentations are visible in the avascular retinal periphery. As in OD, the nasal retinal periphery (so far as visible) is normally vascularized. No retinal defects, exudates or neovascularizations. |

*Conclusion*
Slight peripheral fundus changes ODS, consistent with a diagnosis of uncomplicated DEVR.

*Subject IV-7 (12-11-50)*

*History*
No visual complaints. Birth weight was about 2250 g. No record of neonatal oxygen administration. Patient is one of a pair of dizygotic twins.

*Ophthalmological examination*
| | |
|---|---|
| Visual acuity | VOD: 0.6., uncorrected. |
| | VOS: S − 2.25 0.8. |
| Eye position | Straight. |
| Anterior segments | ODS: Normal. |
| Vitreous | ODS: Normal structure, no cells. |
| Fundi | ODS: Normal appearance of the posterior poles. Central to the temporal equator the small retinal |

vessels show a somewhat stretched course with some multiple ramifications at the level of the equator. Peripheral to the temporal equator, no abruptly terminating vascular branches are visible, but the luminal width of the vessels in this area may have been too small to render them visible with the contact lens. The fundus periphery shows no pigmentations, defects or other lesions of the retina.

*Conclusion*

Slightly abnormal VODS, anisometropia and very slight anomalies of the retinal vasculature of the peripheral fundi. The findings are suggestive, but not conclusive, of a very mild manifestation of DEVR.

*Subject III-4 (31-10-22)*

*History*

No visual complaints. Good general health. Birth weight unknown.

*Ophthalmological examination*

| | |
|---|---|
| Visual acuity | VOD: 1.0, uncorrected. |
| | VOS: 1.0, uncorrected. |
| Eye position | Straight. |
| Intraocular pressure | OD: 14 mm Hg. |
| | OS: 15 mm Hg. |
| Anterior segments | ODS: Normal. |
| Vitreous | ODS: No anomalies apart from slight liquefaction. |
| Fundi | ODS: Slightly abnormal configuration of the retinal vessels in the posterior poles: the temporal branches take a slightly too stretched course from the disc. The maculae seems slightly ectopic. Temporal to the posterior poles there are fairly numerous ramifications of somewhat peculiar orientation. In the fundus OD, a large ramification of the superior temporal artery traverses across the terminal ramifications of the inferior temporal vein (Figure 60). In the temporal retinal periphery the vasculature terminates peripheral to the equator in both eyes. The nasal periphery shows intact vascularization. No exudates, defects or neovascularizations in the peripheral retina. |

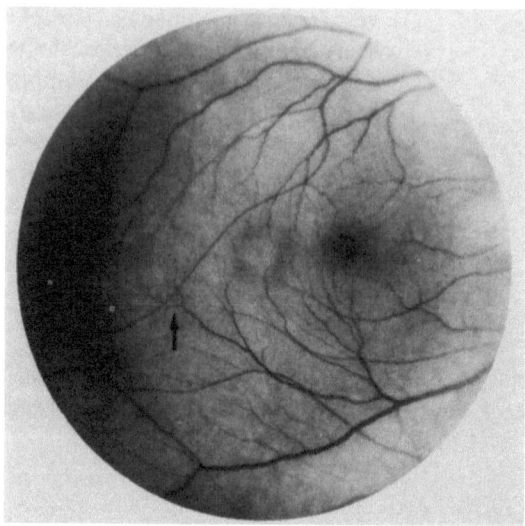

Figure 60 (III-4). OD. Abnormal configuration of retinal vessels temporal to the posterior pole. A ramification of the superior temporal artery traverses across ramifications of the inferior temporal vein (arrow).

## Conclusion
Bilateral retinal vascular changes consistent with a diagnosis of DEVR.

*Subject IV-12 (23-08-55)*

*History*
Poor VOD from the start. In infancy, occlusion treatment OS for a few months, but without success. No strabismus correction by operation or corrective spectacles. No record of premature birth of neonatal oxygen administration.

*Ophthalmological examination*

| Visual acuity | VOD: 2/60. |
| | VOS: S − 0.5 1.0. |
| Cylcoplegic refraction | OD: S − 1.75. |
| | OS: S − 1.0. |
| Eye position | Convergent strabismus OD, about 10°. |
| Anterior segments | ODS: Normal. |
| Vitreous | ODS: Normal structure, no cells. |
| Fundi | OD: Normal disc and macula. Normal pattern of retinal vessels in the posterior pole. Temporal to the posterior pole, numerous vascular branches extend more or less parallel in temporal direction. |

Several smaller ramifications of these vessels, and especially of the venules, are abnormally tortuous near the equator. Between 8 and 10 o'clock, all small retinal vessels terminate abruptly slightly peripheral to the equator, so that the peripheral retina in this sector is entirely avascular.

OS: Normal posterior pole. The vascular pattern of the equatorial retina in the temporal periphery is virtually identical to that in OD. The temporal retinal periphery in the sector between 2 and 4 o' clock, and possibly beyond, is avascular. No pigmentations or defects in the avascular part of the retina.

*Conclusion*

Peripheral retinal vascular changes consistent with a diagnosis of DEVR. Convergent strabismus and amblyopia OD.

*Subject III-5 (31-07-24)*

*History*

Poor VOS from the start. In childhood, examined by several ophthalmologists; corrective spectacles prescribed. Not known whether amblyopia treatment was given. Strabismus operation not performed.

*Ophthalmological examination*

| | |
|---|---|
| Visual acuity | VOD: S + 5.0/Cyl. − 3.5 axis $15°$ 0.8. |
| | VOS: S + 5.5/Cyl. − 4.0 axis $155°$ 0.2. |
| Intraocular pressure | ODS: 14 mm Hg. |
| Eye position | Convergent strabismus OS, about $3°$. |
| Anterior segments | ODS: Normal. |
| Vitreous | ODS: Normal structure, no cells. |
| Fundi | ODS: Normal posterior poles. Temporal to the posterior poles an abnormal number of small vascular branches take a stretched course in temporal direction. Some venous ramifications in the equatorial zone show delicate, corkscrewlike tortuosities. In the area peripheral to the equator in OD and near 3 o'clock in OS, the extreme ramifications of the retinal vessels terminate abruptly. The retina peripheral to these ramifications is avascular in both eyes and in both fundi shows several gross superficial pigmentations. The nasal fundus periphery, so far as visible, |

seems to show a normal retinal vascularization. No retinal defects or neovascularizations.

*Conclusion*

Bilateral peripheral retinal vascular changes consistent with a diagnosis of DEVR. Hypermetropic astigmatism ODS. Convergent strabismus OS and amblyopia OS.

*Subject IV-15 (30-01-61)*

*History*

No visual complaints. No record of premature birth or neonatal oxygen administration. Good general health.

*Ophthalmological examination*

| | |
|---|---|
| Visual acuity | VOD: 1.0., uncorrected. |
| | VOS: 1.0, uncorrected. |
| Eye position | Straight. |
| Anterior segments | ODS: Normal. |
| Vitreous | ODS: Normal structure, but with some delicate whitish particles. |
| Fundi | ODS: Slight ectopia of the maculae in temporal direction. Retinal vessels somewhat stretched and orientated to the 9 o'clock position in OD and to the 3 o'clock position in OS. Due to the parallel course of the vessels and their ramifications, the neuroretina is abundantly vascularized in the mid-periphery near the abovementioned positions. The smaller veins in this area are tortuous. Peripheral to the equator the smallest ramifications terminate rather abruptly (local retinal periphery is avascular). No defects or degenerative areas in the peripheral retina. |

*Conclusion*

Slight changes of the peripheral retinal vasculature, consistent with a diagnosis of DEVR.

*Subject IV-16 (26-11-57)*

*History*

VOS is reported to have always been slightly diminished. In childhood the patient was reportedly examined ophthalmologically but no amblyopia treatment was given. The birth weight was about 3500 g. No record of neonatal oxygen administration. Good general health.

*Ophthalmological examination*

| | |
|---|---|
| Visual acuity | VOD: 1.0, uncorrected. |
| | VOS: S + 1.5/Cyl. − 1.0 axis 175° 0.8. |
| Eye position | Straight. |
| Anterior segments | ODS: Normal. |
| Vitreous | ODS: Normal structure, no cells. |
| Fundi | ODS: In both posterior poles, diminished curvature of the large temporal vessels pericentrally. Both maculae show slight ectopia in temporal direction. Some retinal vessels in the temporal mid-periphery show a rather irregular tortuous course. In the inferior temporal quadrant, it is only just distinguishable that a few peripheral vascular branches terminate abruptly in a few short terminal ramifications distinctly anterior to the equator. The extreme retinal periphery in these quadrants is avascular but otherwise presents a normal appearance. Nowhere else in the fundi are peripheral degenerative changes, exudates or neovascularizations of the retina seen. |

*Conclusion*

Slight bilateral peripheral retinal vascular changes consistent with a diagnosis of DEVR. Slight anisometropia and slightly subnormal VOS.

*Subject III-6 (21-12-25)*

*History*

No visual complaints. No record of premature birth or neonatal oxygen administration.

*Ophthalmological examination*

| | |
|---|---|
| Visual acuity | VOD: S + 0.5. 0.8. |
| | VOS: S + 0.5 0.8. |
| Eye position | Straight. |
| Anterior segments | ODS: Normal. |
| Vitreous | ODS: Normal structure, no cells. |
| Fundi | ODS: The retinal vessels in the posterior pole are slightly stretched, especially in OS (Figure 61). The macular zones ODS contain delicate drusen-like translucencies. Central to the temporal |

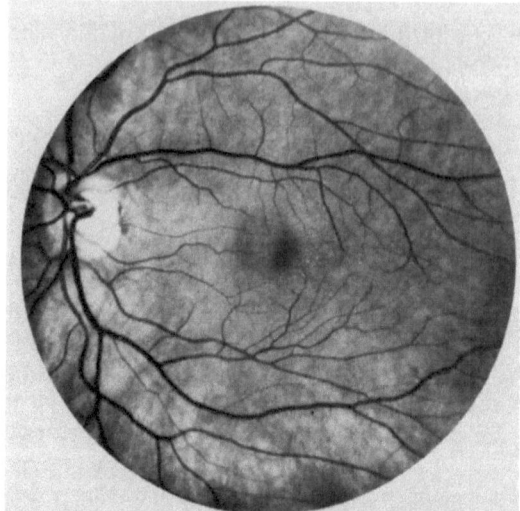

Figure 61 (III-6). OS. Slightly stretched course of the temporal vascular branches.

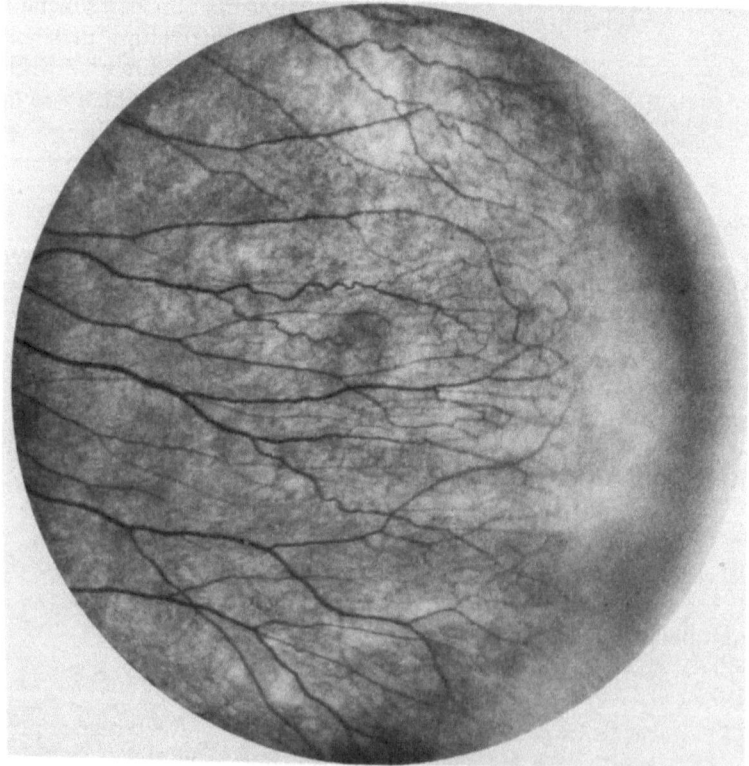

Figure 62 (III-6). OS. Numerous ramifications in the area central to the temporal equator. The retinal periphery is avascular (right side of photograph).

equator ODS, an increased number of vascular ramifications take a more or less parallel course in temporal direction (Figure 62). They terminate abruptly anterior to the temporal equator. The avascular retinal periphery OS shows no unusual features, but in OD it assumes a whitish colour near 4 o'clock. No retinal defects, exudates or neovascularizations.

*Conclusion*
Bilateral retinal vascular changes consistent with a diagnosis of DEVR.

*Subject IV-17 (19-10-58)*

*History*
No visual complaints. Birth weight 4500 g. No neonatal oxygen administration.

*Ophthalmological examination*

| | |
|---|---|
| Visual acuity | VOD: S − 1.0/Cyl. − 0.25 axis 110° 0.8. |
| | VOS: S − 0.5/Cyl. − 0.5 axis 90° 1.0. |
| Eye position | Straight. |
| Anterior segments | ODS: Normal. |
| Vitreous | Normal structure, no cells. |
| Fundi | ODS: Normal posterior poles. Vascular pattern temporal to the posterior poles likewise normal. Peripheral to the equator on the temporal side, some small ramifications of retinal vessels show slight anomalies: some curve abruptly and take a course more or less parallel to the ora serrata, to ramify into terminal branches of insufficient luminal width to be visible. Some other peripheral retinal vessels in this area curve even further and return to the equator, while ramifying into a few short, hardly visible terminal branches. It cannot be established with certainty whether the temporal retinal periphery is vascularized. The fundus periphery OS contains a pigmented cicatrix anterior to the equator near 3 o'clock. No other changes are visible. |

*Conclusion*
Minimal vascular changes in the temporal fundus periphery ODS. Probably a very mild form of DEVR, but the diagnosis cannot be clinched.

*Subject IV-19 (06-04-63)*

*History*
No visual complaints. Birth weight about 4500 g. No neonatal oxygen administration.

*Ophthalmological examination*

| | |
|---|---|
| Visual acuity | VOD: S − 2.75 0.8. |
| | VOS: S − 2.75 0.8. |
| Eye position | Straight. |
| Anterior segments | ODS: Normal. |
| Vitreous | ODS: Normal. |
| Fundi | ODS: Slightly stretched temporal branches of the retinal vessels in the posterior poles, but no distinct ectopia of the maculae. The temporal peripheral retina is avascular ODS, and somewhat whitish OS. Near 3 o'clock and 9 o'clock in OD and OS, respectively, the avascular retina extends in central direction to a level near the equator, where this is bounded by aberrant ramifications of the most peripheral retinal vessals. In OS, these short terminal ramifications form a clearly defined boundary from the avascular retinal periphery, but in OD the transition from vascular to avascular retina is less well-defined. No retinal defects, pigmentations or neovascularizations. |

*Conclusion*

Bilateral retinal vascular changes consistent with a diagnosis of DEVR.

*Subject III-8 (06-04-31)*

*History*

No visual complaints. No record of premature birth of neonatal oxygen administration.

*Ophthalmological examination*

| | |
|---|---|
| Visual acuity | VOD: 1.25, uncorrected. |
| | VOS: 1.25, uncorrected. |
| Eye position | Straight. Slightly nasal corneal reflex OS. |
| Intraocular pressure | ODS: 15 mm Hg. |
| Anterior segments | ODS: Normal. |
| Vitreous | ODS: Normal structure, no cells. |
| Fundi | ODS: The temporal branches of the central retinal artery and vein in the posterior poles show a slightly stretched course in temporal direction. The macula OS seems to show slight ectopia in the same direction. Temporal to the posterior pole ODS, an abnormally large number of vascular branches take a more or less parallel course. Some terminal ramifications of these vessels |

curve slightly in central direction. In the temporal periphery OS it is just distinguishable that the smallest ramifications end rather abruptly, so that the more anterior part of the retina is avascular. No such transition is visible in the temporal periphery OD. No other anomalies in the fundus periphery ODS. A pigmented retinal cicatrix is visible just outside the large vascular branches in the inferior temporal sector of the posterior pole OS.

*Conclusion*
Bilateral retinal vascular changes consistent with a diagnosis of DEVR.

*Subject IV-25 (26-07-63)*

*History*
No visual complaints. Birth weight about 3000 g. No neonatal oxygen administration.

*Ophthalmological examination*

| | |
|---|---|
| Visual acuity | VOD: 1.25, uncorrected. |
| | VOS: 1.25, uncorrected. |
| Eye position | Straight. |
| Anterior segments | ODS: Normal. |
| Vitreous | ODS: Normal structure, no cells. |
| Fundi | ODS: The large vessels in the posterior poles are slightly stretched in temporal direction. The maculae show slight ectopia. The fundus area temporal to the posterior pole ODS contains numerous branches of the temporal retinal vessels arranged more or less parallel. They end in abnormally short terminal ramifications anterior to the equator, so that the retinal periphery in these parts of the fundi is avascular. The avascular retina ODS shows slight white without pressure and delicate pigmentations. No visible retinal defects or exudates. |

*Conclusion*
Bilateral retinal vascular changes consistent with a diagnosis of DEVR.

*Subject IV-26 (27-04-67)*

*History*
No visual complaints. Birth weight about 3000 g. No neonatal oxygen administration.

*Ophthalmological examination*

| | |
|---|---|
| Visual acuity | VOD: S + 0.75/Cyl. − 0.75 axis 125° 0.8. |
| | VOS: Cyl. − 0.25 axis 160° 0.8. |
| Eye position | Straight. |
| Anterior segments | ODS: Normal. |
| Vitreous | ODS: Normal structure, no cells. |
| Fundi | ODS: The retinal vessels in the posterior poles are slightly stretched, but the maculae show no ectopia. Between 7 and 10 o'clock OD and between 2 and 4 o'clock OS, a distinct boundary between avascular and vascular retina is visible peripheral to the equator. This boundary takes a slightly undulating course and is not visible outside the abovementioned sectors. The retinal vessels within these sectors end in delicate multiple ramifications on the central boundary of the avascular retinal periphery. Delicate pigmentations are visible in the avascular retina ODS, but no other changes are observed. |

*Conclusion*

Bilateral peripheral retinal vascular changes consistent with a diagnosis of DEVR.

*Subject IV-33 (09-05-65)*

*History*

As early as December 1979 this boy had been referred to our department with retinal detachment OS, which was probably of long standing because the school medical officer had found reduced VOS 5 months earlier. Two years earlier he had reportedly sustained a blow from a football against the left eye. The relationship with the C family was discovered only in the course of the family study. For this reason the examination of the peripheral fundus was repeated and supplemented by fluorescein angiography. Moreover, two sisters (IV-30 and IV-31), a brother (IV-32) and the father (III-11) were examined. The general history of IV-33 was uncharacteristic. No record of premature birth or neonatal oxygen administration.

*Ophthalmological examination (preoperative, December 1979)*

| | |
|---|---|
| Visual acuity | VOD: S − 0.5 1.25. |
| | VOS: 1/60. |
| Eye position | Straight. |
| Intraocular pressure | OD: 17 mm Hg. |
| | OS: 11 mm Hg. |
| Vitreous | OD: Normal structure, no cells. |
| | OS: Many pigment particles. |

| Fundi | OD: Normal posterior pole. No degenerative changes or defects in the retinal periphery. In the temporal retinal periphery the smaller ramifications of the vessels anterior to the equator are no longer visible. The more central vessels show a normal configuration. |
|---|---|
| | OS: Shifting retinal detachment in both inferior quadrants with a large amount of subretinal fluid. A very small circular retinal defect is visible peripheral to the equator near 1 o'clock. It is localized at the end of a narrow peripheral extension of the retinal detachment. Between the 11 and the 2 o'clock meridian, the retina is in situ. The macula is not included in the retinal detachment. There are several gross pigment deposits in the periphery, but no distinct vascular anomalies are visible. |

*General physical examination*
No abnormal findings were obtained.

*Therapy*
Surgical treatment of the retinal detachment encompassed the following procedures:

10.12.79: Silicone encircling; drainage of subretinal fluid; intravitreous injection of balanced salt solution; episcleral buckle of superior temporal quadrant. Postoperative finding: non-attachment of the retina.

20-12-79: Drainage of subretinal fluid; cryocoagulations of the equatorial sclera; insufflation of an air/SF6 gas mixture; tightening of the encircling loop.
Re-detachment after 6 weeks. Traction of epiretinal membranes. Possibly minute defect inferior and central to the indentation.

24-03-80: Pars plana vitrectomy; internal drainage; episcleral buckle between 4 and 8 o' clock; cryocoagulations and insufflation of an air/SF6 gas mixture.
Re-attachment of the retina (18 months' follow-up).
VOS: 3/60.

| Fluorescein angiogram | OD: The early phase focuses on the area central to the equator, peripheral to which no distinct retinal perfusion is visible. A marginal zone with aberrant terminal ramifications is not visible, nor is fluorescein leakage (Figure 63). |
|---|---|
| | OS: Late exposures of the posterior pole show alterations of the pigmented layer and some fluorescein leakage from retinal vessels, probably as a |

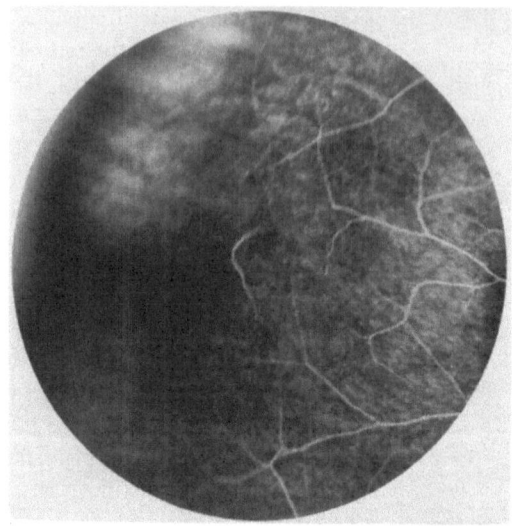

Figure 63 (IV-33). OD. Fluorescein angiogram showing slight aberrant pattern of retinal vessels anterior to the equator. No fluorescein leakage.

result of the retinal detachment and the surgical procedures. The periphery is not clearly visualized.

*Conclusion*

Rhegmatogenous retinal detachment OS. Apparently disturbed perfusion of the temporal retinal periphery OD. The changes are probably a manifestation of DEVR, but the diagnosis is not quite certain.

*Subject III-11 (10-03-25)*

*History*

No visual complaints. No record of premature birth.

*Ophthalmological examination*

| | |
|---|---|
| Visual acuity | VOD: 1.0, uncorrected. |
| | VOS: 1.0, uncorrected. |
| Eye position | Straight. |
| Anterior segments | ODS: Normal. |
| Vitreous | ODS: Normal structure, no cells. |
| Fondi | ODS: Normal posterior poles. Normal configuration of retinal vessels throughout the posterior fundi. In the temporal equatorial zone of both fundi, a few slightly tangentially curved or even reversing retinal vessels are seen near the horizontal meridian. The retina peripheral to this area, so far as visible, seems avascular. However, no dis- |

tinct boundary between vascular and avascular retina is visible. No defects, exudates or degenerative changes in the peripheral fundi.

*Conclusion*

Slight bilateral peripheral retinal vascular changes, which may represent a mild manifestation of DEVR. However, the diagnosis is not certain. Fluorescein angiography might supply more information on the vascular anomalies but, in the absence of subjective symptoms, the patient's motivation for this examination is poor.

*Subject III-19 (07-01-23)*

*History*

This blind 58-year-old man was examined at his home, as he requested. VODS has always been poor, and reading caused great difficulties in primary school. Reported to have had severe encephalitis at age 9. Marked deterioration of visual acuity at about age 20. Lens extraction OS at age 35? This was followed by some improvement in VOS.

*Ophthalmological examination*

| | |
|---|---|
| Visual acuity | VODS: No light perception. |
| Eye position | Divergent strabismus with nystagmoid movements. |
| Anterior segments | No distinct changes. Pupils do not respond to light. Dense cataract OD, and some after-cataract OS. |
| Fundi | OD: No light reflex. |
| | OS: Totally atrophic disc. Many gross pigment deposits in the posterior pole of the retina. No retinal vessels visible. |

*Conclusion*

Bilateral absence of light perception with cataract OD. Situation after lens extraction, total disc atrophy and retinopathy with pigmentations of unknown origin OS. The findings are not consistent with a terminal stage of DEVR.

### 3.5 The D family

*Introduction*

The proband of this family (VI-3) was referred to our department in September 1980 in view of a recent diminution of VOD as a result of retinal detachment. The preoperative fundus examination revealed changes which might be suggestive of DEVR. To clinch this possible diagnosis, the parents and a brother and sister of this patient were examined. When unmistakable symptoms found in the father clinched the diagnosis of DEVR, efforts were made to examine as many family members as possible.

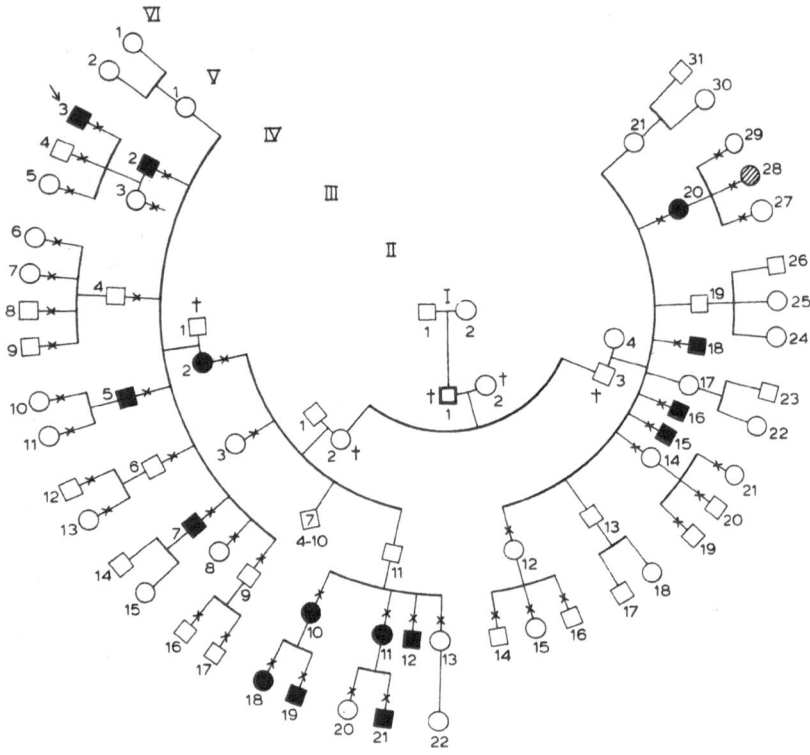

Figure 64. The pedigree of the D family.

*Proband VI-3 (18-02-63)*

*History*

This 17-year-old male was referred by his ophthalmologist in view of a one-week history of diminished VOD. Examination had revealed retinal detachment OD. VOS had always been poor, and VOD was reported never to have been optimal. In infancy, this patient had in this context been examined by another ophthalmologist. Strabismus correction was reported to have been performed at age 4 (type of correction and indication no longer traceable). Amblyopia treatment never given. In spite of the somewhat limited visual acuity, patient attended normal primary and secondary schools. General health has always been good. No record of premature birth or neonatal oxygen administration. No complications during pregnancy. The family history showed that a few paternal cousins once removed had always had poor eyesight.

*Ophthalmological examination*

Visual acuity                    VOD: S − 6.0/Cyl. − 4.0 axis 195° 0.1.
                                 VOS: 1/60.

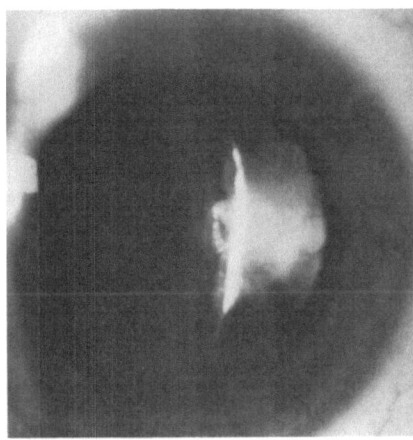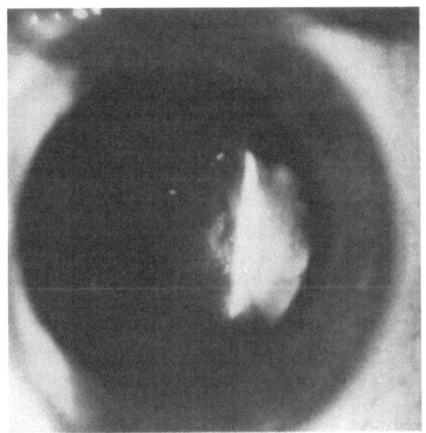

Figure 65 (VI-3). OS. Stereo-photograph. Tissue mass attached to the posterior lens capsule on the temporal side. The lens is locally cataractous.

| | |
|---|---|
| Eye position | Straight. OD seems to have an abnormally wide kappa angle (not exactly assessable due to nystagmus). Pendular nystagmus, especially upon attempts at fixation on small objects. |
| Anterior segments | ODS: Normal. |
| Vitreous | OD: An unmistakable vitreous membrane extends anterior to the temporal periphery.<br>OS: A fibrotic mass in the retrolental space is attached to the posterior aspect of the lens on the temporal side (Figure 65). The posterior capsule and cortex of the lens show a local opacity at 3 o'clock. The vitreous structure ODS shows liquefaction, and delicate white particles are visible. No pigment particles. |
| Fundi | OD: The retina temporal to the posterior pole contains a large exudate, and there are numerous smaller exudates central to it in the posterior pole, temporal and superior to the macular (Figure 66). The macula shows some ectopia in temporal direction. The large retinal vessels in and around the posterior pole are abnormally stretched in the same direction and take a parallel course. A flat retinal detachment extends throughout the fundus periphery between 8 and 11 o'clock, and centrally into the macular region. This sector of the fundus periphery contains an abnormally large number of small ramifications of retinal vessels, terminating abruptly in the equatorial zone. The retina peripheral to this is avascular. |

108

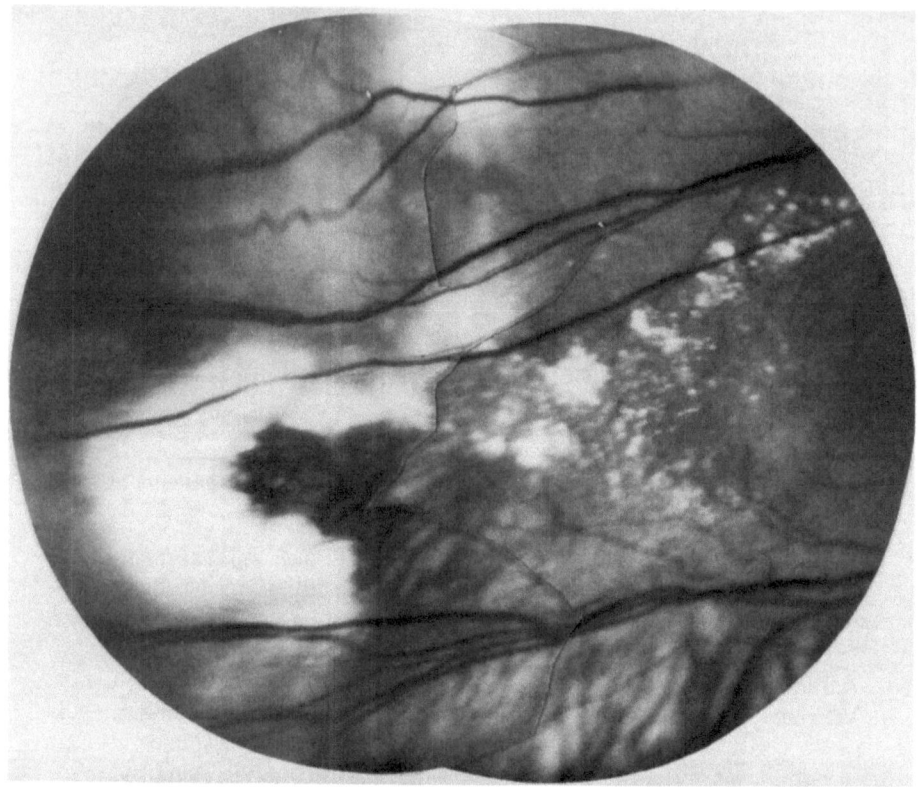

Figure 66 (VI-3). OD. Flat retinal detachment with subretinal and intraretinal exudates temporal to the posterior pole. Note the course of the retinal vessels.

Near the boundary between vascular and avascular retina, several delicate fibrotic structures connect the retina with preretinal vitreous membranes of low density. The nasal retinal periphery seems to be entirely in situ and shows an intact vasculature. There are no gross pigmentations or active neovascularizations. No retinal defects are visible.

OS: A falciform retinal fold extends from the disc into the vitreous space at the 4 o'clock meridian (Figure 67). On the peripheral side this retinal duplicature proves to end in a white tissue mass attached to the posterior lens capsule in the inferior temporal sector and, so far as can be seen, probably also to the pars plana. A few blood vessels are visible in the tissue mass. Near the disc, the retinal vessels are distorted in inferior temporal direction, and several branches are included

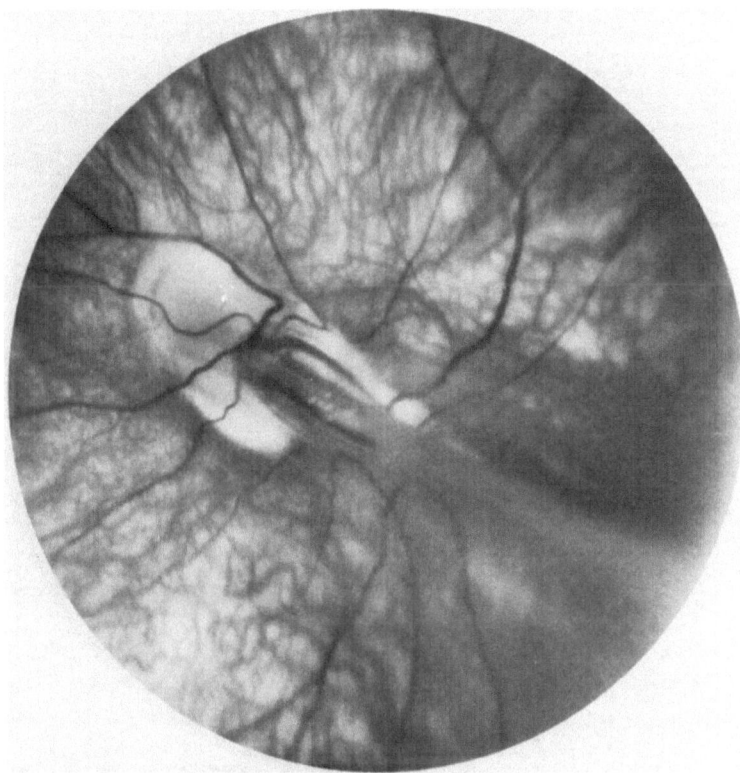

**Figure 67 (VI-3). OS.** A raised retinal fold extends from the disc to the inferior temporal sector. The choroidal vessels are clearly visible.

in the falciform fold. No hyaloid vessels or other remnants of the primary vitreous other than these retinal vessels are visible in the posterior pole. Choriocapillaris and retinal pigmented layer seem underdeveloped in the posterior pole, and consequently the large choroidal vessels and sclea are readily visible in this area. The macula is not visible (probably included in the retinal fold). There are no vascular proliferations apart from the fibrovascular tissue mass. No retinal defects, subretinal or intraretinal exudates or pigmented scars are visible.

Fluorescein angiogram     OD: Dilatation of perimacular capillaries is visible in the early phase. A little later, considerable fluorescein leakage is seen from these vessels and from the capillary bed superior and temporal to

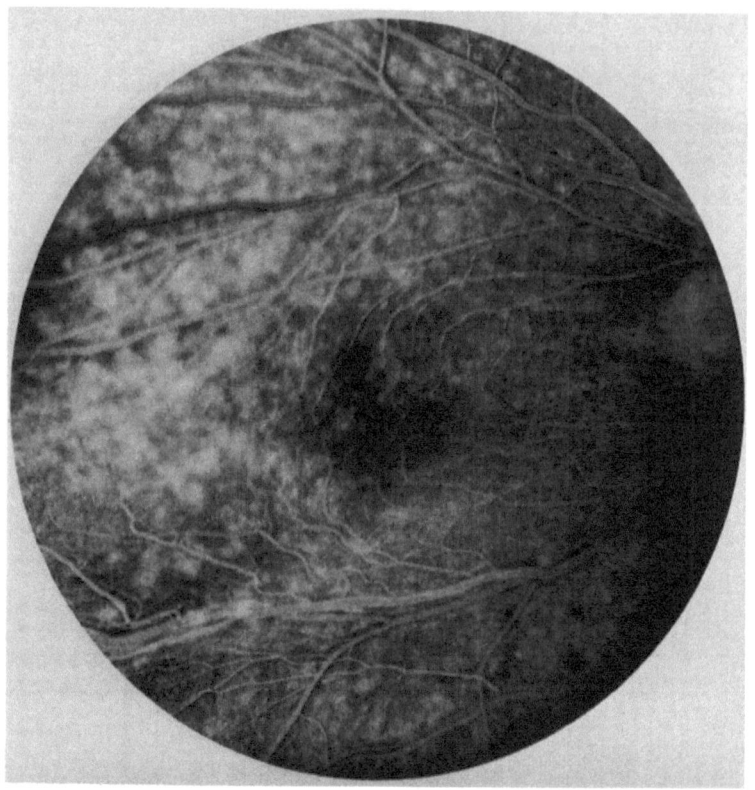

Figure 68 (VI-3). OD. Diffuse fluorescein leakage as early as the arteriovenous phase of the angiogram.

the macula (Figure 68). The retinal circulation time is increased (about 10 sec). Leakage from the retinal vessels in the temporal mid-periphery and on the disc is seen in the late phase.

OS: The late phase shows fairly diffuse leakage from the retinal vascular bed and intensive leakage from the fibrovascular tissue mass in the temporal periphery.

*General physical examination*
No abnormalities were found at general physical examination.

*Laboratory studies:*
Blood                    Haemoglobin: 9.9 mmol/l.
                         Haematocrit: 0.44.
                         Leucocyte count: $5.5 \times 10^9$/l.

| | Differentation: | eosinophils | 21% |
| | | basophils | 1% |
| | | neutrophils | 52% |
| | | lymphocytes | 26% |
| Serum values | Electrolytes: | Na | 139 |
| | | K | 4.2 |
| | | Cl | 99 |
| | | HCO₃ | 29.9 |

Urea: 5.0 mmol/l.
Creatinine: 103 mmol/l.
Alkaline phosphatase: 72 U/l.
SGOT: 15 U/l.
SGPT: 16 U/l.

Coagulation studies Bleeding time (Ivy)' 1 min 55 sec – 1 min 36 sec
– 2 min 33 sec.
Platelets: $224 \times 10^9$ /l.
Quick time: 20 sec.
Thrombotest (Owren): 95%.
Cephalin-kaolin time (Langdell-Margolis): 34 sec.
Fibrinogen content: 2730 mg/l.
Thrombin time: 24 sec.
Conclusion: normal coagulation data.

*Therapy*

The retinal detachment OD was treated by operation a few days after admission. Superior temporal drainage of subretinal fluid, followed by injection of Ringer's solution into the vitreous space via the pars plana. Cryocoagu-

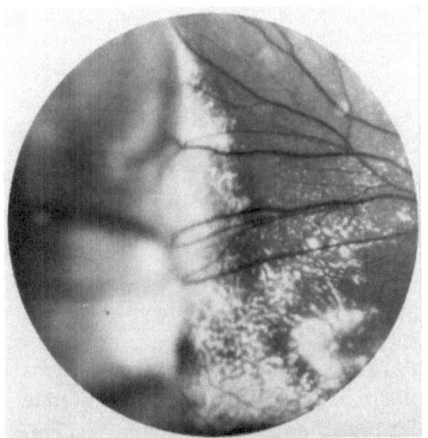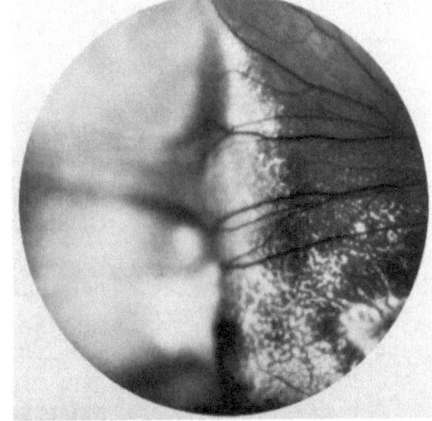

Figure 69 (VI-3). OD. Stereo-photograph. Re-attachment of the retina in the temporal part of the fundus after scleral buckling.

lations in the area of the temporal equator and central to this. A nr. 40 encircling loop was fastened round the eyeball virtually on the equator; in the temporal sector between about 8 and 12 o'clock, a silicone explant was pushed beneath the encircling loop in order to enlarge the indentation in this sector.

*Postoperative course*
A small amount of subretinal fluid was present central to the indentation in the superior temporal quadrant. Some increase in subretinal exudates was observed during a few weeks temporal to the posterior pole (Figure 69). Corrected visual acuity two months after the operation was 0.2. On the indentation of the encircling loop near 10 o'clock, a rather taut serous vesicle of the neuroretina persisted. Visual acuity remained unchanged, and a contact lens was prescribed for OD.

*Visual fields*
Six weeks after the operation, general sensitivity was diminished ODS, with absolute limitation of the nasal visual field. The blind spots cannot be located accurately due to slight nystagmus.

*Conclusion*
Fundus changes consistent with a diagnosis of DEVR, complicated by congenital retinal fold OS and mainly exudative retinal detachment OD, treated by operation.

*Subject V-2 (22-03-34)*

*History*
No visual or ocular complaints other than mild complaints about lacrimation OD. Good general health. Normal birth weight. No neonatal oxygen administration.

*Ophthalmological examination*

| Visual acuity | VOD: S − 3.5/Cyl. − 1.25 axis 80° 0.8. |
| | VOS: S − 2.5/Cyl. − 0.75 axis 130° 0.8. |
| Eye position | Straight; central corneal reflexes. |
| Anterior segments | ODS: Normal. |
| Vitreous | ODS: Some syneresis. Central posterior vitreous detachment anterior to both posterior poles. No cells or pigment particles. |
| Fundi | OD: Slight temporal ectopia of the macula. Temporal to the posterior pole, abnormally numerous retinal vascular branches are seen. The retinal vasculature terminates abruptly in a well-defined zone immediately anterior to the equator. Just |

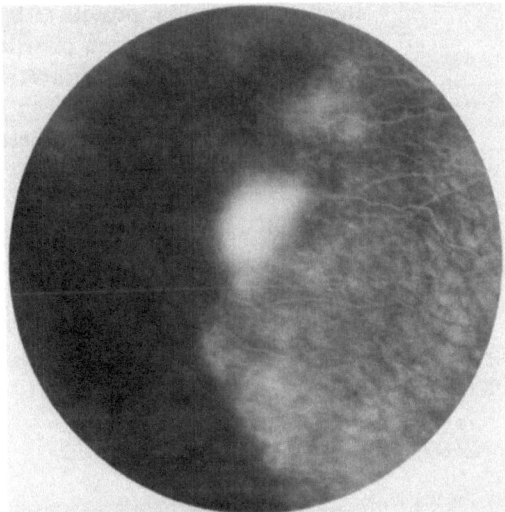

Figure 70 (V-2). OD. Fluorescein angiogram. Non-perfusion of the peripheral retina. Intensive leakage from a small neovascularization.

Fluorescein angiogram

peripheral to this zone on the 3 o'clock meridian there is a small neovascularization which shows some whitish fibrosis. No exudates, retinal defects or distinct signs of traction on the peripheral retina. As in the fundus OD, the retinal periphery in the nasal half, so far as visible, is normally vascularized.

OD: Abruptly ending temporal vasculature. The terminal ramifications of the retinal vessels are slightly dilatated and show fluorescein leakage. An intensively leaking neovascularization is visible on the 10 o'clock meridian (Figure 70). Hyperfluorescent disc in the late phase. No leakage from perimacular capillaries.

OS: The early phase reveals the abrupt termination of the retinal vasculature in the temporal equatorial zone. At one site, a neovascularization peripheral to the line of demarcation has grown into the avascular retina. The capillaries in the peripheral zone of the vascular retina show numerous saccular dilatations. Many capillaries seem to have a loose end unconnected to other parts of the vasculature, and end blindly in such dilatations (Figure 71a). Intensive leakage from the neovascularization occurs after a few seconds, and the peripheral zone of retinal vessels shows less marked leakage (Figure 71b). The late phase of the posterior pole shows a hyperfluorescent disc but no leakage in the macular region.

*Policy*
It was decided to confine activities to periodical follow-ups, and not to coagulate the neovascularizations as long as they remained stationary.

*Conclusion*
Distinct bilateral retinal vascular changes consistent with a diagnosis of DEVR. Small neovascularizations ODS.

*Subject V-5 (26-12-37)*

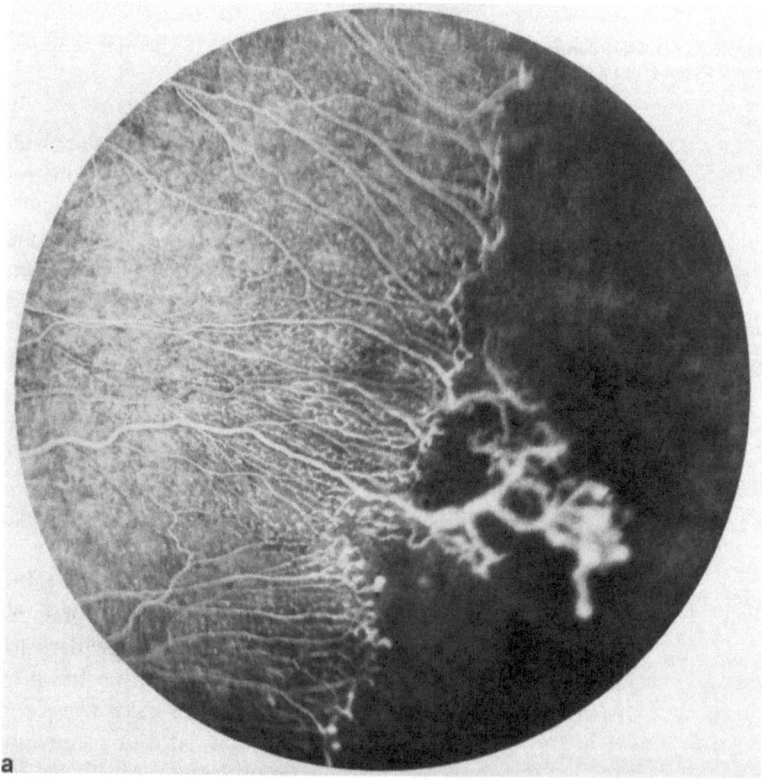

a

Figure 71 (V-2). OS. a) Non-perfusion of the peripheral retina in the early phase of angiography. Neovascularizations in the avascular zone. Note the numerous small outpouchings along the small peripheral ramifications in the retinal vasculature. b) Slight diffuse leakage in the peripheral retinal vascular bed and intensive leakage from the neovascularizations.

*History*

No visual or ocular complaints other than recent recurrent erosion of the cornea OD. Birth weight unknown, but birth reportedly premature (about 8 months). No record of neonatal oxygen administration.

*Ophthalmological examination*

| | |
|---|---|
| Visual acuity | VOD: S − 0.25/Cyl. − 1.25 axis 95° 1.0. |
| | VOS: S − 0.5 0.8. |
| Eye position | Straight; central corneal reflexes. |
| Anterior segments | ODS: Normal. |
| Vitreous | ODS: Normal structure, no cells. |
| Fundi | ODS: Normal vasculature in the posterior poles. No macular ectopia. Immediately temporal, too, no distinctly abnormal configuration of retinal vessels is visible. In the temporal equatorial zone, however, both fundi show several retinal vessels which terminate in short multiple ramifications leaving the peripheral retina apparently avascular. |

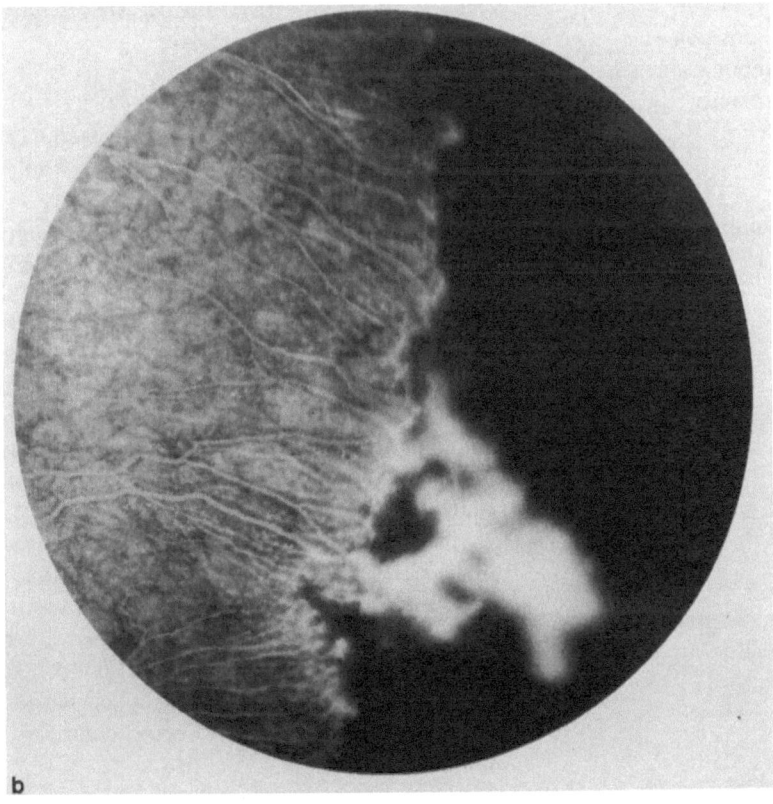

b

At the level of these terminal ramifications, near the 3 o'clock meridian, a small pigmented scar is visible in OS. No degenerative changes in the avascular fundus periphery.

*Conclusion*

Slight bilateral vascular changes in the temporal fundus periphery, consistent with a diagnosis of DEVR.

*Subject V-7 (01-05-42)*

*History*

No visual complaints. Good general health. No record of premature birth or neonatal oxygen administration.

*Ophthalmological examination*

| | |
|---|---|
| Visual acuity | VOD: 1.0, uncorrected. |
| | VOS: S − 0.5/Cyl. − 0.75 axis 10° 0.8. |
| Eye position | Straight; central corneal reflexes. |
| Anterior segments | ODS: Normal. |
| Vitreous | OD: Normal structure, no cells. |
| | OS: Normal structure of retrolental vitreous. The vitreous anterior to the temporal retinal periphery shows delicate opacities and is very mobile. |
| Fundi | OD: Normal posterior pole. The retina posterior to the temporal equator shows some very tortuous venous branches (like corkscrews). The small retinal vessels terminate in a well-defined zone immediately anterior to the equator. Near 9 o'clock, this boundary between vascular and avascular retina deviates in central direction, thus producing a wedge-shaped extension of the avascular retina between the most peripheral vascular ramifications. |
| | OS: Normal posterior pole. As in OD, the temporal retinal periphery is avascular and, near 3 o'clock, shows a wedge-shaped extension in central direction. Some small venous branches are extremely tortuous. Between 1 and 2 o'clock, the avascular retina shows a whitish spot surrounding a minute circular defect. No neovascularizations or exudates. |

*Conclusion*
Bilateral peripheral retinal vascular changes consistent with a diagnosis of DEVR.

*Subject IV-2 (02-10-09)*

*History*
No defined visual complaints. Patient has a history of several operations, e.g. cholecystectomy, operation for rectocele and partial pancreatectomy after pancreatitis. Diabetes mellitus developed after this operation, necessitating insulin medication. As a result of drum perforations after otitis media, hearing is somewhat defective. No record of premature birth.

*Ophthalmological examination*

| | |
|---|---|
| Visual acuity | VOD: S + 3.0/Cyl. − 3.0 axis 108° 0.5. |
| | VOS: S + 3.0/Cyl. − 3.5 axis 98° 0.4. |
| Eye position | Straight. |
| Intraocular pressure | ODS: 18 mm Hg. |
| Anterior segments | ODS: Nuclear cataract causing slight optical disturbance. |
| Vitreous | OD: Normal structure. Posterior vitreous detached. |
| | OS: Normal structure. Posterior vitreous possibly detached. |
| Fundi | ODS: Deep central cupping of both discs. The large vessels in the posterior poles take a decidedly stretched course in inferior temporal direction, causing macular ectopia in the same direction. Near the macula, the centre of the posterior poles comprises a few very small exudates in the retina. The retinal vasculature temporal to the posterior pole is definitely aberrant: numerous ramifications of superior and inferior temporal vessels are packed in this area and show a distinctly parallel course in temporal direction. The ramifications of these vessels all terminate abruptly in the area anterior to the temporal equator. There is a welldefined line of demarcation between the vascular and the avascular retina; near the 9 o' clock meridian OD and near the 3 o'clock meridian OS, this demarcation turns back sharply in central direction. The nasal fundus periphery seems to be completely vascularized. The avascular retinal periphery in both fundi shows white |

without pressure, but no retinal defects, neovascularizations or exudates.

*Conclusion*
Marked bilateral retinal vascular changes consistent with a diagnosis of DEVR.
Slight senile cataract and delicate exudates in both posterior poles, possibly as
a result of iatrogenic diabetes mellitus.

*Subject V-10 (25-12-36)*

*History*
No visual complaints. Birth weight 3000 g. No record of neonatal oxygen administration.

*Ophthalmological examination*

| | |
|---|---|
| Visual acuity | VOD: 1.0, uncorrected. |
| | VOS: 1.0, uncorrected. |
| Eye position | Straight. |
| Intraocular pressure | ODS: 18 mm Hg. |
| Anterior segments | ODS: Normal. |
| Vitreous | ODS: Normal structure. Minute white dust-like particles. |
| Fundi | ODS: The large retinal vessels in the posterior poles are somewhat stretched, but there is no macular ectopia. The smaller arterioles outside the posterior pole take a stretched radial course, especially in the temporal fundus, and the smaller venous branches in the same area often show corkscrew-like tortuosities. It is clearly visible that the retinal vessels end in the equatorial zone of the temporal fundus half. The extreme periphery of the nasal fundus half likewise seems to be avascular, but this cannot be established with certainty. The avascular periphery in both fundi shows some white specks with occasional delicate pigmentations. This region contains a small circular retinal defect on the 10 o'clock meridian OD. |

*Conclusion*
Bilateral peripheral retinal vascular changes consistent with a diagnosis of
DEVR.

*Subject VI-18 (03-05-68)*

*History*
No visual complaints. Good general health. Birth weight 3100 g. No neonatal oxygen administration.

*Ophthalmological examination*

| | |
|---|---|
| Visual acuity | VOD: 1.0, uncorrected. |
| | VOS: 1.0, uncorrected. |
| Eye position | Straight |
| Anterior segments | ODS: Normal. |
| Vitreous | OD: Delicate white particles. Normal structure. |
| | OS: Normal structure, no cells. |
| Fundi | ODS: Normal posterior poles. The retinal vessels show short, brush-like ramifications immediately anterior to the temporal equator. Peripheral to these ramifications, the retina is avascular. No pigmentations, exudates or neovascularizations. The nasal retinal periphery in both fundi seems to be normally vascularized. |

*Conclusion*
Slight bilateral retinal vascular changes consistent with a diagnosis of DEVR.

*Subject VI-19 (01-05-71)*

*History*
No visual complaints. Good general health. Birth weight 3100 g. No neonatal oxygen administration.

*Ophthalmological examination*

| | |
|---|---|
| Visual acuity | VOD: 0.8, uncorrected. |
| | VOS: 0.8, uncorrected. |
| Eye position | Straight; central corneal reflexes. |
| Anterior segments | ODS: Normal. |
| Vitreous | ODS: Normal structure, no cells. |
| Fundi | ODS: Normal posterior poles. No macular ectopia. A rather pale, meandering zone is visible in the temporal equatorial region. Some retinal vessels terminate in this zone in multiple small terminal ramifications. Occasionally, however, a retinal vessel seems to extend past this zone to the retinal periphery. The retinal vessels in the nasal periphery present a normal appearance, as do the more centrally localized vessels. No retinal defects, neovascularizations or exudates. |

*Conclusion*
Slight bilateral peripheral retinal vascular changes consistent with a diagnosis of DEVR.

*Subject V-11 (30-01-43)*

*History*
No visual complaints. Good general health. Birth weight 3000 g. No neonatal oxygen administration.

*Ophthalmological examination*

| | |
|---|---|
| Visual acuity | VOD: 1.0, uncorrected. |
| | VOS: 1.0, uncorrected. |
| Eye position | Straight. |
| Anterior segments | ODS: Normal. |
| Vitreous | ODS: In the anterior portion of the vitreous space OD, a remnant of the hyaloid artery is visible. Delicate white particles in the retrolental vitreous ODS. A thin preretinal vitreous membrane is seen in the temporal fundus periphery. |
| Fundi | ODS: Normal posterior poles. The retinal vasculature terminates in the temporal sector immediately anterior to the equator (Figure 72). |

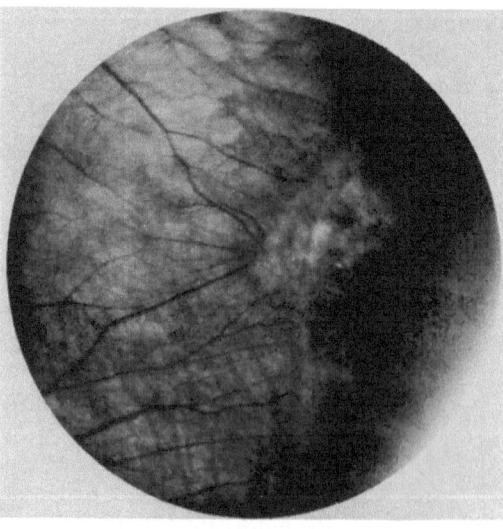

Figure 72 (V-11). OS. Avascular temporal retinal periphery (on the right).

Slightly central to the demarcation between vascular and avascular retina, a thin preretinal vitreous membrane is attached to the retina. In OS, a small white fibrosed neovascularization is visible at the margin of the vascular retina near 2 o' clock. Slightly peripheral to this, the avascular retina shows a few small circular defects.

## Conclusion
Bilateral retinal vascular changes consistent with a diagnosis of DEVR.

*Subject VI-21 (25-06-70)*

## History
An ophthalmologist diagnosed amblyopia OD when this boy was 5 years old. The amblyopia was treated by application of atropine to OS for a few months. Treatment was unsuccessful and therefore discontinued. General health has always been good. Birth weight 3530 g. No record of neonatal oxygen administration.

## Ophthalmological examination

| | |
|---|---|
| Visual acuity | VOD: 0.16, uncorrected. |
| | VOS: 1.0, uncorrected. |
| Eye position | Straight; positive kappa angle. |
| Anterior segments | ODS: Normal. |
| Vitreous | ODS: Normal. |
| Fundi | ODS: The temporal branches of the retinal vessels in the posterior poles are somewhat stretched in temporal direction, causing some ectopia of the maculae in the same direction. The temporal retinal periphery in both fundi is avascular. Central to this avascular part, the vessels end in short ramifications in a rather pale zone of the retina, which at this site seems slightly elevated. No defects, pigmentations or neovascularizations in the peripheral fundi. |

## Conclusion
Bilateral peripheral retinal vascular changes consistent with a diagnosis of DEVR. Amblyopia OD.

*Subject V-12 (26-12-45)*

*History*

This 35-year-old man has had poor VOD from the start, and VOS is reported never to have been normal. At age 3 it was reportedly found that OD was due to an abnormal position; corrective spectacles were prescribed. Amblyopia OD was treated for a while by application of atropine to OS. In childhood, this patient was examined by several ophthalmologists; at age 24, he was examined for the first time (at his own request) at our department. This examination (1969) yielded the following findings:

VOD: S − 7.0/Cyl. − 1.5 axis 0° 1/60.

VOS: S − 7.0/Cyl. 1.0 axis 15° 0.8.

Eye position: Divergent strabismus OD, pendular nystagmus.

Media: Clear.

Chorioretinitis scars in OD.

Until 1980, several follow-ups at our department revealed no changes in visual acuity or fundus features. In 1977 this man was examined at the Leiden University Department of Ophthalmology, where congenital chorioretinitis (probably due to toxoplasmosis) was likewise diagnosed. Apart from complaints about dizziness and hyperhidrosis, general health is reportedly good. No record of premature birth or neonatal oxygen administration. I decided to re-examine this patient in the context of the family study.

*Ophthalmological examination*

| | |
|---|---|
| Visual acuity | VOD: S − 7.0/Cyl. − 1.5 axis 0° 1/60. |
| | VOS: S − 7.5/Cyl. − 1.0 axis 15° 0.6. |
| Eye position | Virtually straight. Despite poor fixation OD, it is demonstrable that the marked nasal displacement of the corneal reflex of this eye is due to an abnormally wide positive kappa angle. OS likewise shows a rather wide positive kappa angle. Latent nystagmus is present. |
| Intraocular pressure | ODS: 16 mm Hg. |
| Anterior segments | ODS: Normal. |
| Vitreous | ODS: Marked syneresis. No cells. Virtually complete detachment of the posterior vitreous. Anterior to the temporal periphery of both fundi, membranes are visible which near the equator are attached to the retina and exert some traction on it. |
| Fundi | OD: Highly abnormal pattern of retinal vessels in the posterior pole: from the disc, the temporal vascular branches are stretched in inferior temporal direction, giving rise to the features of |

dragged disc. The macula shows marked ectopia in the same direction, but there is no congenital retinal fold. Near the equator, a few large chorioretinal cicatrices with many gross pigmentations are visible between 7 and 9 o'clock. From one of these cicatrices, a fibrotic strand traverses the vitreous space to the posterior lens capsule, to which it is attached via some white fibrotic tissue. The retinal vessels in the inferior temporal quadrant of the fundus are distorted in the direction of the equatorial scars, where they terminate in deformed ramifications. The retinal vasculature of the remainder of the temporal periphery is not accurately assessable due to preretinal vitreous opacities. There are no retinal defects, exudates or neovascularizations.

OS: From the disc, the retinal vessels take an abnormally stretched course to the inferior temporal area. There is no real dragged disc, but some macular ectopia exists. Immediately central to the equator, two large pigmented scars are visible near 3 and 4 o'clock. The temporal ramifications of the retinal vessels terminate near these scars, leaving the peripheral retina at this site avascular. In the inferior temporal sector of the equatorial zone, a few small, white occluded retinal vessels are visible. A preretinal vitreous membrane is attached to the retina roughly at the demarcation between the vascular and the avascular part. In the superior temporal sector this exerts some unmistakable traction on the retina. The nasal fundus periphery shows a striking number of vascular ramifications in the equatorial zone, but seems completely vascularized.

Visual fields (Goldmann)    ODS: Absolute limitation of the nasal visual field. Enlarged blind spot, which is displaced in temporal direction.

## Conclusion

Bilateral peripheral retinal vascular changes with deformation of the posterior poles. Peripheral vitreous membranes exerting traction on the retina. Myopia. Visual acuity reduced due to damaged posterior poles and amblyopia OD. The findings are consistent with fairly marked DEVR.

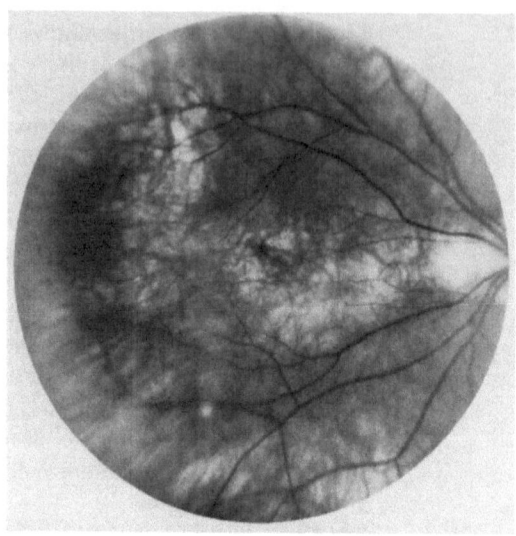

Figure 73 (IV-15). OD. Atrophy of choroid and pigment epithelium, and abnormal configuration of retinal vessels.

*Subject IV-15 (12-12-33)*

*History*

VODS diminished from the start. At age 20, retinal detachment OS was treated by operation. Birth weight unknown, but no record of premature birth or neonatal oxygen administration.

*Ophthalmological examination*

| | |
|---|---|
| Visual acuity | VOD: S − 12.0/Cyl. − 1.0 axis 0° 0.2. |
| | VOS: S − 12.0/Cyl. − 1.0 axis 0° 0.2. |
| Eye position | Straight. |
| Anterior segments | ODS: Slight, optically unobtrusive opacities in the cortex of the lenses. |
| Vitreous | ODS: Normal structure of the retrolental vitreous. No cells. Anterior to the temporal fundus periphery OD, a thin preretinal membrane is seen to extend in posterior direction to a level slightly central to the equator. OS shows almost complete detachment of the posterior vitreous. |
| Fundi | OD: The large retinal vessels in the posterior pole take a slightly stretched course in temporal direction, with slight macular ectopia in the same direction. Throughout the posterior fundus, rather ill-defined areas show marked atrophy of choriocapillaris and pigment epithelium. These also extend into the centre of the posterior pole. |

(Figure 73). The retinal vessels end in aberrant, short terminal ramifications near the temporal equator. The retina peripheral to this is avascular and shows numerous gross pigmentations.

OS: This fundus likewise shows a stretched course of the large retinal vessels in the posterior pole, with some macular ectopia. The large choroidal vessels are clearly visible throughout the posterior pole. Temporal and inferior to the posterior pole begins an area (clearly demarcated on the central side) with even more marked atrophy of choriocapillaris and pigment epithelium, which extends into the extreme periphery. Several pigment deposits are visible in this area (Figure 74). The temporal retinal periphery is avascular. Near the equator there is a well-defined demarcation between the vascular and the avascular retina. The nasal fundus periphery seems to show normal vascularization. Particularly in the temporal fundus periphery, large pigmented scars are visible. Some of these may be a result of diathermy treatment. No distinct notch is visible. As in the fundus OD, there are no visible exudates, neovascularizations or defects of the retina.

Ultrasonography  OD: Eye axis length: 25.5 mm.

OS: Eye axis length: 23 mm, increasing to about 25 mm when measured in the area temporal to the posterior pole.

*Conclusion*
Bilateral peripheral retinal vascular changes consistent with a diagnosis of DEVR.

*Subject IV-16 (24-12-34)*

*History*
VODS but particular VOS low from the start. No record of any treatment in childhood. Strabismus operations (type unknown) in 1970 and 1977. Birth weight unknown, but no record of premature birth or neonatal oxygen administration.

*Ophthalmological examination*
Visual acuity  VOD: S + 4.0/Cyl. − 2.0 axis 130° 0.2.

VOS: S + 4.0 1/60.

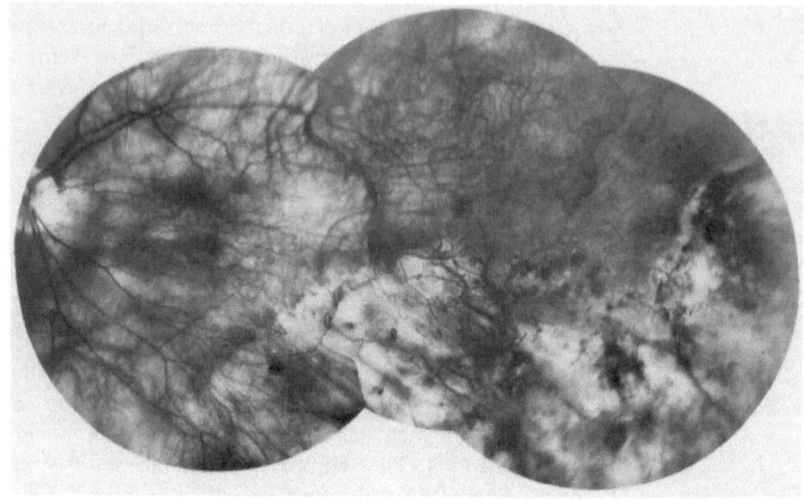

Figure 74 (IV-15). OS. Deformation of retinal vessels and macular ectopia. Extensive zones with atrophy of the choroid and pigment epithelium, encompassing pigment deposits.

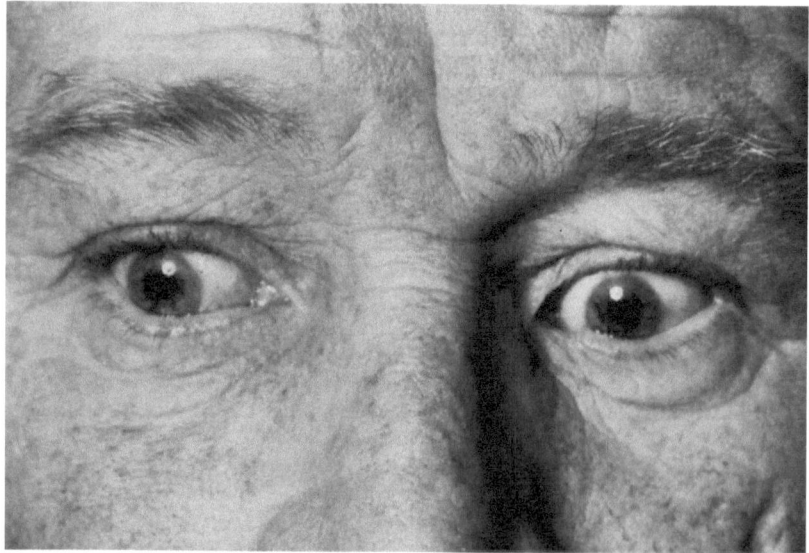

Figure 75 (IV-16). OD: Fixation of the camera at the time of exposure! Note the pseudo-divergent low position of this eye. OS shows no fixation whatever.

| | |
|---|---|
| Eye position | Virtually straight. Marked superior nasal displacement of the corneal reflex at fixation OD. Fixation OS not feasible (Figure 75). |
| Anterior segments | OD: The iris shows some posterior synechiae on the temporal side of the disc. No cells in the aqueous humour, and no Tyndall phenomenon. OS: Normal. |
| Vitreous | ODS: Lacunae with liquefaction, with interspersed fibrous structures. A few peripheral membranes in the temporal periphery of the vitreous space. |
| Fundi | OD: From the disc, the retinal vessels are markedly distorted and stretched in temporal direction (Figure 76a), causing pronounced ectopia of the macula. Immediately temporal and inferior to the macula the retina is slightly raised in a falciform fold, but this is effaced again anterior to the equator near 8 o'clock (Figure 76b). Areas with gross pigmentations are seen on either side of the retinal fold. Similar pigment deposits are |

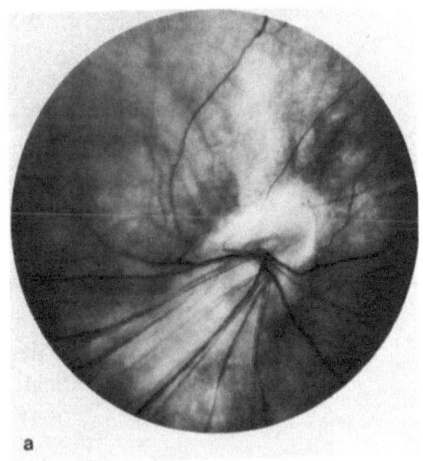

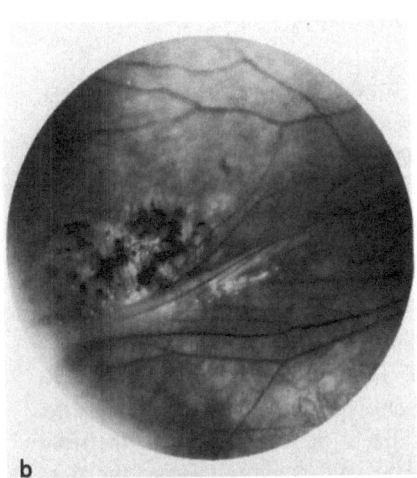

Figure 76 (IV-16). OD. a) Dragged disc. b) Slightly raised retinal fold temporal and inferior to the posterior pole, with gross pigmentations in the adjacent retina.

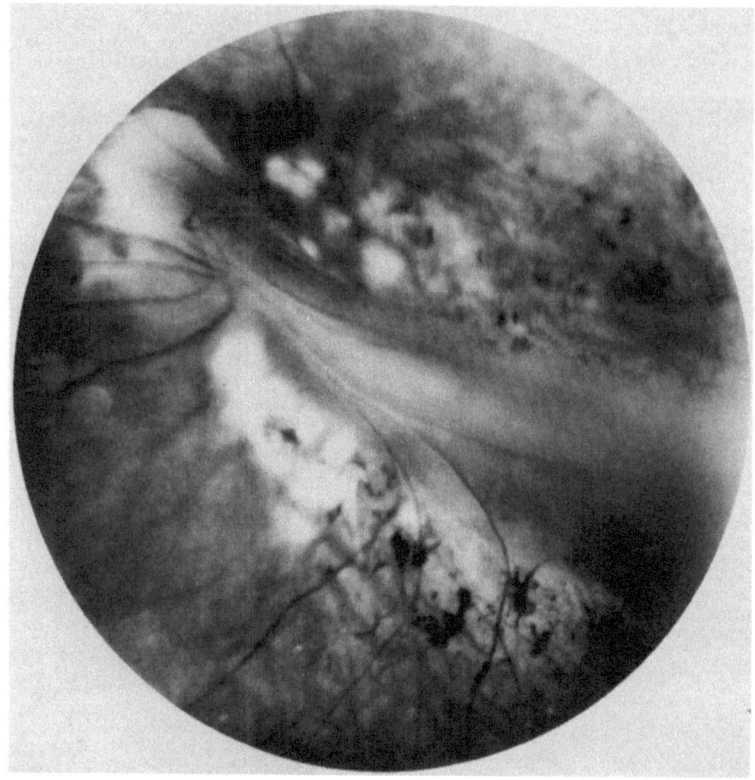

Figure 77 (IV-16). OS. Falciform fold. On either side, atrophic areas in choroid and pigment epithelium with numerous gross pigment deposits in the retina.

visible in the temporal retinal periphery, which also comprises a few exudates. So far as visible, this part of the periphery is avascular. A few preretinal vitreous membranes are seen in the inferior temporal sector.

OS: A falciform fold extends in temporal direction from the disc. Several blood vessels extend from the disc in the fold, and ramifications of these vessels leave the fold to enter the adjacent retina. In the posterior pole, sharply defined white areas of choroidal atrophy and pigment deposits are localized on either side of the fold (Figure 77). The fold roughly follows the 4 o' clock meridian and on the peripheral side ends in the anterior part of the vitreous space in a white

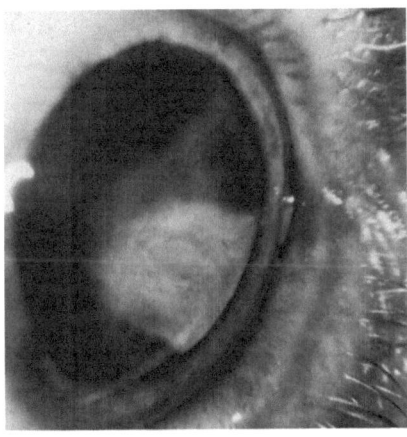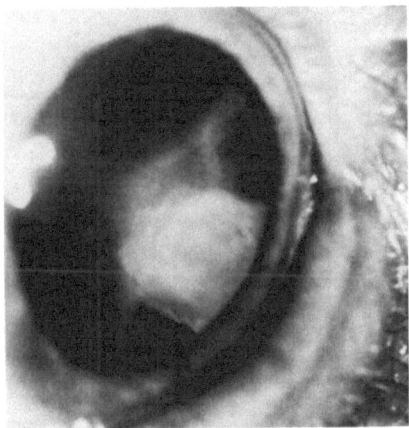

Figure 78 (IV-16). OS. Stereo-photograph. Gliotic tissue mass at the peripheral end of the retinal fold.

tissue mass connected with the pars plana and the posterior lens capsule (Figure 78). The retinal vasculature in the fundus periphery is not clearly visible due to slight vitreous opacities. No retinal defects or neovascularizations are seen.

Ultrasonography      OD: Eye axis length 21—22 mm.
OS: Eye axis length 19 mm.

*Conclusion*
Fundus changes consistent with DEVR, complicated by a large retinal fold OS and a small one OD.

*Subject IV-18 (11-08-38)*

*History*
Very poor VODS from the start. After a few years at a normal primary school, the patient was admitted to a home for visually handicapped children. In 1959, optical iridectomy OD failed to improve visual acuity. VOD has shown some further deterioration in recent years. No congenital anomalies apart from the eyes. Good general health. No record of premature birth or neonatal oxygen administration.

*Ophthalmological examination*
Visual acuity      VOD: 0.5/60, good projection.
VOS: No light perception.
Eye position      Convergent strabismus OS; hardly any fixation OD. Strikingly, there is no nystagmus.

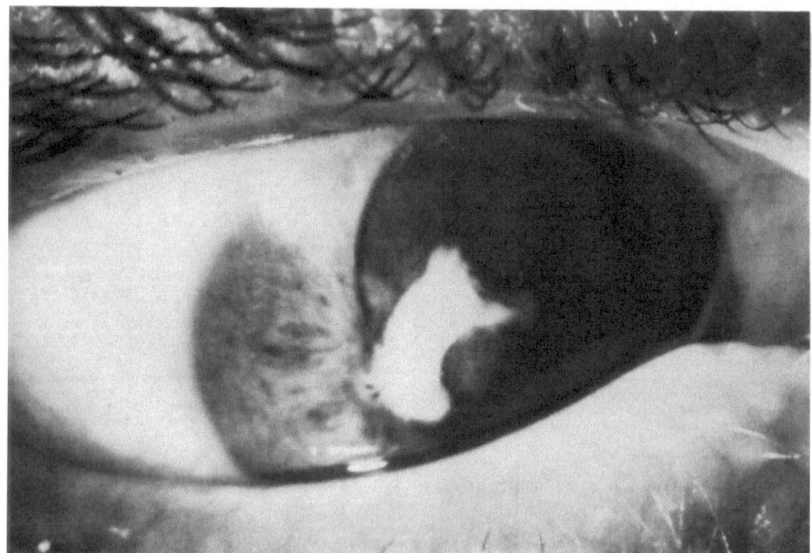

Figure 79 (IV-18). OD. Fibrotic synechiae between the iris and the largely cataractous lens.

Anterior segments

OD: Clear cornea of normal diameter. No cells in the aqueous humour. Large iridectomy defect in the superior nasal quadrant. The inferior temporal quadrant of the iris is connected by posterior synechiae with the anterior lens capsule, which is not ruptured (Figure 79). The lens shows an optically very obtrusive brown cataract, due to which no fundus reflex is visible. Through the iridectomy defect and past the margin of the lens, a feeble red fundus reflex can be observed.

OS: Some microphthalmia. Near the temporal limbus the cornea shows a keratopathy with some calcifications. The remainder of the cornea is clear. Its diameter is 9 mm. The anterior segment is of normal depth, as in OD. The iris shows some atrophic areas. The pupil is of slightly irregular shape, and mydriasis can be achieved only partly due to posterior synechiae. The pupillary aperture comprises white opaque remnants of a totally disintegrated lens (Figure 80). Near the pupillary margin at 8 o'clock, a few delicate blood vessels are visible on and in the fibrotic membrane.

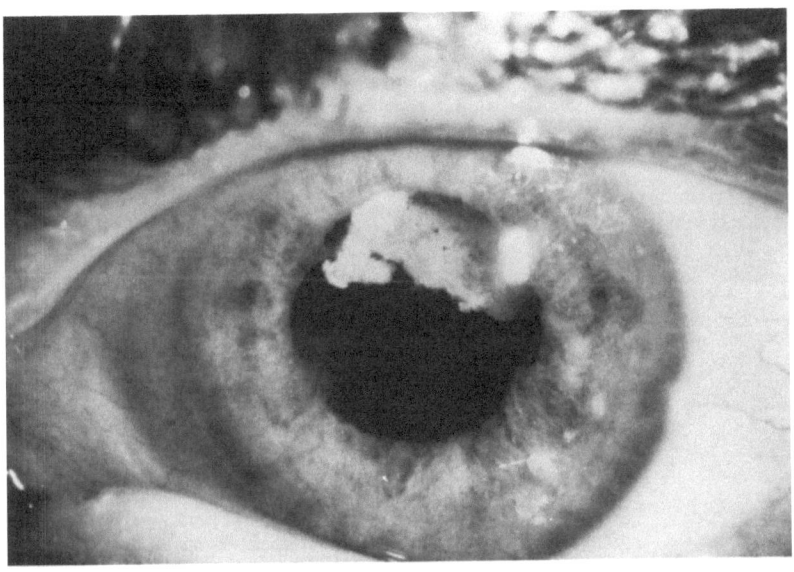

Figure 80 (IV-18). OS. Dehydrated and disintegrated, totally cataractous lens.

| | |
|---|---|
| Vitreous and fundi | ODS: No details are visible in the vitreous space or fundus. Red fundus reflex OS. |
| Ultrasonography | OD: Eye axis length 20 mm (A-scan).<br>OS: Eye axis length 14 mm. |

*Conclusion*
Extensive bilateral anterior segment and fundus changes. The findings are consistent with very severe DEVR.

*Subject IV-20 (15-06-42)*

*History*
No distinct visual symptoms. Birth weight about 3000 g. General health good, apart from relatively mild manifestations of osteochondrosis of the vertebrae (Scheuermann's disease).

*Ophthalmological examination*

| | |
|---|---|
| Visual acuity | VOD: S + 4.0/Cyl. − 3.0 axis 90° 0.8.<br>VOS: S + 3.75/Cyl. − 3.5 axis 83° 0.8. |
| Eye position | Straight. Corneal reflex slightly nasal OD and central OS. |
| Anterior segments | ODS: Normal. |

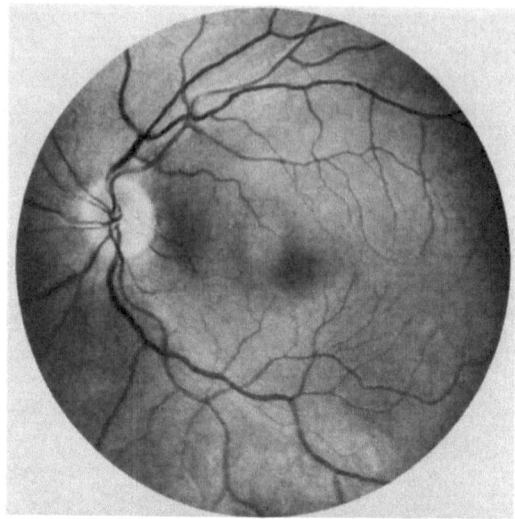

Figure 81 (IV-20). OS. Slight ectopia of the macula.

| | |
|---|---|
| Vitreous | ODS: Very delicate white particles, but otherwise normal structure. Partial detachment of the posterior vitreous membrane anterior to the temporal part of the fundi. |
| Fundi | ODS: Slight temporal ectopia of the maculae in the posterior poles (Figure 81). The configuration of the large vessels in the posterior part of the fundi is hardly aberrant. Between 8 and 10 o' clock in OD and between 2 and 4 o'clock in OS, a few retinal vessels terminate in short multiple ramifications immediately anterior to the equator. The remainder of the fundus periphery ODS is normal. The avascular part of the temporal retinal periphery shows no defects, exudates, pigmentations or neovascularizations. |

*Conclusion*

Slight bilateral vascular changes in the temporal retinal periphery consistent with a diagnosis of DEVR.

*Subject V-28 (14-08-70)*

Figures 67, 76 and 77 published with permission from Graefes Arch Ophthalmol 217: 55–67 (1981). Copyright by Springer-Verlag.

*History*
No visual complaints. Birth somewhat premature, birth weight 2500 g. No neonatal oxygen administration.

*Ophthalmological examination*

| | |
|---|---|
| Visual acuity | VOD: 0.8, uncorrected. |
| | VOS: 1.0, uncorrected. |
| Cylcopegic refraction | OD: S + 1.5. |
| | OS: Emmetropic. |
| Eye position | Straight. Slightly nasal corneal reflex OD. |
| Anterior segments | ODS: Normal. |
| Vitreous | ODS: A few delicate white particles are afloat in the vitreous, which is of normal structure. |
| Fundi | ODS (direct and indirect ophthalmoscopy): Normal retinal vascular pattern in the posterior poles. No distinct ectopia of the maculae. Some conspicuously tortuous retinal vessels are visible central to the equator near 3 o'clock OS. The retinal periphery OD shows no distinct changes. Avascularity of the peripheral retina could not be demonstrated by the method used. |

*Conclusion*
Slight vascular anomalies in the fundus periphery OS and slightly subnormal VOD. The symptoms may represent a very mild manifestation of DEVR, but the diagnosis is not certain.

## 3.6 The E family

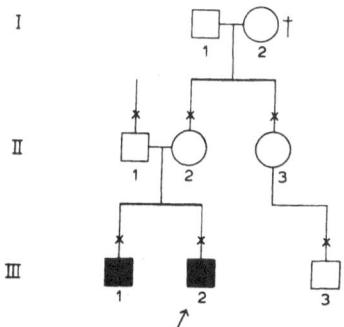

Figure 82. Pedigree of the E family.

*Introduction*

The proband of this family had been known at our out-patient clinic since 1975 as showing diminished VODS and bilateral fundus changes. The possibility of

DEVR was contemplated in 1977, but a superficial study of a few family members failed to disclose changes which could confirm the diagnosis. A fresh family study was performed in 1980, and its findings are reported here.

*Proband III-2 (24-02-68)*

*History*

The eye position was found to be abnormal when the patient was one year old. An ophthalmologist was consulted, who prescribed corrective spectacles and started amblyopia treated by occlusion of the left eye. This was discontinued a year later because the result was disappointing. At age 7 the patient was first examined at our department. General health was good. There was no record of premature birth or neonatal oxygen administration.

*Family history*

No known consanguinity of the proband's parents. His father (II-1) was believed to have poor VOD, and one of the father's brothers reportedly had a lazy eye. The proband's mother had no visual complaints, but her only sister was believed to have a lazy eye.

*Ophthalmological examination (April 1975)*

| Visual acuity | VOD: S − 4.5/Cyl. − 3.5 axis 50° 0.1. |
|---|---|
| | VOS: S − 4.5/Cyl. − 4.0 axis 165° 0.5. |
| Cycloplegic refraction | OD: S − 4.0/Cyl. − 4.0 axis 15°. |
| | OS: S − 4.0/Cyl. 4.5 axis 145°. |
| Anterior segments | ODS: Normal. |
| Vitreous | OD: Preretinal vitreous structures. |
| Fundi | ODS: Aberrant vascular pattern in the posterior poles and atrophy of the choroid. |
| Diagnosis: | Unknown. |

*Therapy*

Prescription of corrective spectacles as dictated by refraction. No further therapy.

*Course*

In view of gradually increasing myopia, the prescription of the corrective spectacles was modified several times. Visual acuity remained unchanged.

*Ophthalmological examination (August 1980)*

| Visual acuity | VOD: S − 6.5/Cyl. − 4.0 axis 20° 0.12. |
|---|---|
| | VOS: S − 8.0/Cyl. − 4.0 axis 165° 0.6. |

| | |
|---|---|
| Eye position | Straight. Due to distinct nasal displacement of the corneal reflex OD, this eye is pseudodivergent. |
| Anterior segments | ODS: Normal. |
| Vitreous | OD: Some liquefaction and syneresis. Numerous delicate pigment particles. Probably posterior vitreous detachment. |
| | OS: Some liquefaction, No cells or particles. |
| Fundi | OD: The retinal vessels show marked distortion from the disc to the inferior temporal sector. In the posterior pole there is consequently a conspicuous parallel course of the large vascular branches, among which a markedly deformed and ectopic macula is visible. The fundus shows pigment paucity and the choriocapillaris is underdeveloped so that the pattern of the large choroidal vessels is clearly visible (Figure 83). In the |

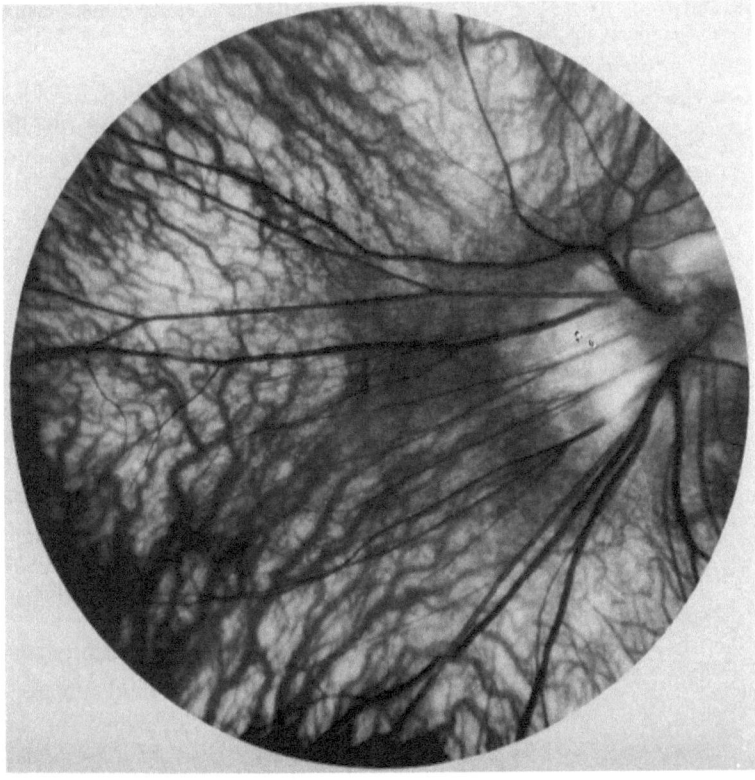

Figure 83 (III-2). OD. Abnormally stretched course of the temporal retinal vascular branches. Ectopia of the macula.

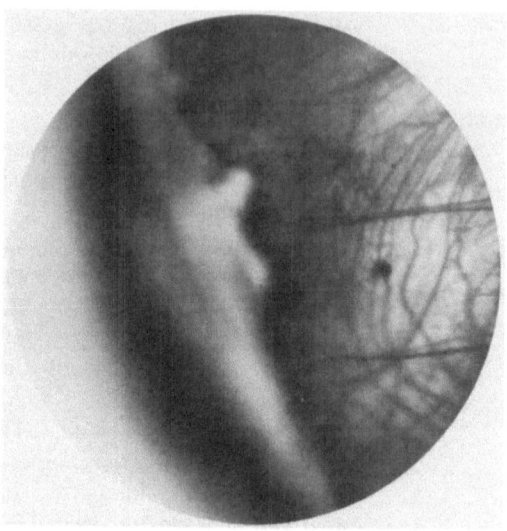

Figure 84 (III-2). OD. Raised white fibrotic ridge with attachment of vitreous membrane in inferior temporal quadrant.

inferior temporal quadrant central to the equator, a raised whitish fibrotic ridge extends parallel to the ora serrata (Figure 84). At this ridge, vitreous membranes are attached to the retina, and along the central margin there is some local retinoschisis with a few small defects in the inner part of the neuroretina. Traction from the peripheral fibrotic structures has stretched the retinal vessels. The preretinal vitreous structures make it impossible to establish whether the retina peripheral to the equator is avascular. A few small exudates are visible in this area. In the nasal fundus periphery, where fewer vitreous opacities are present, the vessels in the retina show a distinctly aberrant course. Peripheral to tortuous vessels which end in irregular multiple ramifications, the retina is entirely avascular. No neovascularizations are visible.

OS: The vessels from the disc are distorted in inferior temporal direction, with marked ectopia of the macula in the same direction. The retinal vessels in the posterior pole show a parallel and stretched course (Figure 85). Conspicuous avascularity of the peripheral retina in all quadrants.

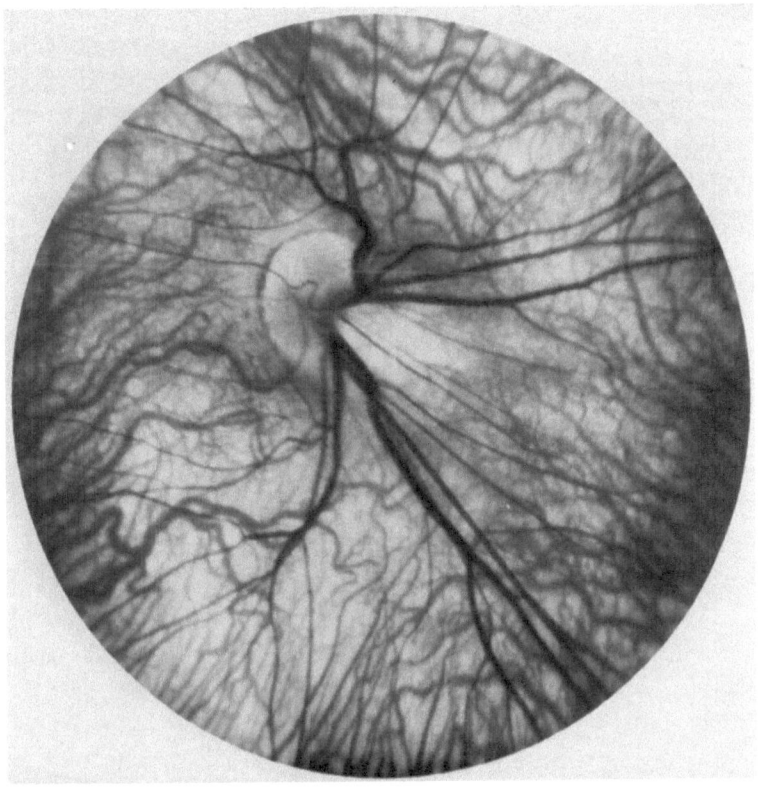

Figure 85 (III-2) OS. The same features of retinal vessels and choroid as in posterior pole OD.

Most vessels terminate in irregular ramifications in the equatorial zone, but in the nasal half of the fundus the vessels extend slightly further in anterior direction. Retinal exudates are seen at several sites in the mid-periphery (Figure 86). No distinct neovascularizations. Several gross superficial pigment deposits in the vascular part of the retina. Especially near the temporal equator, vitreous membranes exert unmistakable traction on the retina. No retinal defects or areas of retinoschisis.

Visual fields (Goldmann)     ODS: The 1–4 isopter shows some limitation of the nasal visual field. No other distinct changes. The blind spot cannot be determined with certainty.

138

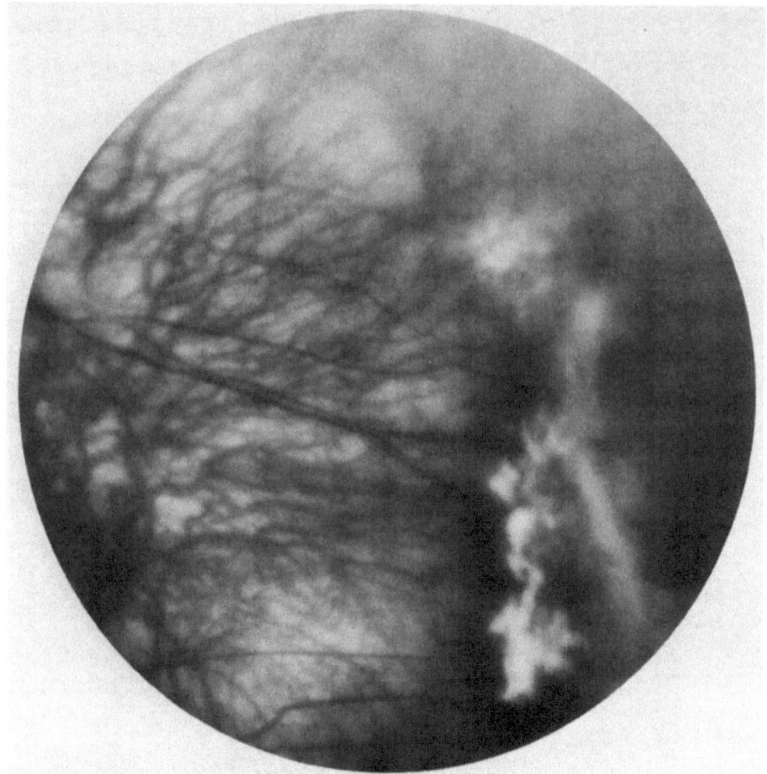

Figure 86 (III-2). OS. Small intraretinal exudates and attachment of vitreous membrane to equatorial retina.

*Conclusion*
Bilateral fundus changes characteristics of fairly severe DEVR.

*Policy*
In view of the unmistakable traction on the retina ODS, the risk of retinal detachment is far from imaginary. The exudates, especially in OS, also require watching.

*Subject III-1 (03-04-66)*

*History*
No visual complaints. Good general health. Birth weight about 3000 g.

*Ophthalmological examination*

| Visual acuity | VOD: S + 2.0 1.25. |
| | VOS: S + 3.25/Cyl. − 0.5 axis 0° 1.0. |

| | |
|---|---|
| Eye position | Straight. |
| Anterior segments | ODS: Normal. |
| Vitreous | ODS: Normal structure, no cells. |
| Fundi | ODS: Normal posterior poles. Some evident vascular anomalies near the equator in the temporal quadrants. The retinal vessels in this area divide into short terminal ramifications. The retina peripheral to these ramifications is avascular. The vasculature of the nasal periphery, so far as visible, is entirely normal. No pigmentations, exudates, retinal defects or neovascularizations. |

*Conclusion*
Slight bilateral peripheral retinal vascular changes consistent with a diagnosis of DEVR.

*Although no symptoms of DEVR were found in the following family members, the results of their examination are nevertheless presented in view of their ophthalmological particulars.*

*Subject II-1 (14-02-36)*

*History*
Reduced visual acuity and strabismus OD from the start. An 8-year history of complaints about numbness in the right leg. No distinct exacerbations or visual complaints. Extensive neurological examination led to a tentative diagnosis of multiple sclerosis.

*Ophthalmological examination*

| | |
|---|---|
| Visual acuity | VOD: S + 6.0 0.1. |
| | VOS: S + 3.75 1.0. |
| Eye position | Divergent strabismus OD, about $25°$. |
| Anterior segments | ODS: Normal. |
| Vitreous | ODS: Normal. |
| Fundi | OD: The temporal side of the disc is somewhat pale. Normal vasculature of the large vessels in the posterior pole and normal macula. Normal vascular pattern in the peripheral funuds. No peripheral changes at the indentation either. |
| | OS: The disc presents a normal appearance. The vasculature of the retina is normal in the posterior pole and in the periphery. |
| Visual fields (Goldmann) | OD: Central sensitivity decreased. No limitation of visual field. |

|                          | OS: Normal.                        |
| Visual evoked responses  | OD: No potentials recordable.      |
|                          | OS: Normal.                        |
| Colour vision            | OD: Distinctly disturbed.          |
|                          | OS: Normal.                        |

*Conclusion*

Amblyopia as a result of anisometropia. Opticopathy OD, possible as a result of multiple sclerosis. No symptoms of DEVR.


*Subject II-2 (03-12-33)*


*History*
No visual complaints. Good general health.

*Ophthalmological examination*

| Visual acuity    | VOD: 1.0, uncorrected. |
|                  | VOS: 1.0, uncorrected. |
| Eye position     | Straight. |
| Anterior segments | ODS: Unmistakable opacities of the posterior cortex of both lenses. Their centre is fairly clear. |
| Vitreous         | ODS: Normal structure; dust-like particles. |
| Fundi            | OD: Normal posterior pole. In the equatorial zone, the temporal fundus shows no distinct vascular anomalies. At 11 o'clock just outside the equator there is a small circular defect. The retina peripheral to the equator shows no vascular ramifications, but assessment of details in this area is difficult due to the lens opacities. |
|                  | OS: Normal posterior pole. The peripheral vascular pattern is not anomalous, but assessment of the vascularity of the extreme periphery is again impossible. Some pigmentations are visible in the superior temporal part of the mid-periphery. |

*Conclusion*

No distinct vascular anomalies consistent with DEVR, but some slight degenerative changes in the peripheral fundus. Assessment of small details in the fundus is impossible due to some media opacities.

### 3.7 The F family

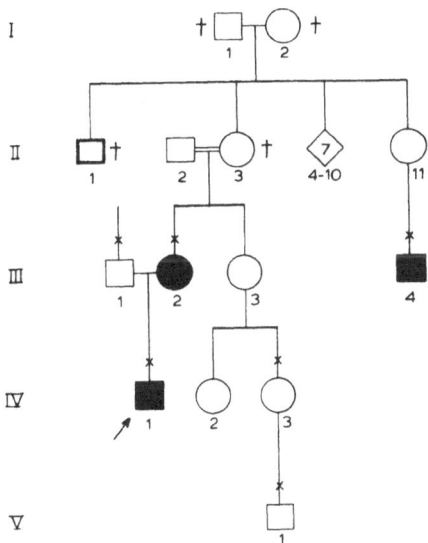

Figure 87. Pedigree of the F family.

*Introduction*

The proband of this family was traced in view of a publication (Hamburg 1963) which reported some clinical data on him. The combination of a so-called pseudoglioma in one eye and congenital retinal fold in the other was suggestive of a diagnosis of DEVR, and gave me sufficient motivation to examine this patient and his immediate relatives. The fact that histological data were available — one eye having been enucleated at the time — was an additional motivation for re-examination.

*Proband IV-1 (19-08-61)*

*History*

The parents observed eye abnormalities about a month after birth. Ophthalmological examination disclosed a retrolental tissue mass in OD, probably associated with total retinal detachment. The fundus OS showed a congenital retinal fold. Enucleation OD was performed six weeks after birth because a malignant tumour could not be excluded. The microscopic speciment presented no indications of a retinoblastoma.

Pregnancy and parturition had been uneventful. Birth weight was 3000 g and no neonatal oxygen administration is on record. During the first few weeks post partum there were a few days of fever and some regurgitation of food. These symptoms disappeared spontaneously. A cardiological examination was made, allegedly in view of a heart murmur, but no congenital heart defect was found.

General health in childhood was good. In view of his visual handicap the patient attended school at an institution for visually handicapped children.

*Ophthalmological examination (January 1981)*

| | |
|---|---|
| Visual acuity | VOS: S − 12.0/Cyl. − 2.0 axis 110° 1/60 − 1/30 |
| Eye position | Pronounced pendular nystagmus. |
| Anterior segments | OD: Prosthesis. |
| | OS: Clear cornea. Normal depth of anterior chamber. Gonioscopy reveals no abnormality of the iridocorneal angle. The aqueous humour contains no cells. The iris is not atrophic and has no synechiae. The lens shows some subcapsular opacities on the temporal side, which are optically not very obtrusive. |
| Vitreous | OS: The retrolental vitreous is of normal structure, without cells. The posterior part of the vitreous space is optically empty due to posterior vitreous detachment. |

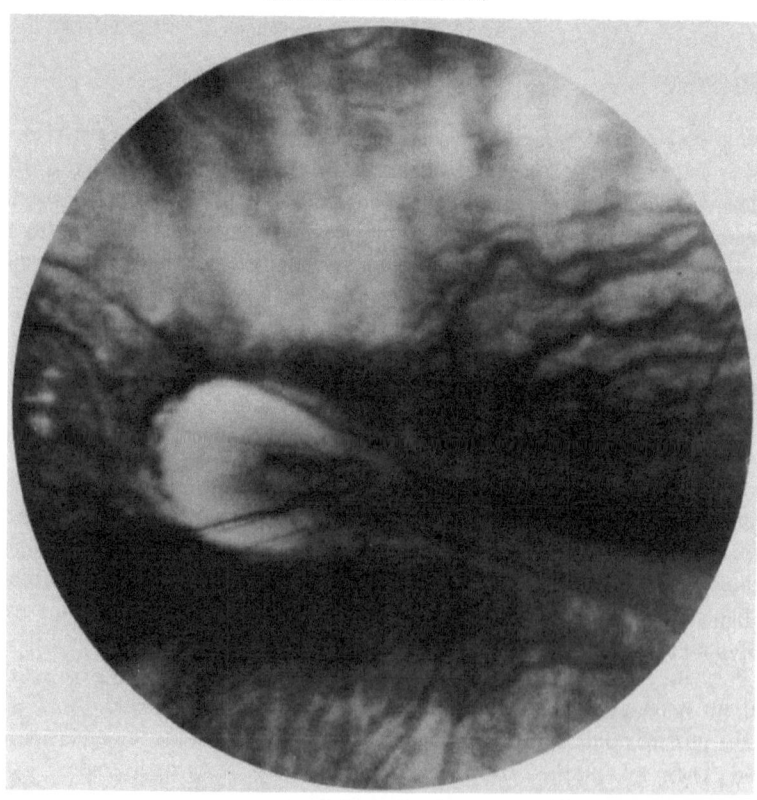

Figure 88 (IV-1). OS. Falciform retinal fold.

| Fundi | OS: From the disc, a falciform retinal fold extends through the centre of the posterior pole to the inferior temporal fundus periphery (Figure 88). The retinal fold ends in a local mass of white tissue which is attached to the lens equator near 4 o'clock and the pars plana. The vascular branches on the disc are distorted in the direction of the fold. The macula cannot be identified. Temporal to the posterior pole, there are small areas of RPE atrophy and gross pigmentations near the base of the retinal fold. This area also comprises some candlewax-like exudates in the retina. No neovascularizations or retinal defects. The retina anterior to the temporal equator outside the fold seems avascular. Due to nystagmus and a few media opacities it is impossible to assess minute details in the fundus. |
|---|---|

*Pathology*

The report on the pathological examination of the enucleated eye is presented in Chapter 4 (see also Figures 119 and 120).

*Conclusion*

History and clinical findings suggest a bilateral congenital proliferative retinopathy, which has led to total retinal detachment OD and a falciform retinal fold OS. The anomalies may be consistent with severe DEVR.

*Subject III-1 (18-09-28)*

*History*

The proband's father had several attacks of fairly severe iridocyclitis of both eyes. No abnormalities at general physical examination. A sister is reported to have a lazy eye, but otherwise the family history reveals no ophthalmological abnormalities. No record of consanguinity between III-1 and III-2.

*Ophthalmological examination*

| Visual acuity | VOS: S − 1.0 1.0. |
|---|---|
| | VOS: S − 1.75 1.0. |
| Eye position | Straight. |
| Anterior segments | ODS: The aqueous humour contains no cells and shows no positive flare. Slight pigment film on the anterior lens capsule. No synechiae. |
| Vitreous | ODS: Normal structure, but contains a considerable number of cells. |

144

| | |
|---|---|
| Fundi | OD: Normal posterior pole. Extreme retinal periphery slightly whitish, especially on the temporal side; no distinctly visible retinal vessels. In the equatorial zone, however, the configuration of the retinal vessels is normal. No pigmentations exudates or defects of the retina.<br>OS: Mydriasis and examination by mirror contact lens was avoided at the patient's request. So far as can be seen, posterior pole and mid-periphery show no anomalies. |

## Conclusion

Mild residual symptoms of uveitis ODS. Peripheral retinal vascular branches are not clearly visible in OD. No unmistakable symptoms of DEVR.

*Subject III-2 (29-06-27)*

## History

VODS in the proband's mother is alleged to have always been subnormal. Good general health apart from arthrosis of the fingers of both hands. Meningitis in childhood, with subsequent recovery without residual symptoms. Normal birth weight.

## Family history

This woman's parents (II-2 and II-3) are reportedly consanguineous, but both are reported to have always had good eyesight. Her only sister (III-3) and her offspring show no anomalies. One of her uncles (II-1) is reported to have been virtually blind from early infancy. One of her maternal cousins has had poor eyesight from the start. There is a record of strabismus in one of her mother's brothers and in her mother's father (I-1).

## Ophthalmological examination

| | |
|---|---|
| Visual acuity | VOD: S + 3.5/Cyl. − 2.0 axis 120° 0.5.<br>VOS: S + 3.75/Cyl. − 2.0 axis 80° 0.3. |
| Anterior segments | ODS: The retrolental vitreous is of normal structure and shows no cells. |
| Fundi | OD: The disc seems normal. The configuration of retinal vessels in the posterior pole is normal, as is the macula. The temporal fundus periphery, however, shows anomalies: between the 7 and the 12 o'clock meridian, a sector of retinoschisis extends in central direction to slightly beyond the equator. Small ramifications of retinal vessels are visible in the most central part of the retino- |

schisis, but most of the area peripheral to the equator comprises no visible vessels. The configuration of the retinal vasculature along the central demarcation of the retinoschisis is somewhat aberrant: some venous branches curve slightly back. No striking tortuosities, and no abnormally large number of small venules and arterioles in this area. No pigmentations or defects in the peripheral retina.

OS: From the disc, the temporal retinal vessels take a slightly stretched course in temporal direction, but no other anomalies are visible in the posterior pole. Retinoschisis is seen in the superior temporal quadrant of the peripheral fundus. Its central demarcation is roughly the equator. The pattern of retinal vessels in the temporal equatorial zone is not aberrant. Peripheral to the equator, however, no ramifications of retinal vessels are visible in the retinoschisis; nor are any visible in the inferior temporal quadrant. Assessment of small details in the extreme periphery is impossible due to slight vitreous opacities anterior to this region. No retinal defects, pigmentations or neovascularizations are found.

*Conclusion*

Subnormal VODS. Bilateral retinoschisis in the temporal fundus periphery, combined with slight retinal vascular anomalies, especially in OD. The findings may well be a result of DEVR.

*Subject III-4 (18-12-32)*

*History*

Diminished VODS from early infancy. Patient attended normal primary school and could read with difficulty using the left eye, which was better than the right. At age 13, VOS diminished acutely due to a retinal haemorrhage (no longer any light perception). The patient was transferred to a home for the visually handicapped. Secondary glaucoma OS at age 18; two subsequent glaucoma operations. VOD has gradually diminished in recent years. Good general health. Birth weight believed to have suggested slightly premature birth (some 2000 g). No record of neonatal oxygen administration.

*Ophthalmological examination*

Visual acuity                    VOD: 1/60.

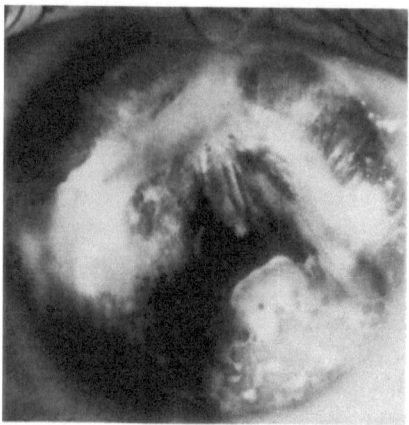 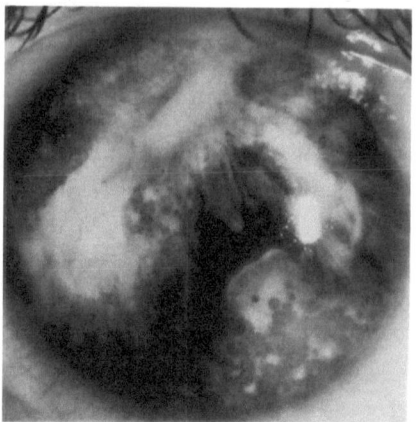

Figure 89 (III-4). Stereo-photograph. Anterior segment OS.

|  | VOS: No light perception. |
|---|---|
| Eye position | Straight; pendular nystagmus. |
| Intraocular pressure | OD: 14 mm Hg. |
|  | OS: 22 mm Hg. |
| Anterior segments | OD: Slight band keratopathy near the inferior limbus of the cornea. Cornea otherwise clear. A few posterior synechiae. Local subcapsular posterior cataract on the temporal side. The lens shows a few dense local opacities in the anterior cortex, and some nuclear cataract. |
|  | OS: Cornea of normal diameter. Near the limbus on the superior and on the nasal side, scars of the glaucome operations are visible. There is some nasal and temporal band keratopathy. The temporal inferior quadrant of the cornea is likewise dystrophic due to extensive synechiae (Figure 89) between endothelium and iris in this sector. The iris shows many white fibrotic scars and is atrophic. An opaque tissue mass is visible through a small pupillary aperture in the deformed iris. |
| Vitreous | OD: A few membranes are visible in the central and retrolental vitreous space. On the posterior side of the lens capsule in the inferior temporal quadrant, a white tissue mass is attached near the lens equator. |
| Fundi | OD: The large vascular branches on the disc are deformed, and distorted in inferior temporal |

direction. From the disc, a large falciform retinal fold extends through the centre of the posterior pole to the temporal fundus periphery (Figure 90). The protrusion of the fold in the vitreous space increases as the fold approaches the fundus periphery. Near 8 o'clock, the peripheral end of the retinal fold is enveloped in a white gliotic tissue mass, which with the slit-lamp can be observed on the posterior side of the lens in the inferior temporal quadrant. The macula is not identifiable: it is apparently enveloped in the retinal fold. The posterior fundus shows striking anomalies of the choroid and the pigmented layer of the retina. In large areas, mostly inferior and temporal to the disc, these structures are virtually invisible; one looks through the neuroretina almost directly upon the sclera. Many gross pigment deposits are seen adjacent to these areas (Figure 90). More delicate pigmentations are seen immediately anterior to the retina in the vitreous space at several sites in the fundus periphery. Some of them seem to be localized in a thin layer of retinoschisis. Some white proliferative tissue is localized on the retina anterior to the equator in the inferior nasal quadrant. No distinct vascular structures are visible in this area. Due to nystagmus and some media opacities, the degree of vas-

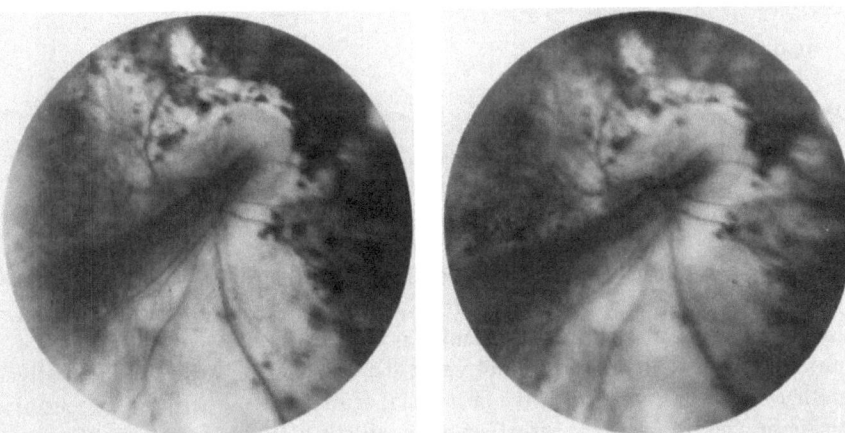

Figure 90 (III-4). OD. Stereo-photograph. Falciform retinal fold and extensive atrophic changes of choroid and pigment epithelium in the posterior pole.

cularization of the peripheral retina cannot be established with certainty.

*Conclusion*

Congenital retinal fold OD and total vitreous organizations OS. The findings are consistent with a diagnosis of severe DEVR.


**3.8 The G family**

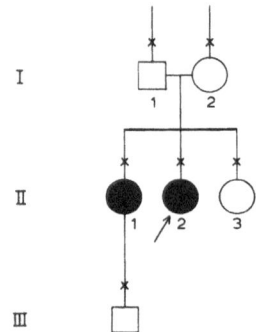

Figure 91. Pedigree of the G family.

*Introduction*

The proband of this family had been known at our department since 1971 as showing severe bilateral ophthalmological changes regarded as a possible consequence of congenital toxoplasmosis. The patient was brought to my attention in view of a falciform retinal fold in the left eye.

*Proband II-2 (23-09-62)*

*History*

The following data were supplied by the patient and her parents, and retrieved from previous examinations at our department. When the patient was about 10 months old, the parents noticed an anomalous eye position. According to the mother, the district nurse had previously remarked on this, but little attention had been paid. Ophthalmological examination at the Royal Victorian Eye Hospital in Melbourne (the family was living in Australia at the time) disclosed bilateral fundus changes interpreted as congenital dysplasia of unknown cause. In her pre-school years she could manage very well, mostly with the left eye which had the best visual acuity. During her primary school years in The Netherlands, visual acuity gradually deteriorated so that, at age 8, she was transferred to a home for the visually handicapped. The patient had been delivered by forceps extraction under general anaethesia. She is reported to have been placed in an incubator on the day after birth, with mild neonatal oxygen administration. Birth weight 3500 g. No premature birth. The mother was febrile during a few days in the latter half of the pregnancy, but the cause of this is unknown. No paternal or maternal family history of eye diseases. One of the mother's brothers reportedly has a possibly congenital heart condition.

*Ophthalmological (1971, age 9)*

| | |
|---|---|
| Visual acuity | VOD: No light perception. |
| | VOS: 4/60, correction not feasible. |
| Intraocular pressure | OD: Not exactly determinable. |
| | OS: 6/7.5 (Schiøtz tonometer). |
| Eye position | Pendular nystagmus. |
| Anterior segments | OD: Subnormal corneal diameter. Severe band keratopathy. Anterior chamber shows funnel-shaped depression. Pupil distorted in nasal direction and of irregular shape. Atrophy of the iris and extensive posterior synechiae. A totally white opaque lenticular mass is visible in the pupillary aperture. |
| Vitreous | OD: Inspection not feasible. |
| | OS: Many cells and some membranes. |
| Fundi | OD: Inspection not feasible. |
| | OS: From the disc, a falciform fold extends through the centre of the posterior pole in temporal direction. The large vessels on the disc are distorted in the same direction, and partly follow the course of the fold (Figure 92). Some gross pigmentations are visible slightly superior to the fold in the posterior pole. The choroid and the pigmented layer show marked atrophy near the disc. In the extreme temporal periphery, the raised retinal fold ends in a greyish tumour-like mass with a wrinkled surface. |
| ERG | OD: No recordable potentials. |
| | OS: Diminished photopic and scotopic responses. |
| Ultrasonography | OD: The vitreous space is almost entirely filled by opacities in which the retina cannot be identified. |

*General physical examination*
This examination (at the paediatric department) revealed no abnormalities.

150

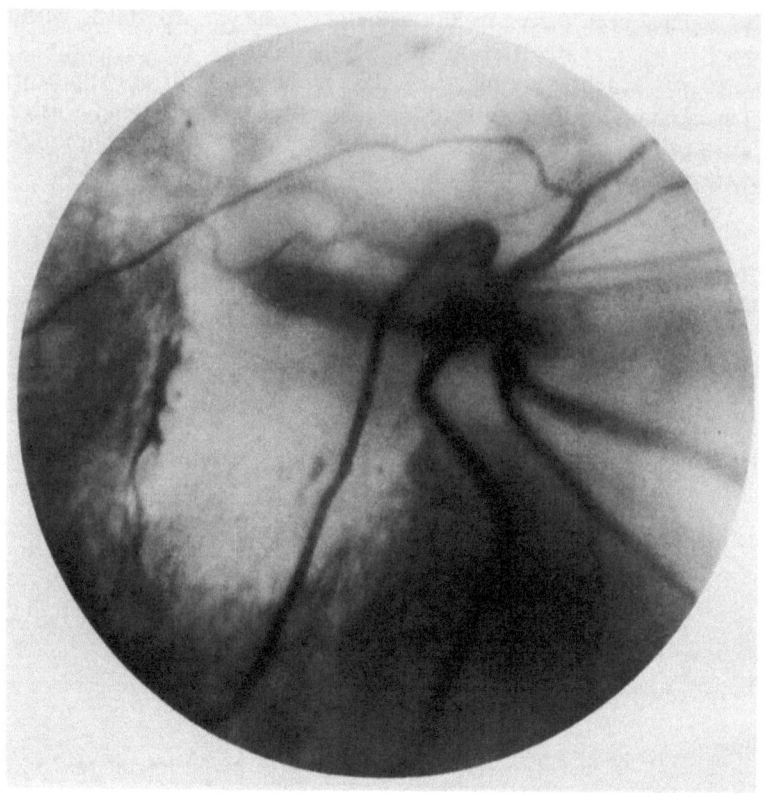

Figure 92 (II-2). OS. Disc with central portion of a falciform retinal fold.

*Laboratory studies*

| | |
|---|---|
| Blood | ESR 5 mm in the first hour. |
| | Hb 7.9 mmol/l. |
| | Haematocrit 0.39. |
| | WBC 6000, with normal differentiation. |
| Serum | Urea: 4.13 mmol/l. |
| | Creatinine: 60 μmol/l. |
| Enzymes | Normal SCOT, SGPT and alkaline phosphatase values. |

*Serological tests*

| | |
|---|---|
| Toxoplasmosis | Complement fixation test 1:4. |
| Immunofluorescence | 1:128. |
| Toxocara | Complement fixation test negative. |
| Ascaris | Complement fixation test negative. |
| Syphilis | All tests negative. |

Rheumatic disease          AST 75 U.
                           Rose test 1:32.
                           Latex negative.

*Radiological examination*

Skull                      Some circumscribed calcifications are visible in
                           the right parietal and occipital regions. Findings
                           consistent with a previous toxoplasmosis.
Teeth                      OPT: Some hypoplastic teeth in the permanent
                           dentition.
Chest                      No significant changes.
Paranasal sinuses          No significant changes.

*Diagnosis (1971)*
Falciform retinal fold as a result of congenital toxoplasmosis.

*Course*
Between age 11 and age 13 this patient was repeatedly seen at our department
with symptoms of uveitis OS. The aqueous humour showed a positive flare in
varying degrees, and cells were sometimes seen. Upon exacerbations she was
treated by mydriatics, local application of Decadron (dexamethasone) and
also, briefly, with oral prednisone. Unfortunately, secondary glaucoma developed and patient lost light perception OS also, at age 15.

*Ophthalmological examination (1981)*
OD as described above. OS is small, like OD, and also shows a reduced corneal
diameter (9 mm). The pupil is narrow and irregular. The iris shows numerous
posterior synechiae. In the pupillary aperture, a white mass is visible in a
shrunken lens capsule. Inspection of the vitreous space is impossible.

*Conclusion*
Although the changes had been previously interpreted as consequences of
congenital toxoplasmosis, the extensive vitreous proliferations, the falciform
retinal fold, the extensive pigment scars and the irritation of the anterior segment are all features which can be encountered in DEVR. This diagnosis was
confirmed when the anomalies in the eyes of this patient's sister (II-1) were
found.

*Subject II-1 (22-12-58)*

*History*
No visual complaints. Good general health. The patient is four months pregnant.
Her birth weight was 3750 g. No record of neonatal oxygen administration.

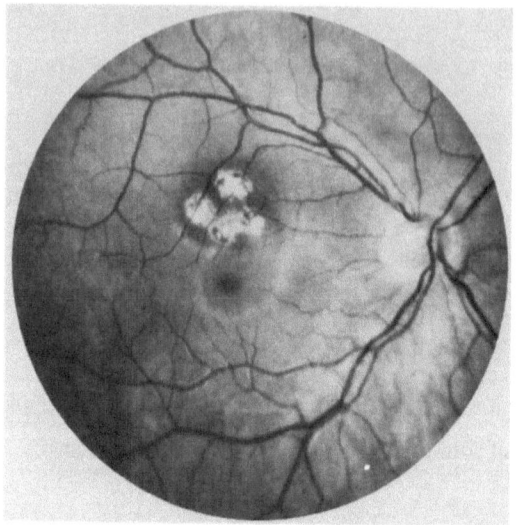

Figure 93 (II-1). OD. Some chorioretinal scars in the posterior pole.

*Ophthalmological examination*

| | |
|---|---|
| Visual acuity | VOD: S − 2.0/Cyl. − 1.5 axis 0° 1.0. |
| | VOS: S − 2.25/Cyl. − 1.5 axis 30° 1.0. |
| Eye position | Straight. |
| Vitreous | ODS: Normal structure, no cells. |
| Fundi | OD: Normal configuration of the large retinal vessels in the posterior pole. Immediately superior to the macula there are four small circular scars, characterized by atrophy of RPE and pigment deposits in the neuroretina (Figure 93). The temporal fundus periphery shows a pale, band-like zone which between 7 and 11 o'clock extends in the equatorial zone and slightly meanders. In this pale retinal zone, the retinal vessels are clearly seen to terminate in short multiple ramifications (Figure 92). The retina peripheral to this zone is of slightly darker colour and avascular. The nasal fundus periphery presents a normal appearance. No retinal defects, exudates or neovascularizations are seen. |
| | OS: Entirely normal posterior pole. No band-like pale zone as in OD. However, a striking finding is that the retinal vessels end in terminal ramifications in the temporal equatorial zone. The peri- |

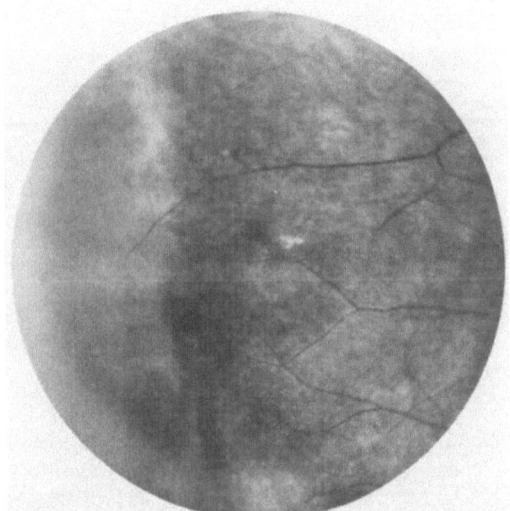

Figure 94 (II-1). OD. Pale band-like zone in the temporal equatorial zone.

pheral retina contains not a single vessel anterior to the equator between the 1 and the 5 o'clock meridian.

*Conclusion*

Symptoms of incomplete vascularization of the peripheral retina ODS, consistent with a diagnosis of DEVR.

*Subjects I-1 and I-2*

The proband's parents were both examined ophthalmologically. As in virtually all patients described in this study, the fundi were examined by slit-lamp biomicroscopy. However, this technique failed to identify any symptoms of DEVR in either parent. Consanguinity between the parents was not on record and is highly unlikely, because they come from different parts of The Netherlands. No eye diseases were known in the families of the two parents.

It must be assumed that one of the parents possesses the DEVR gene, but that in this case the condition is not penetrant. It cannot be excluded that fluorescein angiography of the peripheral fundus might have disclosed minor anomalies in one of the parents. However, fluorescein angiography could not be performed.

### 3.9 The H family

*Introduction*

The proband of this family was referred to our department in June 1980 with

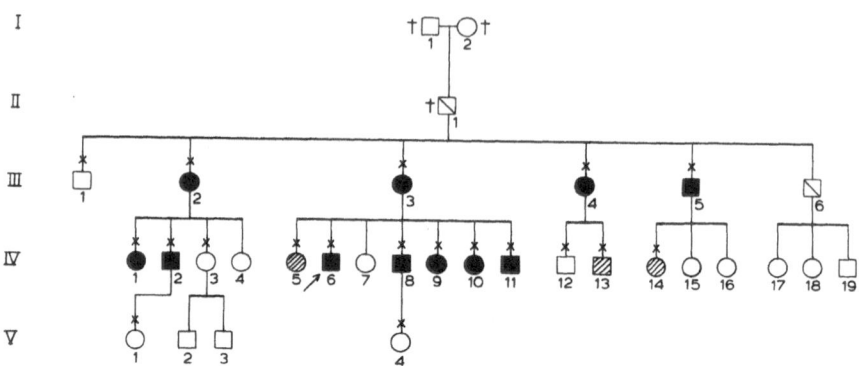

Figure 95. Pedigree of the H family.

a recently detached retina. In this patient I found fundus changes suggestive of DEVR, and consequently an ophthalmological family study was carried out.

*Proband IV-6 (28-08-54)*

*History*
This 25-year-old man was referred to our department by his ophthalmologist, with retinal detachment OS. Vision of this eye had deteriorated in the past five days. No recent history of any traumatic injury. According to the patient the left eye was lazy and had always shown low visual acuity. No record of amblyopia treatment. No record of premature birth or neonatal oxygen administration. General health reported to be good. The patient had had meningitis and bilateral otitis media at age 2.

*Family history*
The patient's mother (III-3), uncle (III-6) and grandfather (II-1) had been surgically treated for retinal detachment.

*Ophthalmological examination*

| Visual acuity | VOD: S − 2.25/Cyl. − 1.0 axis 5° 0.8. |
|---|---|
| | VOS: 2/60, correction not feasible. |
| Cycloplegic refraction | OD: S − 2.25/Cyl. − 1.0 axis 5°. |
| | OS: S − 2.25/Cyl. − 2.5 axis 170°. |
| Eye position | Virtually straight. No nystagmus. |
| Anterior segments | ODS: Normal. |
| Vitreous | OD: No cells or membranes. Some liquefaction. |
| | OS: Numerous pigment particles. Some lique-faction. Preretinal membranes in the posterior vitreous space. |

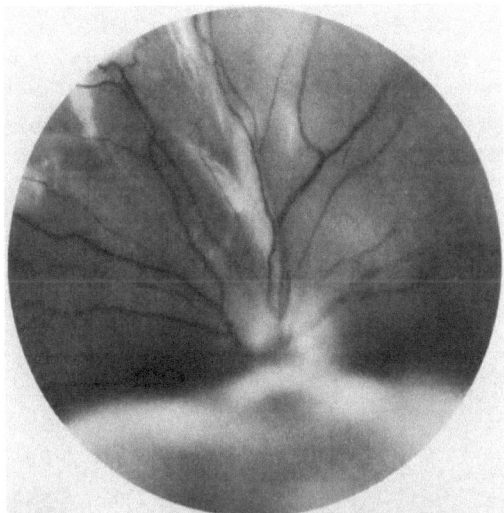

Figure 96 (IV-6). OS. Total retinal detachment.

Fundi

OD: In the posterior pole, the temporal retinal vessels take a slightly stretched course from the disc in temporal direction, with hardly noticeable ectopia of the maculae in that direction. The disc is normal. Temporally, no retinal vessels are visible anterior to the equator. It is difficult to see where the most peripheral ramifications end. At 11 o'clock, a small circular defect anterior to the equator is surrounded by local whitish degeneration in the avascular retinal periphery.

OS: Total movable retinal detachment, protruding slightly in the vitreous space in the superior and central parts, but markedly in the inferior part of the fundus (Figure 96). Despite the retinal detachment, it is evident that the vascular pattern of the retina is aberrant. Especially in the nasal and superior temporal quadrants, the vessels are tortuous and terminate in a well-defined zone which demarcates an avascular retinal periphery. The latter part comprises two small, nearly circular defects in the superior nasal quadrant (Figure 97). No exudates or distinct neovascularizations.

Fluorescein angiogram

OD: The retinal vessels outside the posterior pole are not readily distinguishable due to poor con-

156

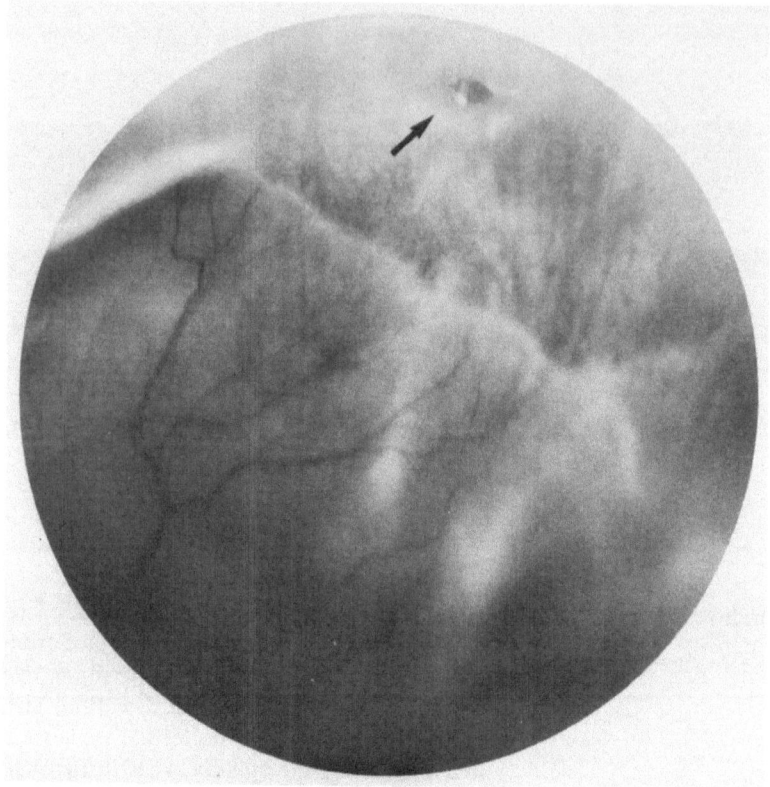

Figure 97 (IV-6). OS. Defect in avascular part of retinal periphery (arrow). Note the well-defined demarcation between vascular and avascular retina.

trast with the choroidal fluorescence. However, the equatorial retina proves to be non-perfused (Figure 98). The late phase shows no fluorescein leakage in the posterior pole and the temporal part of the retina.

OS: The perfusion of the periphery of the detached retina terminates abruptly in the nasal and superior temporal quadrants. The most peripheral capillaries show irregular dilatations and loops. Intensive fluorescein leakage from these vessels is observed (Figure 99). The late phase of the posterior pole shows fluorescein staining of the subretinal fluid and some leakage from the disc.

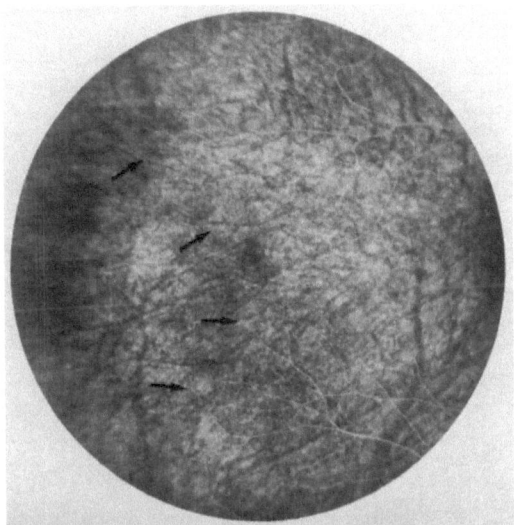

Figure 98 (IV-6). OD. The late phase of the fluorescein angiogram shows the hardly visible termination of retinal vessels near the equator (arrows). The retinal area on the left is avascular. No fluorescein leakage.

## General physical examination

The patient's habitus is somewhat gracile and leptosome. Height 183 cm, weight 69 kg. Blood pressure 120/70. Pulse rate 60/min, regular. No anomalies apart from thoracic kyphoscoliosis.

## Dental examination

Chronic periapical inflammation of M2Sd. No congenital abnormalities of the teeth and jaws.

## Laboratory studies

| | |
|---|---|
| Blood | ESR 12 mm in the first hour. |
| | Haemoglobin 9.8 mmol/l. |
| | Haematocrit 0.48. |
| | WBC 7300/mm$^3$. |
| | Differentation: 58% neutrophils |
| | 35% lymphocytes |
| | 2% eosinophils |
| | 5% monocytes. |
| Serum | Electrolytes: Na 135, K 4.4, Cl 98 mmol/l. |
| | Urea 7.5 mmol/l. |
| | Creatinine 82 mmol/l. |
| | Glucose 4.2 mmol/l. |
| Urine | Specific gravity 1032. |
| | Glucose negative. |

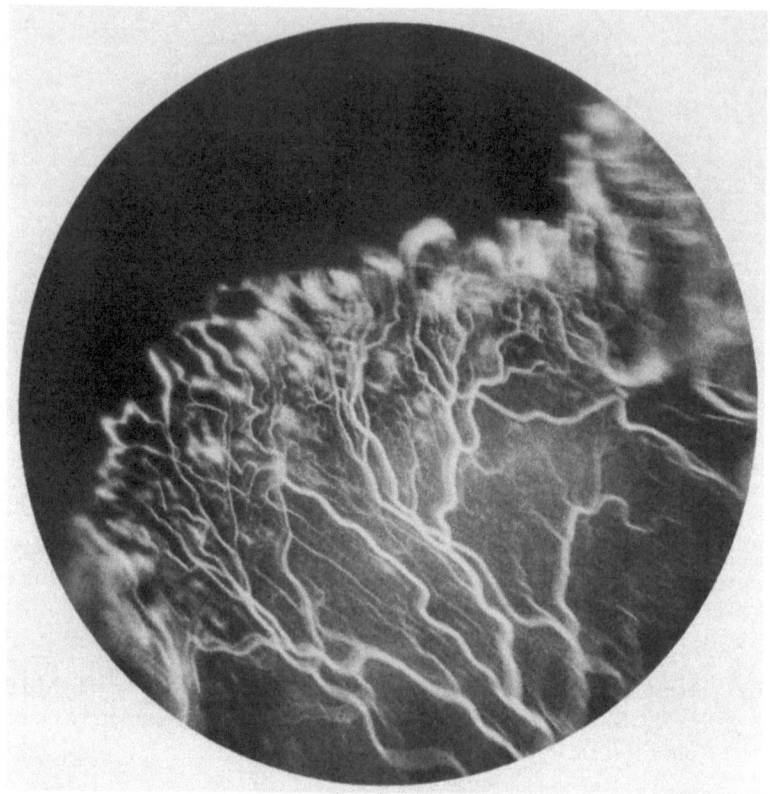

Figure 99 (IV-6). OS. Fluorescein angiogram of the periphery of the detached retina near 12 o'clock. Unmistakable non-perfusion of the peripheral retina and some leakage from a broad zone of aberrant ramifications.

| | |
|---|---|
| | Acetone negative. |
| | Urobilin trace. |
| | Porphobilin negative. |
| Coagulation studies | Bleeding time (Ivy) 4 min 3 sec. |
| | Platelets 159 000/mm$^3$. |
| | Thromboplastin time (Quick) 19 sec. |
| | Thrombotest (Owren) 41%. |
| | Cephalin-kaolin time 32 sec. |
| | Fibrinogen content 4785 mg/l. |
| | Thrombin time 18 sec. |
| | Fibrin degradation products 15 mg/l. |
| | Ethanol gelation test negative. |
| Conclusion | No anomalies. |

*Therapy and course*

In view of the preretinal vitreous membranes and the rigid retinal folds, a vitrectomy was performed. A silicone encircling band was applied to the equator (nr. 40). Using the Ocutome system, many tough pigmented membranes were removed from the vitreous via the pars plana. Puncture of the superior temporal sclera yielded a large amount of viscous fluid. A mixture of 80% air and 20% SF6 gas was insufflated via the pars plana. The retina failed to efface properly: a superior temporal fold persisted. Cryocoagulation round the clock peripheral to the encircling band.

Total retina re-detachment OS within a week of this procedure. No open retinal defect was visible. Again, pars plana vitrectomy, gas insufflation and drainage. A long silicone explant was inserted beneath the encircling band in both inferior quadrants. Within two weeks of this operation, subretinal fluid had accumulated again and total retinal re-detachment occurred. Peripheral to the buckle, a small circular defect seemed to have developed at 4 o'clock.

Six weeks after the first operation a third vitrectomy was performed.

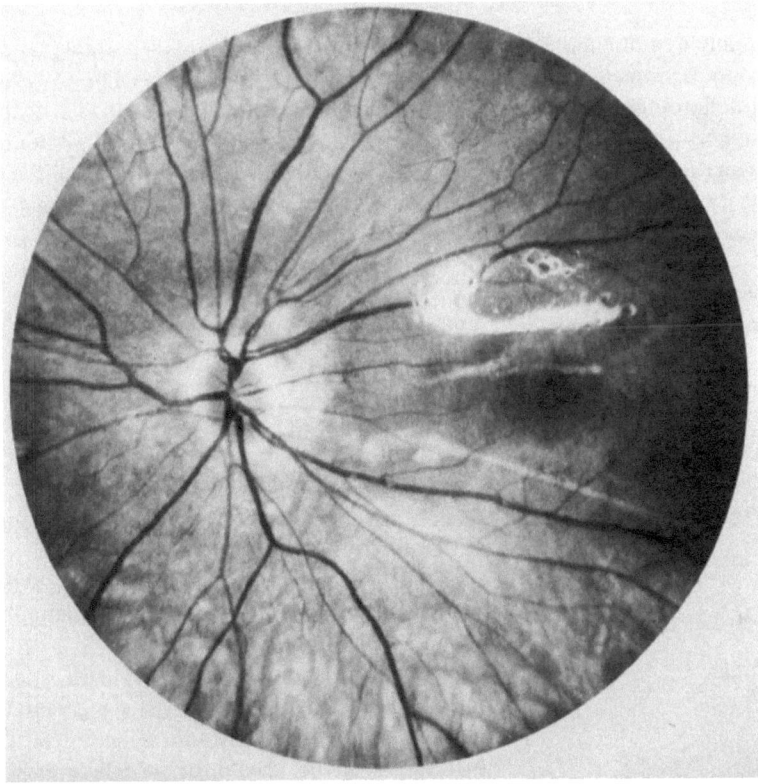

Figure 100 (IV-6). OS. Attached retina after intravitreous injection of silicone oil. The reflex superior to the macula comes from the posterior surface of the oil bubble.

There were no longer many membranes in the central vitreous space, but some membranes were present on the retina itself. The latter could not be removed with the vitrectomy apparatus. A drainage aperture was made in the sclera and 4 ml silicone oil was gradually injected. As a result the retina effaced almost entirely. After this operation the entire retina was in its proper position (Figure 100).

The retinal defect in OD was surrounded by two rows of coagulates with the Argon laser. The situation remained unchanged over a follow-up period of 6 months, apart from the development of a slight subcapsular posterior cataract in OS. VOS was 0.12 with correction S − 1.0.

## Conclusion
Rhegmatogenous retinal detachment OS with bilateral vascular anomalies of the retinal periphery consistent with a diagnosis of DEVR.

*Subject III-3 (20-01-23)*

## History
The left eye of this 57-year-old mother of the proband is reportedly lazy and has poor visual acuity. Virtually total retinal detachment OD in 1979. Her ophthalmologist reported a fair-sized circular retinal defect in the temporal periphery. In this area, a double sponge was applied to the sclera. After cryo-coagulations the retina re-attached itself. A few degenerative spots in the periphery of the left eye were treated by Xenon coagulation. General health believed to be good. No record of premature birth.

## Ophthalmological examination

| | |
|---|---|
| Visual acuity | VOD: S − 3.0/Cyl. 1.25 axis 65° 0.5. |
| | VOS: S − 7.0/Cyl. − 3.0 axis 115° 2/60. |
| Intraocular pressure | OD: 17 mm Hg. |
| | OS: 14 mm Hg. |
| Anterior segments | ODS: Normal. |
| Eye position | Divergent strabismus OS (narrow angle). |
| Vitreous | OD: Some liquefaction but otherwise normal structure. Some pigment particles. |
| | OS: Some liquefaction. Some pigment particles. A delicate vitreous membrane is seen anterior to the temporal fundus periphery. |
| Fundi | OD: A small area of choriocapillaris and pigmented layer atrophy and some pigmentations are seen on the temporal side of the disc. The retinal vessels in the posterior pole take a slightly stretched course in temporal direction. Some temporal ectopia of the macula. Near the equator |

between 9 and 11 o'clock, a buckle surrounded by coagulation scars is visible. No visible defect. The temporal retinal vessels terminate in delicate ramifications anterior to the equator. No exudates or neovascularizations.

OS: The disc implantation is askew in inferior temporal direction, but no signs of dragged disc. As in OD, there is some diffuse atrophy of the choriocapillaris and pigmented layer so that the choroidal vessels and sclera are clearly visible. The temporal branches of the retinal vessels take a slightly stretched course to the inferior temporal periphery, with some macular ectopia in the same direction. Many coagulation scars are seen anterior to the equator. Peripheral to these, no retinal vessels but only some whitish spots are seen in the temporal fundus. No retinal exudates, defects or neovascularizations.

*Conclusion*
Bilateral peripheral retinal vascular changes consistent with a diagnosis of DEVR. Amblyopia OS due to anisometropia. Surgically treated rhegmatogenous retinal detachment OD.

*Subject IV-5 (30-06-52)*

*History*
No visual complaints. Good general health. Birth weight 3500 g.

*Ophthalmological examination*

| | |
|---|---|
| Visual acuity | VOD: S − 1.25 0.8. |
| | VOS: S − 1.25 0.8. |
| Eye position | Straight. |
| Anterior segments | ODS: Normal. |
| Vitreous | ODS: Normal structure, no cells. |
| Fundi | OD: Normal posterior pole. No ramifications of retinal vessels are visible in the extreme temporal periphery. No exudates, defects or neovascularizations. |
| | OS: Normal posterior pole. A few vascular ramifications seem to terminate abruptly anterior to the temporal equator. At 12 o'clock near the equator there are some irregular dilatations of small vessels. |

Fluorescein angiography     OD: The early phase shows some curved and reversing vascular branches in the temporal equatorial zone.
OS: Temporal periphery shows the same features as in OD. The vascularization of the retina peripheral to these branches is not properly assessable. No leakage from the peripheral vessels of in the posterior pole.

## Conclusion

This patient shows minimal vascular anomalies in the peripheral retina ODS, but a positive diagnosis of DEVR cannot be established with certainty.

*Subject IV-8 (06-08-57)*

*History*
No visual complaints.

*Ophthalmological examination*

Visual acuity     VOD: 1,0, uncorrected.
VOS: 1.0, uncorrected.

Eye position     Straight.

Anterior segments     ODS: Normal.

Vitreous     ODS: Normal structure, no cells.

Fundi     OD: The temporal aspect of the disc is somewhat pale. Normal vasculature in the posterior pole. Anterior to the equator the peripheral ramifications of the retinal vessels terminate rather abruptly. The demarcation of the avascular retinal periphery deviates in central direction at 9 o' clock, giving rise to a wedge-shaped outpouching of the avascular periphery between the most peripheral ramifications. In the equatorial zone there are some curved and reversing venous branches at 12 o'clock. No retinal defects, exudates, pigmentations or neovascularizations.
OS: Features of posterior pole and fundus periphery virtually identical to those in OD.

## Conclusion

The symptoms are consistent with mild, uncomplictated DEVR.

*Subject IV-9 (06-03-59)*

*History*
No visual complaints. Good general health. Birth weight 3650 g.

*Ophthalmological examination*

| | |
|---|---|
| Visual acuity | VOD: Cyl. $-$ 0.5 axis $0°$ 1.25. |
| | VOS: S $+$ 0.25/Cyl. $-$ 0.25 axis $10°$ 1.0. |
| Eye position | Straight. |
| Vitreous | ODS: Normal structure, no cells. |
| Fundi | ODS: The superior and inferior vessels in and about the posterior pole are slightly stretched in temporal direction. No distinct macular ectopia. In the temporal periphery the retinal vessels terminate immediately peripheral to the equator. Some venous ramifications central to the equator are tortuous. No other complications. |

*Conclusion*
Mild asymptomatic DEVR.

*Subject IV-10 (14-08-60)*

*History*
No visual complaints. Good general health. Birth weight 3300 g.

*Ophthalmological examination*

| | |
|---|---|
| Visual acuity | VOD: S $+$ 0.25/Cyl. $-$ 0.5 axis $0°$ 1.0. |
| | VOS: S $-$ 0.25 1.0. |
| Eye position | Straight. |
| Anterior segments | ODS: Normal. |
| Vitreous | ODS: Minute dust-like particles. Normal structure. |
| Fundi | OD: Normal posterior pole. In the temporal zone between 8 and 11 o'clock, numerous slightly stretched, more or less parallel vascular ramifications terminate fairly abruptly near the equator. A pigmented scar is localized just within the avascular retina at 9 o'clock. |
| | OS: Normal posterior pole. Retinal vessels end temporally in the equatorial zone. The superior temporal part of the non-perfused retinal periphery comprises a snailtrack-like lesion in which a few minute defects are distinguishable. No complications such as exudates or neovascularizations in either fundus. |
| Fluorescein angiogram | OD: The early exposures show the equatorial |

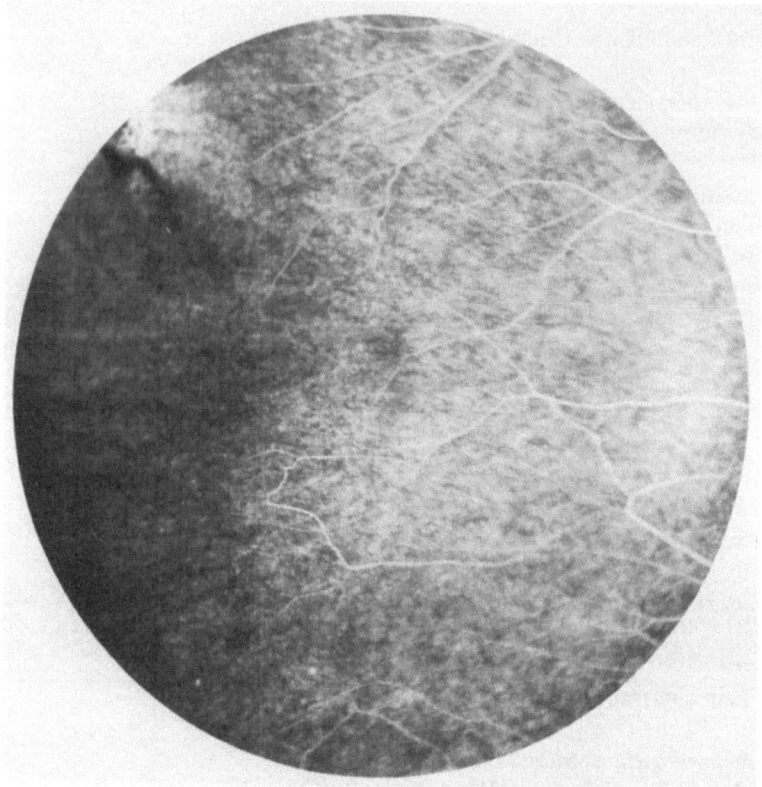

Figure 101 (IV-10). OD. Late phase of the fluorescein angiogram shows non-perfusion of the temporal retinal periphery. A well-defined zone of terminal ramifications is absent, and there is no fluorescein leakage in the retina.

zone near 9 o'clock. No distinct anomalies of the choroidal circulation. The retinal vessels end at the level of the equator, some showing a curvature near their termination. The scar is clearly visible as a pigmented layer defect. Strikingly, the late phase shows no leakage from the peripheral vascular ramifications (Figure 101). The late phase of the posterior pole shows slight hyperfluorescence of the disc, but no leakage from the perimacular capillaries.

OS: Late exposures of the equatorial zone at 3 o'clock show non-perfusion of the retina anterior to the equator. No leakage from the most peripheral branches of the retinal vessels, nor from vessels in the posterior pole.

*Conclusion*
Unmistakable non-perfusion of the temporal retinal periphery ODS, consistent
with a diagnosis of DEVR.

*Subject IV-11 (02-04-62)*

*History*
No visual complaints. Birth weight 3700 g. No neonatal oxygen administration.

*Ophthalmological examination*

| | |
|---|---|
| Visual acuity | VOD: S — 4.25 0.8. |
| | VOS: S — 6.0 0.8. |
| Eye position | Slight exophoria. |
| Anterior segments | ODS: Normal. |
| Vitreous | ODS: Normal structure, no cells. |
| Fundi | OD: The temporal vascular ramifications in the posterior pole take a slightly stretched course in temporal direction. In the central part of the posterior pole the retina shows a few minute white spots, probably very small exudates. In the temporal mid-periphery a fair number of retinal vessels take a more or less parallel, radial course and terminate abruptly near the equator. The nonperfused retinal periphery shows features of white without pressure at some sites. The nasal fundus periphery is normally vascularized. No retinal defects. |
| | OS: The vascular pattern of the posterior pole is virtually identical to that in OD, but without paramacular exudates. The pattern of the temporal equatorial zone is likewise highly similar to that in OD. The superior temporal avascular retinal periphery comprises some areas of whitish degeneration without distinct defects. |
| Fluorescein angiogram | OD: Late phase: abnormal vascular pattern of ramifying more or less parallel vessels central to the equator. No fluorescein leakage. |
| | OS: Early phase of the equatorial zone (3 o'clock). The retinal vessels terminate equatorially in ramifications. Normal perfusion of the peripheral choroid. Two pigment epithelium defects immediately peripheral to the extreme ramifications of the retinal vessels (Figure 102). Late exposures |

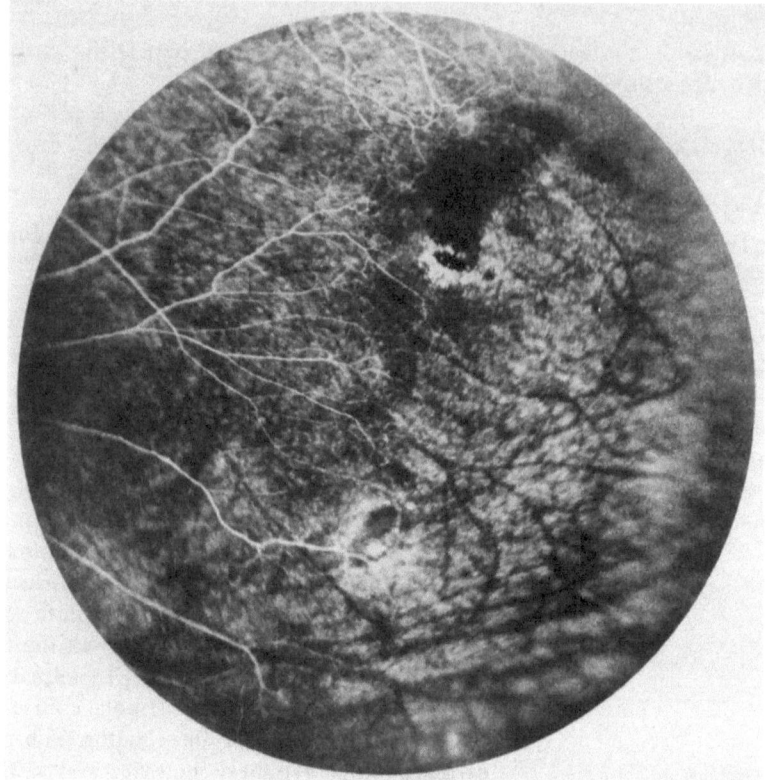

Figure 102 (IV-11). OS. Non-perfusion of the temporal retinal periphery. No fluorescein leakage in the marginal zone.

show no leakage from peripheral vessels and from perimacular capillaries.

*Conclusion*
Unmistakable absence of retinal vasculature in the peripheral retina consistent with a diagnosis of DEVR.

*Subject III-2 (30-11-21)*

*History*
No visual complaints. Good general health. Birth weight about 3000 g.

*Ophthalmological examination*
Visual acuity            VOD: S − 0.5/Cyl. − 2.25 axis 170° 0.6.
                                      VOS: S − 0.25/Cyl. − 1.75 axis 5° 1.0.

| | |
|---|---|
| Eye position | Straight. Very nasal corneal reflex especially in OD. |
| Intraocular pressure | ODS: 20 mm Hg. |
| Anterior segments | ODS: Normal. |
| Vitreous | ODS: Normal structure, no cells. |
| Fundi | OD: Vessels in the posterior pole are distinctly stretched in temporal direction, with some macular ectopia in that direction. The retinal vessels temporal to the posterior pole are tortuous. An abrupt transition from vascular to avascular retina is visible anterior to the temporal equator. The avascular zone is visible up to the superior nasal sector. Some of the most peripheral ramifications show delicate telangiectases. A few gross pigmentations are visible in the temporal sector of the avascular retina. |
| | OS: The pattern of the large vessels in the posterior pole is not distinctly abnormal. Nor is there evident macular ectopia. Near the equator in the superior temporal quadrant, a pale zone is visible in which the abundantly ramifying small retinal vessels terminate. The retina peripheral to this zone is avascular. The entire fundus, but especially the periphery, shows pigment paucity (as in OD) so that the large choroidal vessels are clearly visible. No retinal defects, pigmentations or neovascularizations are visible. |

*Conclusion*

Bilateral peripheral retinal vascular changes consistent with a diagnosis of DEVR.

*Subject IV-1 (02-05-46)*

*History*

Treatment of amblyopia OD during childhood. Surgical correction of convergent strabismus at age 31. Birth weight about 3500 g. Good general health. Three months pregnant.

*Ophthalmological examination*

| | |
|---|---|
| Visual acuity | VOD: S − 1.75/Cyl. − 0.5 axis 15° 0.8. |
| | VOS: S − 3.25/Cyl. − 0.75 axis 165° 1.0. |
| Eye position | Convergent strabismus OD, about 3°. Central corneal reflexes. |

| Anterior segments | ODS: Normal. |
| Vitreous | ODS: No abnormality apart from slight syneresis. |
| Fundi | OD: Normal posterior pole. The temporal fundus periphery shows white without pressure and no retinal vascularization. Central to the equator the temporal sector does show retinal vessels. No well-defined demarcation between vascular and avascular retina. |
| | OS: Normal posterior pole. White without pressure in the avascular temporal retinal periphery. Anterior to the temporal equator, a few retinal vessels show delicate multiple ramifications which are short and terminate slightly more anteriorly. Some of them curve back in central direction. No retinal defects, pigmentations or neovascularizations in either fundus. |

*Conclusion*

Bilateral peripheral retinal vascular changes consistent with a diagnosis of DEVR.

*Subject IV-2 (23-07-47)*

*History*

No visual complaints. Good general health apart from bouts of migraine. Birth weight about 4500 g.

*Ophthalmological examination*

| Visual acuity | VOD: S − 0.25/Cyl. − 0.25 axis 15° 1.0. |
| | VOS: Cyl. − 1.0 axis 15° 0.8. |
| Eye position | Straight. Positive kappa angle ODS. |
| Anterior segments | ODS: Normal. |
| Vitreous | OD: Some pigment particles; normal structure. |
| | OS: Normal. |
| Fundi | OD: The large vessels in and about the posterior pole show some stretching in inferior temporal direction, with slight macular ectopia in the same direction. In the mid-periphery between 8 and 10 o'clock a relatively large number of vascular branches are seen, several of which terminate in short, brush-like ramifications near the equator. Peripheral to them, the avascular retina comprises a few small pigmentations. |

OS: Less deformation of the large vessels in the posterior pole than in OD. Minimal temporal macular ectopia. The pattern of the peripheral retinal vasculature closely resembles that in OD. At 6 o'clock in the periphery there is a snail-track with an atrophic area in the neuroretina.

*Conclusion*
Anomalies of the retinal vessels in the posterior pole and periphery ODS, consistent with a diagnosis of DEVR.

*Subject III-4 (22-06-24)*

*History*
VOD poor from the start. No record of ophthalmological treatment. General health: several attacks of otitis media, biliary complaints and migraine. Birth weight unknown. No record of premature birth or neonatal oxygen administration.

*Ophthalmological examination*

| Visual acuity | VOD: S − 4.0 2/60. |
| | VOS: S − 3.5/Cyl. − 1.5 axis 5° 0.8. |
| Eye position | Straight. Extremely nasal corneal reflex OD, giving the impression of divergent strabismus. Central corneal reflex OS. |
| Anterior segments | OD: Moderate subcapsular posterior cataract. |
| | OS: Normal. |
| Vitreous | OD: Distinct syneresis. No particles or cells. A faire number of very thin vitreous membranes anterior to the nasal periphery of the retina. |
| | OS: Distinct syneresis. No particles or cells. |
| Fundi | OD: The large vessels show marked distortion from the disc in temporal direction. The macula shows ectopia in the same direction and is deformed. An area of pigment epithelium atrophy with sharply defined, irregular margins is seen temporal to the posterior pole. A few gross pigmentations are seen near the temporal equator. The retinal vessels in this area are tortuous and show some diliatations, and they terminate peripheral to the equator. A few small exudates are visible at 9 o'clock. The nasal fundus periphery is likewise affected. Thin membranes are visible anterior to the inferior nasal retinal periphery, and there |

may be local retinoschisis in this area. The nasal retinal periphery also seems avascular, but it is difficult to establish this due to the media opacities. No evidence of defects or neovascularizations.

OS: The vessels of the posterior pole take a slightly stretched course in temporal direction. Only slight macular ectopia. The temporal equatorial zone comprises a slightly aberrant pattern of small vascular branches, some of which curve back in central direction. Peripheral to the equator, no retinal vessels are visible between 2 and 4 o'clock. No retinal defects or neovascularizations.

## Conclusion

Distinct bilateral peripheral retinal vascular changes consistent with a diagnosis of uncomplicated DEVR.

## Subject IV-13 (27-05-59)

### History

No visual complaints. Anxious young man who, like his brother (IV-12) is mentally underendowed. Both brothers show low implantation of the ears. No record of premature birth or neonatal oxygen administration.

### Ophthalmological examination

| | |
|---|---|
| Visual acuity | VOD: 1.0 with corrective spectacles. |
| | VOS: 1.0 with corrective spectacles. |
| Eye position | Straight. Central corneal reflexes. |
| Anterior segments | ODS: Normal. |
| Vitreous | ODS: Normal. |
| Fundi | OD: Contact lens examination is difficult due to insufficient cooperation. No distinct fundus changes observed. |
| | OS: Examination with the contact lens less difficult. Normal posterior pole. The vasculature central to the temporal equator seems slightly aberrant. Possibly avascular retina anterior to the equator. No evidence of retinal defects, exudates or neovascularizations. |

### Conclusion

Probably mild peripheral fundus anomalies OS, consistent with a diagnosis of uncomplicated DEVR. However, the diagnosis is not certain.

*Subject III-5 (05-12-25)*

*History*
No visual complaints. Good general health. Birth weight about 3500 g.

*Ophthalmological examination*

| | |
|---|---|
| Visual acuity | VOD: S − 0.25/Cyl. − 0.75 axis 100° 1.0. |
| | VOS: Cyl. − 0.5 axis 95° 1.0. |
| Eye position | Straight. |
| Intraocular pressure | OD: 14 mm Hg. |
| | OS: 16 mm Hg. |
| Anterior segments | ODS: Normal. |
| Vitreous | ODS: Posterior vitreous detachment. Normal structure. No cells or particles. |
| Fundi | OD: Normal posterior pole. Normal vascularization of the nasal fundus periphery. In the temporal mid-periphery, a few vascular branches curve back and have aberrant brush-like ramifications. Peripheral to them, the retina is avascular and shows some gross pigmentations and a few cobblestones. No retinal defects, exudates or neovascularizations. |
| | OS: Normal posterior pole. Some tortuosity of retinal vessels in the temporal mid-periphery. A few small vessels have aberrant multiple ramifications or delicate telangiectases. An avascular retinal periphery is visible between 11 and 5 o'clock. No retinal defects, pigmentations or exudates. |

*Conclusion*
Bilateral peripheral retinal vascular changes consistent with a diagnosis of DEVR.

*Subject IV-14 (13-06-56)*

*History*
No visual complaints. Good general health. Birth weight about 3000 g.

*Ophthalmological examination*

| | |
|---|---|
| Visual acuity | VOD: S − 1.0 0.8. |
| | VOS: S − 1.0/Cyl. − 0.5 axis 115° 1.0. |
| Eye position | Straight. |
| Anterior segments | ODS: Normal. |

172

| Vitreous | ODS: Normal. |
|---|---|
| Fundi | ODS: The vascular pattern seems to be slightly stretched in temporal direction, possibly with minimal macular ectopia. Normal vascularization of the nasal fundus periphery. Some slight anomalies of the retinal vessels are visible in the equatorial zone near 9 o'clock in OD and near 3 o' clock in OS. A few venous branches curve back and show short ramifications in central direction. An avascular zone is visible in the temporal retinal periphery ODS. Fundus features otherwise normal. |

*Conclusion*
Very slight vascular anomalies in both fundi. It is not certain whether these represent a minimal manifestations of DEVR.

*Subject III-6 (05-03-34)*

*History*
This man was not examined. According to his ophthalmologist there had been retinal detachment OD at age 17. Type of operative treatment unknown. Reportedly, there were multiple retinal defects. Most recently measured visual acuity: VOD: S + 1.0 0.3. VOS: S − 2.0 1.2. The retina is attached in both eyes. Many pigmented scars in the fundus OD. Nothing is known about possible retinal vascular anomalies.

*Subject II-1 (15-06-1889)*

*History*
This meanwhile deceased man was reported to have had fairly good eyesight. Operation on the retina about 1964, but exact data could not be retrieved.

### 3.10 The I family

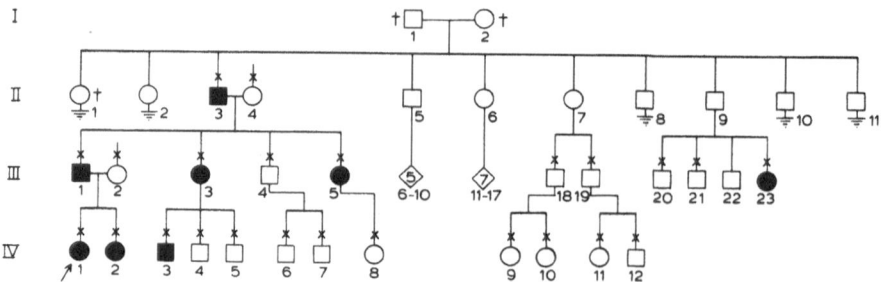

Figure 103. Pedigree of the I family.

*Introduction*

The female proband of this family was known at the out-patient clinic of the ophthalmological department of the Canisius-Wilhelmina Hospital as showing unilateral deformation of the vasculature of the posterior pole of the retina. Although no real retinal fold had formed, a mild form of falciform detachment was considered. The unilaterality of the condition and the negative family history initially seemed not to be suggestive of a hereditary condition.

*Proband IV-1 (01-11-76)*

*History*
Divergent strabismus OS was noticed a few months after the birth of this now 4-year-old girl. Pregnancy and parturition had been uneventful. Birth weight was 3000 g, and there was no neonatal oxygen administration. No general abnormalities apart from some motor retardation.

*Ophthalmological examination (at age 3)*

| | |
|---|---|
| Visual acuity | VOD: 1.0. |
| | VOS: 0.3. |
| Eye position | Straight, but marked pseudostrabismus OS due to a very wide positive kappa angle (Chapter 4, Figure 104). |
| Anterior segments | ODS: Normal. |
| Cycloplegic refraction | OD: Emmetropic. |
| | OS: S + 2.0/Cyl. − 2.0 axis 0°. |
| Vitreous | OD: Normal structure. |
| | OS: Many pigment particles and thin preretinal membranes. |
| Fundi | OD: Contact lens examination was impossible in this very young girl. The fundus was examined by indirect ophthalmoscopy, but this gave no adequate view of the peripheral retinal vasculature. The disc and macula appear to be normal. Normal configuration of the retinal vessels throughout the posterior fundus. A number of white spots are visible anterior to the equator near 9 o'clock; these may be small exudates. |
| | OS: The retinal vessels take a distinctly stretched course from the disc to the inferior temporal quadrant. Consequently there is pronounced macular ectopia in that direction. The parallel pattern of radial retinal vessels is also seen in the region temporal to the posterior pole. These ret- |

inal vessels disappear from sight anterior to the equator, where several pigment deposits are localized in the retina near 3 o'clock. No exudates or neovascularizations are seen.

### Conclusion

Bilateral anomalies in the temporal retinal periphery, suggestive of DEVR.

### Subject III-1 (16-07-44)

### History

The proband's father has never had visual complaints and has never been ophthalmologically examined. Birth weight was 2250 g, but no neonatal oxygen administration. Good general health.

### Ophthalmological examination

| | |
|---|---|
| Visual acuity | VOD: Cyl. — 0.5 axis 90° 1.25.<br>VOS: 1.25, uncorrected. |
| Eye position | Straight. Central corneal reflexes. |
| Intraocular pressure | ODS: 13 mm Hg. |
| Anterior segments | ODS: Normal. |
| Vitreous | ODS: Slight syneresis. No cells or particles. Posterior vitreous detachment. |
| Fundi | OD: The temporal retinal vascular branches take a slightly stretched course from the disc in temporal direction. The macula consequently shows slight ectopia in that direction. In the temporal quadrant central to the equator, there are abnormally numerous retinal vessels with a near-parallel course. The smallest ramifications terminate immediately anterior to the equator, so that the temporal retinal periphery is avascular. The well-defined demarcation between vascular and avascular retina deviates in central direction at 9 o'clock, giving rise to a wedge-shaped notch in the avascular peripheral retina between the most peripheral ramifications of the superior and the inferior temporal vessels. A few glittering white ramifying preretinal structures are visible at this site. These are probably small, partly fibrosed neovascularizations arising from the most peripheral ramifications of the retinal vessels. No retinal defects, exudates or neovascularizations.<br>OS: The posterior pole presents the same appear- |

ance as in OD. The temporal retinal periphery is avascular, and the central demarcation of the avascular part shows a notch near 3 o'clock. Again there is white preretinal fibrosis, not larger than one disc diameter. No other complications are visible.

Visual fields (Goldmann)  ODS: Absolute limitation of the nasal visual field to about 30°.

*Conclusion*
Bilateral peripheral retinal vascular changes consistent with a diagnosis of DEVR.

*Subject IV-2 (27-12-78)*

*History*
The parents have noticed nothing abnormal about the eyes of this 2-year-old girl. Birth weight was 3050 g.

*Ophthalmological examination*

Visual acuity          Not yet properly determinable.
Eye position           Straight.
Anterior segments      ODS: Normal.
Vitreous               ODS: No abnormal structures at ophthalmo-scopy.
Fundi                  ODS: Normal vasculature of the posterior pole. Tortuous, irregularly dilatated vascular loops are visible in the temporal equatorial region. They form a zone which more or less parallels the ora serrata. No retinal vessels are clearly visible anterior to this zone. So far as visible, there are no preretinal neovascularizations, membranes, retinal defects or exudates.

*Conclusion*
Slight but unmistakable DEVR.

*Policy*
No therapy indicated. In view of the patient's extreme youth, periodical follow-ups on visual acuity and fundi are advisable.

*Subject II-3 (14-01-08)*

*History*

No visual complaints. Patient uses anticoagulants in view of cerebral circulatory disorders. No record of premature birth.

*Ophthalmological examination*

| | |
|---|---|
| Visual acuity | VOD: S + 0.5 0.8. |
| | VOS: S + 1.0 0.6. |
| Eye position | Straight. |
| Intraocular pressure | ODS: 10 mm Hg. |
| Anterior segments | ODS: Slight posterior cortical cataract of both lenses. |
| Vitreous | ODS: Normal structure, no cells. Posterior vitreous detachment OS. |
| Fundi | OD: Slightly stretched retinal vessels in the posterior pole. Slight temporal ectopia of the macula. Temporal to the posterior pole, the small veins in particular are somewhat tortuous. Anterior to the equator the retinal vessels end in a clearly defined zone which is the central demarcation of the avascular peripheral retina. This is visible between 7 and 11 o'clock. Between 9 and 11 o'clock, retinoschisis in this region extends to slightly central to the equator. A few small retinal vessels are visible in the centre of this retinoschisis. The remainder is avascular, and this avascular part comprises a small circular defect. No visible retinal exudates or neovascularizations. |
| | OS: The posterior pole shows a vasculature which resembles that in OD, but without distinct macular ectopia. The retinal periphery is avascular between 1 and 5 o'clock. No complications. |

*Conclusion*

Bilateral peripheral retinal vascular changes consistent with a diagnosis of DEVR.

*Subject III-3 (04-05-46)*

*History*

Acute iridocyclitis at age 31, with smooth recovery after treatment. General physical examination failed to disclose the cause of this inflammation. At present no visual complaints. Birth weight was 1500 g, but no record of neonatal oxygen administration.

*Opthalmological examination*

| | |
|---|---|
| Visual acuity | VOD: 1.0, uncorrected. |
| | VOS: 1.25, uncorrected. |
| Eye position | Straight. |
| Anterior segments | ODS: Normal. |
| Vitreous | ODS: Normal structure, no cells. |
| Fundi | ODS: Normal posterior pole. Temporal retinal sector avascular. Especially in OS, this sector is somewhat whitish but there are no defects, pigmentations or exudates. The avascular retina is demarcated on the central side by delicate terminal ramifications of retinal vessels. The vascular pattern central to the equator is virtually normal, so that the changes are not very conspicuous. |

*Conclusion*

Subtle vascular changes in the temporal retinal periphery ODS, consistent with a mild manifestation of DEVR.

*History*

No visual complaints apart from a possibly viral inflammation OD, which was cured by treatment and did not relapse. Birth weight 2500 g. No neonatal oxygen administration.

*Ophthalmological examination*

| | |
|---|---|
| Visual acuity | VOD: 1.25, uncorrected. |
| | VOS: 1.0, uncorrected. |
| Eye position | Straight. |
| Anterior segments | ODS: Normal. |
| Vitreous | ODS: Normal. |
| Fundi | ODS: Normal posterior pole, normal pattern of vasculature also in the more peripheral areas of the posterior fundus. Peripheral to the temporal equator, however, the retinal vessels terminate in multiple ramifications; consequently the retina anterior to the midline between equator and ora serrata, near the horizontal meridians, is avascular. No other changes are visible in the avascular temporal retinal sectors. |

*Conclusion*

Slight vascular anomalies in the temporal retinal periphery ODS, consistent with DEVR.

*Subject III-5 (07-10-51)*

*History*

This woman has worn spectacles (subsequently contact lenses) for correction of myopia since age 7. No abnormalities other than the myopia believed to have been diagnosed. Birth weight some 3000 g. Good general health.

*Ophthalmological examination*

| | |
|---|---|
| Visual acuity | VOD: S − 4.0 0.6. |
| | VOS: S − 4.5 0.6. |
| Eye position | Straight. Corneal reflex OD decidedly nasal and slightly too high. Corneal reflex OS only nasal. The consequence is divergent pseudostrabismus and deorsumvergence OD. |
| Anterior segments | ODS: Normal. |
| Vitreous | ODS: Moderate syneresis. Posterior vitreous detachment OD. No cells. |
| Fundi | OD: The retinal vessels of the posterior pole take a distinctly stretched course in temporal direction. Marked temporal and slightly inferior ectopia of the macula. The area central to the temporal equator shows an abundance of mostly radial retinal vessels which, slightly more anteriorly, end in a well-defined zone of irregular terminal ramifications. The retina peripheral to this zone is quite avascular. Near 9 o'clock, a relatively large arteriole and venule take a radial course as far as the demarcation of the avascular retina, where a partly fibrosed fan-shaped neovascularization is localized on the retinal surface, immediately peripheral to the demarcation of the avascular retina. No visible retinal defects or exudates. |
| | OS: The vessels in the posterior pole show more pronounced distortion in temporal direction than in OD, giving rise to the features of dragged disc. In most of the temporal periphery the retinal vessels terminate anterior to the equator, thus demarcating an avascular peripheral zone. At 3 o'clock, a small fibrosed neovascularization is visible just outside the zone of the most peripheral retinal vessels. Slightly central to this structure, the vascular retina contains small exudates. The nasal fundus periphery shows a normal retinal vasculature. At the extreme periphery in the |

superior nasal quadrant, several pigmentations are seen in a zone parallel to the ora serrata. No visible retinal defects.

*Conclusion*

Unmistakable symptoms of DEVR with small, partly fibrosed retinal neo-vascularizations in both fundi.

*Subject III-18*

I found unmistakable anisometropia in this 37-year-old man. VODS was good, and the fundi showed no symptoms of DEVR. His two daughters (IV-9 and IV-10) showed amblyopia OS due to anisometropia. In these girls, too, no distinct anomalies were found in the fundus periphery.

*Subject III-23 (07-02-58)*

*History*

No visual complaints. Birth weight 4000 g.

*Ophthalmological examination*

| | |
|---|---|
| Visual acuity | VOD: S $-$ 5.75/Cyl. $-$ 0.5 axis 7° 1.0. |
| | VOS: S $-$ 4.75/Cyl. $-$ 0.5 axis 0° 1.0. |
| Eye position | Straight. |
| Anterior segments | ODS: Normal. |
| Vitreous | ODS: Normal. |
| Fundi | ODS: Blond fundi. The choriocapillaris seems very thin so that the course of the large choroidal vessels is clearly visible. In the posterior pole the disc, macula and configuration of retinal vessels are normal. Between the posterior pole and the temporal equator ODS, a fair number of retinal vessels are seen, some of which are decidely tortuous. These vessels terminate in short ramifications anterior to the equator. The peripheral retina is avascular in the temporal sectors, and in OS slightly whitish. No retinal defects, exudates or neovascularizations. |

*Conclusion*

Slight bilateral peripheral retinal vascular changes consistent with a diagnosis of DEVR.

CHAPTER 4

## RESULTS AND DISCUSSION OF THE FAMILY STUDIES

This chapter discusses the results of the nine family studies presented in the previous chapter, and compares them with data on DEVR in the literature.

### 4.1 Numbers of affected and probably affected persons in the various families

The nine families included a total of 75 persons in whom DEVR was diagnosed. In 12 additional persons, symptoms were found which were probably due to DEVR but could not be identified as such with certainty. In most cases this diagnostic uncertainty was caused by the extreme slightness of symptoms or by imperfect visibility of the lesions due to a variety of causes. In some of the 12 persons the diagnosis was not entirely certain because neonatal oxygen administration was on record, so that the possibility of retrolental fibroplasia could not be totally excluded.

This chapter designates as "affected family members" only those who are included in the abovementioned group of 75 persons (marked in full black in the pedigree). The text or the tables explicitly refer to persons in whom the diagnosis is probable but not entirely certain (Hatched markings in the pedigree).

The numbers of persons with DEVR encountered in the various families are listed in Table 1.

Table 1. Distribution of subjects with evident or probable DEVR in the nine families studied.

| Family | Number of subjects with evident DEVR | Number of subjects with probable DEVR |
|--------|--------------------------------------|---------------------------------------|
| A | 17 | 4 |
| B | 4 | — |
| C | 13 | 4 |
| D | 15 | 1 |
| E | 2 | 0 |
| F | 3 | 0 |
| G | 2 | — |
| H | 11 | 3 |
| I | 8 | — |
| Total | 75 | 12 |

Table 2. Sex distribution of subjects with evident or probable DEVR.

|  | Total | Male | Female |
|---|---|---|---|
| Number of subjects with evident DEVR | 75 | 39 | 36 |
| Number of subjects with probable DEVR | 12 | 6 | 6 |
| Total | 87 | 45 | 42 |

## 4.2 Age and sex distribution of the affected and probably affected persons

The sex distribution of the affected and probably affected persons in the various families is indicated in Table 2. As expected on the basis of the postulate of autosomal dominant transmission (see also Chapter 5), the sex distribution approximates a 1:1 ratio.

The age distribution of the affected and probably affected persons in the nine families is indicated in Table 3, on the basis of the person's age at the time of examination in the context of this study. Whenever an individual was examined several times over a longer period, the age at the first examination by me is indicated in the table. The table shows predominance of adolescents and young adults, whereas young children and aged individuals are underrepresented.

## 4.3 Visual acuity

A considerable number of the affected persons had shown unilateral or sometimes bilateral diminution of visual acuity in childhood. A large number, however, had never had any visual complaints. In the latter category my examination sometimes revealed unilateral or bilateral subnormality of visual acuity, but normal VODS was often found. That mild manifestations of DEVR often cause no or hardly any diminution of visual acuity has already been demonstrated by Gow and Oliver (1971), by Laqua (1980) and by Ober et al. (1980).

Table 3. Age distribution of subjects with evident or probable DEVR.

| Age in years | Number of subjects with evident DEVR | Number of subjects with probable DEVR |
|---|---|---|
| 0– 9 | 3 | – |
| 10–19 | 19 | 3 |
| 20–29 | 19 | 7 |
| 30–39 | 8 | – |
| 40–49 | 9 | – |
| 50–59 | 13 | 2 |
| 60–69 | 2 | – |
| 70–79 | 2 | – |

Table 4. Best-corrected visual acuity of 144 eyes with evident DEVR.

| Visual acuity | Number of eyes | % |
|---|---|---|
| 1.0 or better | 57 | 40 |
| 0.6–0.8 | 45 | 31 |
| 0.3–0.5 | 10 | 7 |
| 0.1–0.2 | 8 | 6 |
| 1/60–5/60 | 12 | 8 |
| light perception – 4/300 | 3 | 2 |
| no light perception | 9 | 6 |

Table 4 shows the distribution of visual acuity values in 144 eyes of affected members of the various families. For patients whose visual acuity changed in the course of the study, the last known value is recorded. The table shows that relatively few eyes had severely reduced visual acuity: in only 32 of the 144 eyes (22%) was visual acuity 0.2 or less.

A striking finding was the frequent difference in visual acuity between the eyes of the same individual. Poor visual acuity in one eye and good visual acuity in the other is not uncommon. This difference in function distinguishes DEVR from most other hereditary retinal anomalies, in which a high correlation of the visual acuity of the two eyes is usually found. This fact also implies that many instances of DEVR are classified as unilateral conditions, and that consequently the possibility of a hereditary affection is overlooked.

One of the consequences of the frequent presence of a marked difference in function between the two eyes is that the number of persons with a serious visual handicap as a result of DEVR is smaller than might be expected in view of Table 4.

A relatively large number of individuals with poor visual acuity in one eye had fair or good eyesight in the other.

In this study, visual acuity was as a rule determined for each eye separately, and rarely binocularly.

In order to gain some impression of the degree of visual handicap, the visual acuity in the better eye of 72 persons with evident DEVR was listed. Table 5 shows the distribution on this basis. Only 8 of the 72 affected persons (11%) had a serious visual handicap (visual acuity 0.2 or less).

Table 5. Visual acuity of the better eye in 72 subjects with evident DEVR.

| Visual acuity | Number of subjects | % |
|---|---|---|
| 1.0 or better | 34 | 47 |
| 0.6–0.8 | 25 | 35 |
| 0.3–0.5 | 5 | 7 |
| 0.1–0.2 | 3 | 4 |
| 1/60–5/60 | 2 | 3 |
| light perception – 4/300 | 2 | 3 |
| no light perception | 1 | 1.4 |

## 4.4 Refraction

The refraction of 126 eyes of 75 affected persons was determined subjectively or cycloplegically. Of course this was impossible in eyes with intensive media opacities.

The spherical equivalent of the refraction anomaly of these 126 eyes (spherical value $- \frac{1}{2} \times$ cylindrical value in diopters) was calculated. The distribution of the spherical equivalents (rounded up to whole diopters) of these 126 eyes is presented in Table 6, which shows that myopia is more frequent than hypermetropia, and that the myopic anomaly as a rule exceeds the hypermetropic anomaly.

Astigmatism of 1 diopter or more was found in 43 of the 126 eyes (34%). In 21 eyes (17%) astigmatism was 2 diopters or more.

Anisometropia also proved to be quite common: refraction ODS was determined in 57 affected persons; 18 (32%) showed anisometropia of 1 diopter or more, either in spherical or cylindrical value.

In summary it can be stated that our patients with DEVR relatively frequently showed myopia, and especially myopic astigmatism, as well as anisometropia.

Although reports so far published on DEVR do not always specify the refraction in all cases, myopic astigmatism would seem to be quite common in other studies as well.

Only incidentally did I perform biometric measurements, and it is therefore impossible to establish to which extent the refraction anomalies found correlated with changes in eye axis length.

To my mind, the above described refraction anomalies in DEVR closely resemble those of retrolental fibroplasia (RLF), in which myopia, astigmatism and anisometropia occur frequently (Reese and Stepanik, 1954; Fletcher and

Table 6. Spherical equivalents of 126 eyes with evident DEVR.

| Spherical equivalent (D) | Number of eyes |
|---|---|
| − 10 or more | 5 |
| − 9 | − |
| − 8 | 5 |
| − 7 | − |
| − 6 | 3 |
| − 5 | 1 |
| − 4 | 7 |
| − 3 | 11 |
| − 2 | 9 |
| − 1 | 8 |
| 0 | 55 |
| + 1 | 8 |
| + 2 | 4 |
| + 3 | 8 |
| + 4 | 2 |

Brandon, 1955; Hittner et al., 1979). The close similarity in clinical features between the two conditions is suggestive of a similar pathogenesis of the refraction anomalies found in them.

## 4.5 Amblyopia

In 11 of the 75 affected persons, unilateral diminution of visual acuity was found which could not be ascribed to anomalies in the posterior pole of the fundus but apparently resulted from amblyopia (V-33, V-29 and V-41 in the A family; III-5 and IV-12 in the C family; VI-21 in the D family; IV-6, III-3, III-4 and IV-1 in the H family; IV-1 in the I family). The majority of the patients mentioned showed anisometropia.

These findings seem to warrant the conclusion that amblyopia is a not uncommon complication of DEVR, and that anisometropia plays an important role in its pathogenesis.

So far as I know there are no previous reports on amblyopia as a complication of DEVR. This complication has important diagnostic as well as therapeutic implications: when examining children with amblyopia, DEVR should be considered as a possible cause of the anomaly, especially when there is anisometropia as well. Since symptoms in the posterior pole of the fundus are often absent in DEVR, the diagnosis can be easily overlooked.

Therapeutically, early diagnosis and treatment of amblyopia in young children with DEVR is important (see also Chapter 6).

## 4.6 Nystagmus

Unmistakable pendular nystagmus was observed in 4 persons (VI-3 in the D family. III-4 and IV-1 in the F family; II-2 in the G family). Visual acuity was severely diminished in all.

Unilateral latent nystagmus was found in one person (V-12 in the D family), in the eye with poor visual acuity. The presence of pendular nystagmus suggests that the lesions of the posterior pole have developed in the first years of life.

In the literature I found 7 patients with DEVR who showed nystagmus (Gow and Oliver, 1971; Slusher and Hutton, 1979; Laqua, 1980; Dudgeon, 1980). All showed poor visual acuity.

## 4.7 Eye position

The position of the visual axes (eye position) was examined in 70 of the 75 DEVR patients. Strabismus was found in 15: convergent in 9 and divergent in 6. Some had undergone a strabismus operation in the past, and the primary eye position could no longer be traced.

Pseudostrabismus due to an abnormal kappa angle was frequently found. This phenomenon results from an abnormal position of the macula. At examination the kappa angle was not measured but the position of the corneal fixation on a lamp was recorded for each eye separately. This corneal reflex often showed an abnormal position: nasal or superior nasal displacement in nearly all cases. This corresponded with the temporal or inferior temporal ectopia of the macula in DEVR.

The position of the corneal reflex was not recorded for all persons with evident DEVR. With eyes which have no or poor fixation, moreover, it is impossible to gain an impression of the kappa angle. Of the 95 eyes of DEVR patients, 24 (25%) showed an abnormal position of the corneal reflex which suggested an increased positive kappa angle. The degree of enlargement of the kappa angle differed widely. Not infrequently the size of this angle in the two eyes differed significantly. (Figure 104).

Displacement of the corneal reflex is a readily observable symptom of importance in the diagnosis of DEVR. In the examination of family members its presence is often the first indication of pathology.

## 4.8 Intraocular pressure

Intraocular pressure was determined by applanation in 26 DEVR patients. It exceeded 20 mm Hg in 2 of the 52 eyes : IV-16 in the A family (OD 21 mm

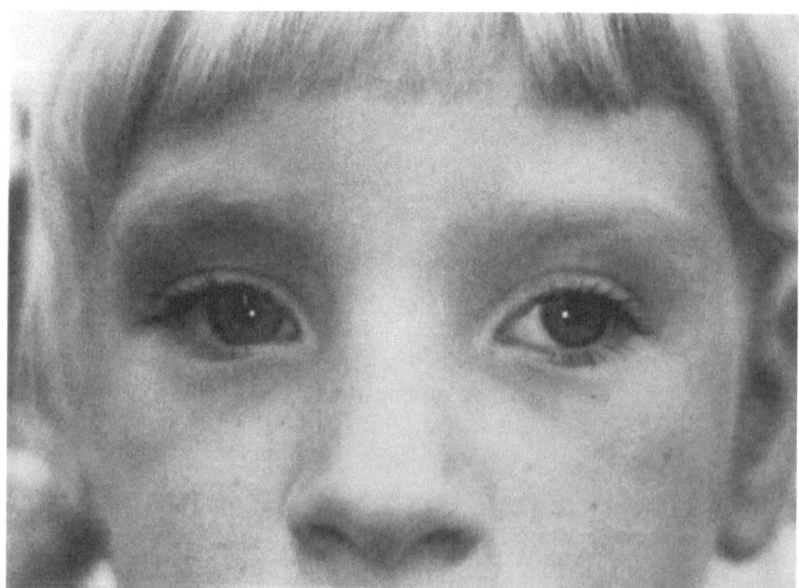

Figure 104. Pseudodivergent position OS due to enlarged positive kappa angle (IV-1 I).

Hg) and III-4 in the F family (OS 22 mm Hg). In both cases this value was measured in an eye without light perception, showing marked changes in the anterior segment and vitreous.

Two patients had a history of secondary glaucoma in an eye with poor function (III-4 in the F and II-2 in the G family). The literature incidentally mentions secondary glaucoma as a complication of DEVR (Laqua, 1980). In none of the members of the various families I examined did I find indications of primary glaucoma.

## 4.9 Anterior segment

Anomalies of the anterior segment were uncommon; they were found only in eyes with severe changes in fundus and vitreous and poor visual acuity.

Various stages of band keratopathy were observed in a few eyes without light perception (IV-18 in the D, III-2 in the B and III-4 in the F family) or with very poor visual acuity (III-4 in the F family). A diminished corneal diameter was found only in eyes with extensive vitreous organizations (IV-18 D and II-2 G).

One affected family member showed a very slight haze in the cornea ODS. At slit-lamp examination this patient's endothelium showed no further anomalies, and VODS was good.

No corneal anomalies were found in the remaining DEVR patients.

A shallow anterior chamber was found only in a few eyes with very marked changes (III-4 D and II-2 G).

In no case were gonioscopic anomalies of the iridocorneal angle observed which might suggest a developmental disorder in this area. In some eyes with marked changes, many secondary anomalies had developed in the iridocorneal angle due to synechiae. Gonioscopy of such eyes was often impossible due to band keratopathy.

Irritation of the anterior segment, manifested by the presence of cells and a flare in the aqueous humour, was likewise found only in eyes with partial or total retinal detachment (V-25 A, V-16 A, III-5 B and II-2 G). In most cases this irritation seemed not very intensive but often it was nevertheless not possible to suppress it entirely by local application of mydriatics and corticosteroids.

Synechiae, often associated with some atrophy of the iris, were observed only in advanced stages of the disease. They were usually posterior synechiae (V-25 A, V-16 A, IV-16 D, III-2 B and II-2 G), although anterior synechiae were occasionally found (III-4 F).

I myself never found rubeosis iridis, but there are two reports on this complication in DEVR, in both cases after operative treatment of retinal detachment (Criswick and Schepens, 1969; Laqua, 1980). The presence of rubeosis iridis is not unexpected because DEVR is a potentially proliferative retinopathy;

Cataract as a complication of DEVR also seems to be confined to severe cases. A few patients showed a local opacity of the posterior lens capsule at the site of attachment of a vitreous strand (VI-3 D, VI-1 F and III-4 F). The opacity was always localized in the temporal sector of the posterior lens capsule, and showed little tendency to progression.

In eyes in which extensive vitreous organizations had developed, as a rule with total retinal detachment, the lens had become totally cataractous (V-25 A, V-16 A, IV-16 A, IV-18 D, III-2 B. II-2 G and III-4 F). In several of these eyes the lens had shrunken due to dehydration, and sometimes disintegrated. Glittering calcifications were often visible in the opaque lens mass.

Some persons showed cataractous changes in the lenses which, unlike those in the abovementioned cases, seemed to be unrelated to DEVR. Most of these persons were middle-aged or older and showed bilateral mild-to-moderate cortical opacities or nuclear sclerosis of the lenses (IV-10 A, IV-13 A, II-3 I, IV-15 D, IV-2 D).

No eye examined showed evidence of congenital cataract or congenital malformation of the lens.

To summarize: the findings obtained in 146 eyes of 75 DEVR patients and 24 eyes of 12 probably affected persons warrant the conclusion that DEVR is not accompanied by primary developmental disorders of the anterior segment of the eye, and that changes in this part of the eye as a rule develop only as a complication of marked changes in the fundus and vitreous space. This conclusion is supported by similar observations in DEVR studies so far published.

## 4.10 Vitreous

The available literature gives varying interpretations of the incidence and significance of vitreous changes in DEVR. In their original publication, Criswick and Schepens (1969) mentioned extensive changes in the vitreous and in fact speculated on the possible importance of vitreoretinal adhesions in the pathogenesis of ischaemia of the peripheral retina. Gow and Oliver (1971) attached less importance to vitreous involvement in the family members they studied than did Criswick and Schepens (1969). Ober et al. (1980) considered vitreous changes not to be essential for a diagnosis of DEVR, and Laqua (1980) maintained that DEVR is not so much a vitreoretinopathy as rather an affection of the small peripheral retinal vessels.

For more exact determination of the incidence and pathogenesis of vitreous changes in DEVR, I performed extensive vitreous examinations and classified the changes found (Table 7).

The vitreous was studied in 148 eyes of 74 evident DEVR patients. In a number of these eyes visual inspection of the vitreous space was impossible due to cataract or retrolental membranes. Although it was beyond doubt that extensive vitreous organizations were present in such cases, often associated

Table 7. Vitreous findings in 148 eyes with evident DEVR.

| Vitreous findings | Number of eyes | % |
|---|---|---|
| Syneresis and liquefaction | 31 | 21 |
| Delicate white particles | 22 | 15 |
| Pigment cells | 8 | 5 |
| Vitreous haemorrhage | 3 | 2 |
| Preretinal membranes and opacities | 23 | 16 |
| Membranes in various parts of the vitreous | 25 | 13 |
| Local glious mass | 5 | 3 |
| Extensive retrolental organizations with total retinal detachment | 7 | 5 |
| Normal vitreous | 77 | 52 |

with total retinal detachment, other intravitreous changes could of course not be established. In 147 of the 148 eyes examined, the assessment of the vitreous was based on clinical observations; in one eye (IV-1 F) it was based on histological findings.

*Syneresis and liquefaction*

The vitreous fibrils in a number of eyes had condensed to form ropey structures separated by optically empty lacunae. In most instances these changes were associated with abnormal mobility of the vitreous as a result of reduced viscosity. Such features were seen in 31 of the 148 eyes (21%) in varying degrees. Some syneresis and liquefaction of the vitreous is frequently observed in older individuals (Goldmann, 1964). It is therefore plausible that the changes found in several older persons in this study are not related to DEVR. However, a few younger family members showed distinct vitreous syneresis which was probably related to DEVR.

*Delicate white particles*

In 22 eyes (15%) the vitreous contained very delicate white particles which were not very conspicuous at slit-lamp examination. Their origin remains obscure.

*Pigment cells*

Pigment cells of a brown colour and much larger than the abovementioned particles were found in 8 eyes (5%) with evident DEVR. Most of these eyes showed rhegmatogenic retinal detachment (III-5 B and IV-6 H) or had been previously treated for retinal detachment or peripheral retinal defects (III-3 H). One eye in which the vitreous contained pigment cells showed a retinoschisis in which defects were localized (II-2 E); two eyes showed no retinal defects (IV-2 H and IV-1 H).

*Vitreous haemorrhages*

Vitreous haemorrhages were rarely observed in this study. Some pre-retinal blood was found in the immediate vicinity of the vascular proliferations in III-5 B. In V-16 A, retrolental haemorrhages OD had been previously observed during the period of loss of light perception in this eye. Histological examination disclosed a vitreous haemorrhage in OD in IV-1 F. Our findings show that vitreous haemorrhages are rare in DEVR, and confined to very severe cases.

*Preretinal opacities and membranes*
Delicate membranes or opacities were found in the preretinal vitreous space in 23 eyes (16%), as a rule in the temporal fundus periphery. The changes ranged from delicate astructural opacities to well-defined membranes. The latter often attached to the central side of the retina. It seems likely that such membranes are often identical to the posterior vitreous membrane which in the periphery has detached itself from the retina, as already postulated by Criswick and Schepens in 1969. In some eyes, such preretinal membranes showed spotty opacities, probably representing a film of proteins originating from leaking vessels in the equatorial retina.

*Membranes in various parts of the vitreous space*
In 6 eyes (4%), membranes were found in various parts of the vitreous space in the absence of fibrovascular organizations throughout this space. These eyes as a rule showed extensive fundus changes, usually with partial or total

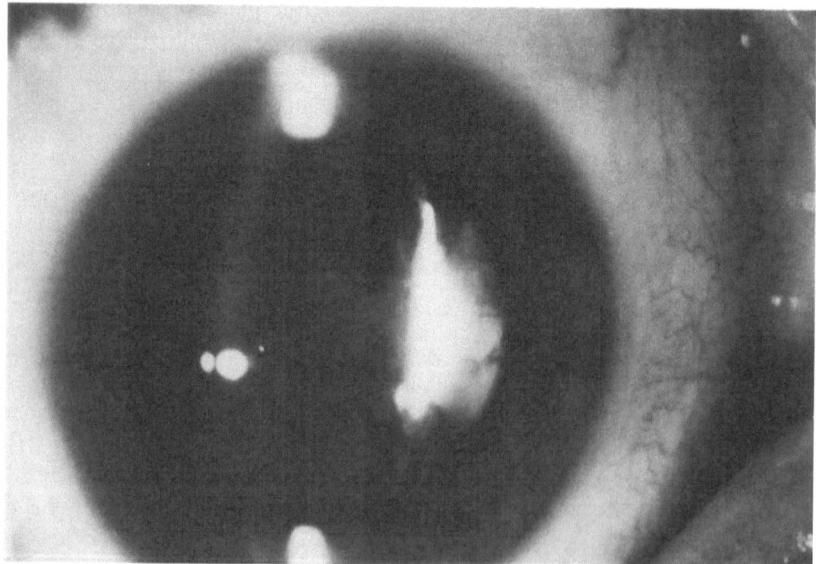

Figure 105. Mass of white proliferative tissue connected with the peripheral part of a falciform retinal fold in the inferior temporal fundus quadrant OS (V-24 A).

retinal detachment. The small number of eyes with vitreous changes of this type is probably explained by the relatively rapid progression to total vitreous organizations.

## Local massive organizations

Local masses of proliferative tissue were found in 5 eyes, without exception in the extreme temporal periphery of the fundus and firmly attached to the pars plana and often also to the posterior lens capsule. In most cases, the peripheral end of a raised falciform retinal fold ended in such a white mass (Figure 105). The appearance and localization of these tissue masses, which prove to be highly vascularized at fluorescein angiography, suggest that they originate from local retinal neovascularizations. A striking feature is the stationary character of these local vitreous organizations. Neither their history nor their appearance indicated progression.

## Marked retrolental vitreous organizations with total retinal detachment.

In 7 eyes, none of which had light perception, extensive vitreous organizations and cataract made it impossible to inspect the vitreous space. Although the position of the retina could not be clinically established in these eyes, it must be assumed that in all cases the neuroretina had become totally detached from the pigmented layer. One eye (OD of IV-1 F) was examined histologically (see page 215). In three eyes (ODS of II-2 G, OS of V-25 A), ultrasonography disclosed the presence of tissue organizations throughout the vitreous space. Nearly all publications on DEVR mention eyes with similar catastrophic manifestations of the condition.

## Normal vitreous

Although widely diverse vitreous changes were frequently found in DEVR, the vitreous proved to be entirely normal in more than 50% of all cases. I was unable to find any vitreous changes in 77 (52%) of the eyes of evident DEVR patients. The absence of vitreous changes in so many patients suggests that the development of the secondary vitreous is undisturbed, unlike that in, for example, Wagner's syndrome.

It seems to me that the vitreous changes in DEVR are secondary to the retinal vascular disorders.

Undoubtedly, the massive vitreous organizations observed in severe cases are a direct result of vascular proliferations from the retina. The pathogenesis of the more subtle changes in the vitreous space is less obvious. It seems to me that chronic leakage from retinal vessels can be held responsible, at least in part, for these changes.

### 4.11 Fundus

#### 4.11.a Biomicroscopic changes

The following is an orderly account of the fundus changes observed at contact lens examination. A survey of these changes, indicating their incidence in the eyes of evident DEVR patients, is presented in Table 8.

Table 8. Biomicroscopically visible fundus changes in 141 eyes with evident DEVR.

| Changes | Number of eyes | % |
|---|---|---|
| Abrupt termination of retinal vessels in the temporal equatorial zone | 118 | 84 |
| Increased number of small vascular branches between posterior pole and temporal equator | 89 | 63 |
| Tortuous peripheral venous branches | 56 | 40 |
| Neovascularizations | 10 | 7 |
| Deformation of retinal vessels in posterior fundus | 84 | 60 |
| Macular ectopia | 67 | 48 |
| Dragged disc | 7 | 5 |
| Intraretinal or subretinal exudates | 16 | 11 |
| Retinal pigmentations | 32 | 23 |
| Retinal haemorrhages | 2 | 1 |
| Retinal defects | 15 | 11 |
| White changes of the peripheral retina | 30 | 21 |
| Atrophic areas of choroid and pigmented layer of the retina | 20 | 14 |
| Retinoschisis | 7 | 5 |
| Retinal detachment*(not falciform) | 6 | 4 |
| Falciform fold | 7 | 5 |

*Only cases of treated or untreated retinal detachment in which examination of the fundus was feasible

*Abrupt termination of retinal vessels in the temporal equatorial zone*
The area in which these changes were usually most clearly visible was the equatorial zone of the temporal half of the fundus, in the sector between 7 and 10 o'clock in OD and between 2 and 5 o'clock in OS.

The phenomenon, which is highly characteristic of DEVR, can usually be established by biomicroscopy. Since the capillary bed of the retina is not visible in biomicroscopy, the phenomenon can only be observed in the small arterial and venous branches of the retina in the equatorial zone. Abrupt termination of such vessels in the equatorial zone is a characteristic feature of DEVR. Also characteristic is that several adjacent vessels terminate in the same zone (Figure 106).

Abrupt termination of the retinal vasculature was biomicroscopically observed in 84% of the eyes with evident DEVR. In the remaining 16%, media opacities precluded examination of the retinal periphery.

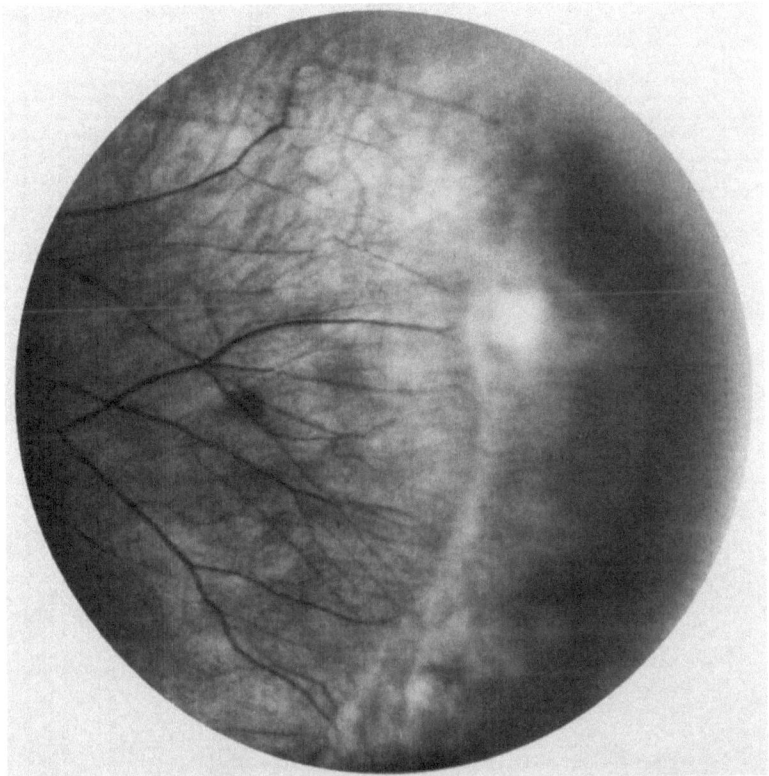

Figure 106. Abrupt termination of retinal vessels in the temporal equatorial zone OS. Small fibrotic neovascularization near the demarcation between vascular and avascular retina (V-11 D).

### Increased number of arterioles and venules

A frequent symptom of DEVR is an abnormally large number of vascular ramifications in the area between the posterior pole and the temporal equator (Figure 107). These vessels often take a decidely parallel course, the angle between the various ramifications being narrow.

### Tortuous venules

Not infrequently, the small venous vessels in the same area posterior to the temporal equator are abnormally tortuous. This tortuosity contrasts with the conspicuous straightness of the arterioles in the same retinal area (see Chapter 3, Figure 62).

### Neovascularizations

The presence of neovascularizations in the retina or in the preretinal vitreous space is not unusually frequent in DEVR. Such neovascularizations as are found, are nearly always localized at the demarcation between the vascular

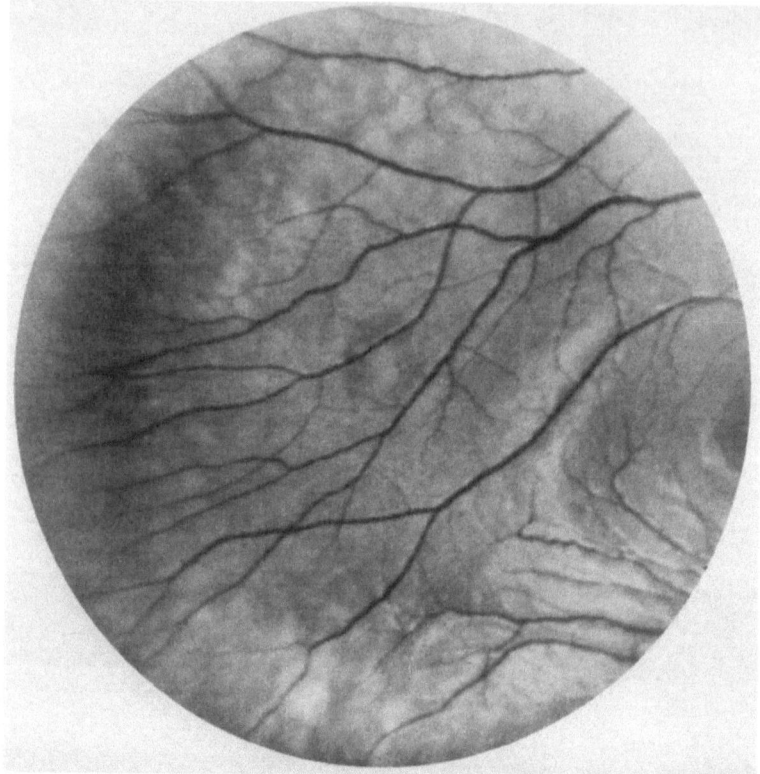

Figure 107. Increased number of vascular branches in the retina temporal to the posterior pole OD. The course of these vessels is strikingly parallel (IV-12 C).

and avascular retina. The fact that extensive neovascularizations are relatively rare is probably explained by the rapid progression of these vessels to total ·vitreous organizations. Small neovascularizations hardly raised above the retinal surface, however, were often sclerosed and seemed to show no marked tendency to grow (Figure 106).

Neovascularizations were biomicroscopically found in 10 eyes (7%). Most studies on DEVR describe peripheral neovascularization. This was a conspicuous phenomenon in the family described by Gitter et al. (1978). It seems to me to be beyond doubt that the autosomal dominant condition described by these authors is identical to DEVR.

### Deformation of retinal vessels in the posterior fundus

Deformation of the retinal vasculature in the posterior pole of the eye is a frequent symptom, which is of great diagnostic importance. The phenomenon can be observed in varying degrees, which range from hardly distinguishable changes to markedly aberrant vascular configurations. The most distinct deformation is shown by the superior and inferior temporal vessels, whose curvature round the centre of the posterior pole is diminished. These vessels take an abnormally stretched course in temporal direction, thus reducing the distance to the macula (Figure 108).

In the more severe cases the central segments of these vessels show distortion in the direction of the horizontal meridian while they are still on the disc. Deformation of retinal vessels in and about the posterior pole was observed in 60% of the eyes examined.

### Macular ectopia

The above described changes were often associated with macular ectopia in temporal direction. In most cases the macula showed not only temporal but also slight inferior ectopia. The degree of ectopia varied widely and was evidently related to the deformation of the vasculature (Figure 108). The degree of macular ectopia can also differ considerably between the two eyes in one individual. In our study, macular ectopia was found in 48% of the eyes with evident DEVR. The anomaly is responsible for the development of an abnormally wide positive kappa angle.

### Dragged disc

In a few eyes the retinal vessels on the disc were so grossly deformed as to produce the features of so-called dragged disc. In these cases virtually all major

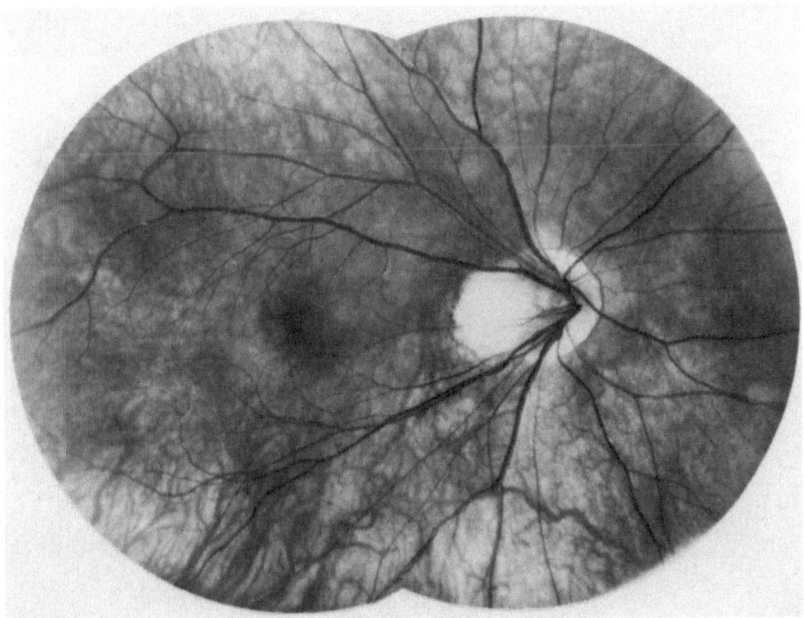

Figure 108. Deformation of retinal vessels in the posterior pole (III-2 B).

ramifications of the central retinal artery and vein traversed the temporal part of the lamina cribrosa (see Chapter 3, Figure 76a).

### Intraretinal and subretinal exudates

Intraretinal or subretinal exudates were found in only 16 eyes. In most cases, small intraretinal exudates were localized mainly in the equatorial zone of the temporal half of the fundus (Figure 109), usually in the immediate vicinity of the extreme peripheral zone of retinal vessels.

Large subretinal exudates evidently raising the neuroretina were found in only a few eyes. Exudates of this type can extend well into the posterior pole of the eye (see also Chapter 3, Figure 16).

The presence of exudates in eyes with cataract and total vitreous organizations is likely but of course cannot be established clinically.

Since Criswick and Schepens (1969) reported intraretinal and subretinal exudates in the majority of their patients, these exudates have been regarded as a frequently present symptom of DEVR.

The fact that only a minority of DEVR patients show exudates makes the designation "dominant exudative vitreoretinopathy" somewhat misleading. This should be borne in mind diagnosing the disease.

### Retinal pigmentations

Retinal pigmentations were frequently found in this study. In most cases they were very small pigment deposits evenly distributed over what seemed to be

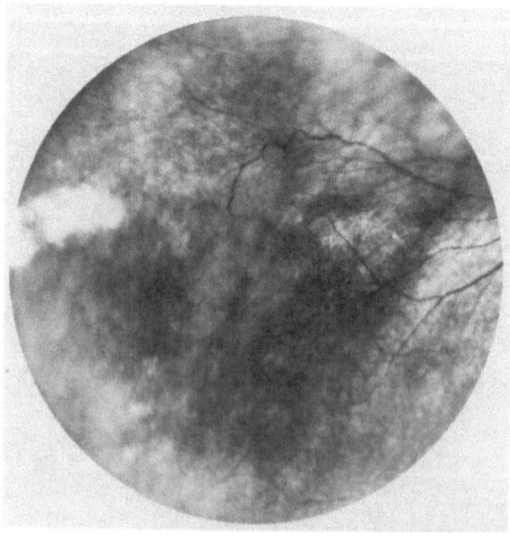

Figure 109. Intraretinal exudates in the temporal fundus periphery OD (IV-9 A).

the superficial part of the neuroretina. They were nearly always confined to the avascular retinal periphery. Such pigmentations are not very obtrusive, and biomicroscopy is indispensable as a means to diagnose these subtle changes, which can be found in the mildest manifestations of DEVR.

The gross pigment deposits which can be found in the periphery as well as in the posterior pole of the retina are more conspicuous. These pigmentations are not confined to the avascular retina. Another difference is that they are usually found in more severe cases of DEVR. In several instances of falciform retinal fold I found such gross pigmentations in the attached retinal parts adjacent to the fold (Figure 110).

*Retinal haemorrhages*
Intraretinal haemorrhages were rare. In one case, intraretinal and preretinal haemorrhages were observed in the immediate vicinity of neovascularization (III-5 B). In another eye with a minor retinal haemorrhage, no neovascularizations were found.

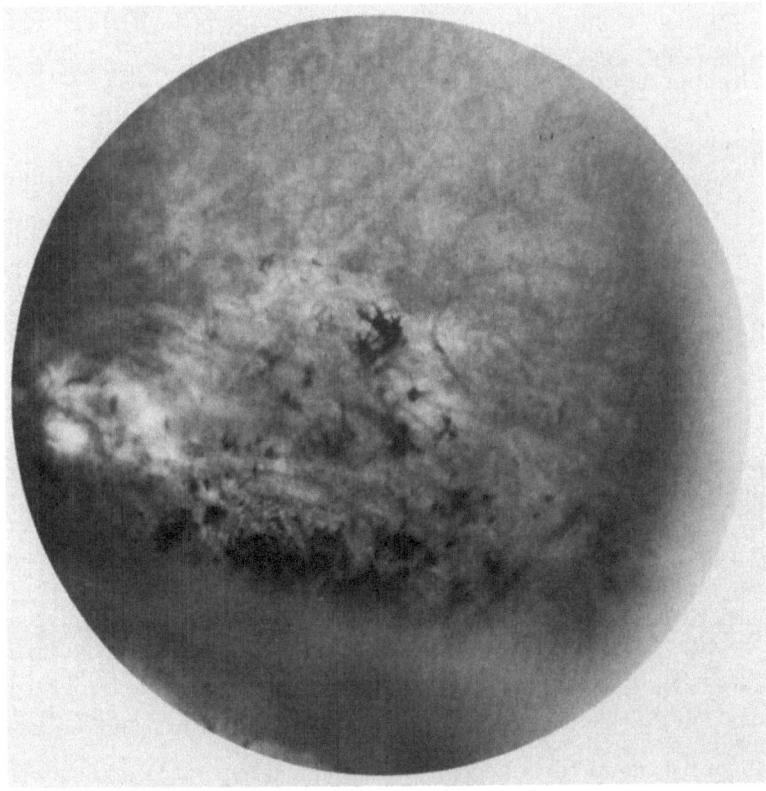

Figure 110. Pigment deposits in the retina superior to a falciform fold (IV-6 D).

*Retinal defects*

In 15 eyes of patients with evident DEVR I found retinal defects or evidence of previously treated retinal defects, sometimes associated with retinal detachment.

The defects in most fundi were small circular defects, nearly always localized in the non-perfused part of the retina. Both solitary and multiple defects were seen, and many were surrounded by some retinal white. In no case was there any association with lattice degeneration, and this is consistent with the fact that the defects were as a rule localized in the avascular retina.

The appearance and localization of the defects indicates an atrophic pathogenesis due to the changes in retinal perfusion. The presence of small retinal defects in DEVR has not been previously described.

Unlike the horseshoe ruptures known as a complication of DEVR (Criswick and Schepens, 1969; Laqua, 1980), the atrophic retinal holes are found in eyes with only slight changes and without traction from the vitreous.

Retinal tears were rare in our study. In one female patient I found a very large retinal rupture with a length of almost one quadrant, which had led to total retinal detachment (III-5 B). This patient's mother (II-2 B) showed a fair-sized horseshoe tear central to the equator in the vascular retina; this, however, had not caused retinal detachment.

*Various white changes in the peripheral retina*

In a number of eyes the retinal periphery showed a fairly evenly distributed whitish appearance, or sometimes minute white specks. These changes were mainly seen in the avascular retina. The phenomenon of white without pressure or white with pressure was also observed in several eyes. A few eyes showed oblong whitish zones which resembled snailtracks. In a few eyes, finally, pale discoloration of the retina was observed in the temporal equatorial zone at the level of the terminal ramifications of the retinal vessels.

*Atrophic areas of choroid and pigmented layer*

Atrophic changes of the choroid and pigmented layer of the retina were seen in the peripheral as well as in the posterior fundus. Their appearance ranged from small, sharply defined lesions, with or without surrounding pigmentations, to larger areas of less distinct demarcation (Figure 110). These atrophic changes were found especially in severe cases of DEVR. Their pathogenesis was often uncertain. Their localization along the base of a falciform fold suggests a reactive development in response to structural changes of the neuroretina. But their presence in areas with an intact neuroretina is entirely inexplicable.

Abnormal chorioretinal hypopigmentation and hyperpigmentation were a conspicuous finding in the family recently described by Kaufman et al. (1982). However, the ocular symptoms of this disorder, which was termed autosomal dominant vitreoretinochoroidopathy (AD-VRC) seem to be different from those of DEVR.

*Retinoschisis*

This was found in 7 eyes, and in all cases was confined to the peripheral retina. The lesions were usually localized in the temporal half of the fundus. The peripheral part of the retinoschisis was often localized in the avascular retina. The more central part of the retinoschisis sometimes did show vessels. In a few eyes, small defects were visible in the inner layer of the cleft retina.

*Retinal detachment*

Retinal detachment is the most serious complication of DEVR. Its clinical features may vary widely. It can be tractional, rhegmatogenous or exudative in origin. Our study has clearly shown that these three mechanisms may be involved in combination in the individual case.

Rhegmatogenous retinal detachment was seen in three patients with evident DEVR (III-5 B, IV-6 H and III-3 H); in one patient (IV-33 C) the diagnosis of DEVR was likely but not certain. Another member of the H family whom I had not examined, proved to have had rhegmatogenous retinal detachment with multiple defects (III-6 H), and the nature of the retinal detachment in II-1 H was unknown. More or less small circular defects were found in two of our patients with rhegmatogenous retinal detachment (IV-6 H and IV-33 C).

The rhegmatogenous retinal detachment in III-5 B presented entirely different features. In this girl, pronounced traction of vitreous membranes had produced a very large rupture. Retinal detachment with a rupture of this size is rare in DEVR, but has been previously described (Laqua, 1980).

In the case of rhegmatogenous retinal detachment with small retinal defects without conspicuous vitreous changes, however, the diagnosis of DEVR is much more difficult. It is quite likely that the cause of this type of retinal detachment is not recognized unless the vasculature of the peripheral retina is examined in detail in patient and family.

In our patients, rhegmatogenous retinal detachment as a rule occurred during puberty or adolescence. The history of III-3 H indicates that this complication can incidentally also occur in middle age. Laqua (1980) also mentioned a case of rhegmatogenous retinal detachment in a 44-year-old patient with DEVR. Retinal detachment accompanied by formation of subretinal exudates without retinal defect was observed in 3 patients, all of whom also showed vitreous anomalies; in all, it was likely that traction on the retina had contributed to its detachment (V-16 A, III-5 B and VI-3 D).

Formation of extensive subretinal exudates without distinct vitreous changes, as for example in Coats' disease, seems to be exceedingly rare in DEVR. Only in VI-3 D were the vitreous changes limited, and should subretinal exudation be regarded as the main cause of the retinal detachment.

Tractional retinal detachment can manifest itself in several ways in DEVR. In some eyes the traction is confined to a local sector in the peripheral retina. It may lead to a local, flat detachment of the peripheral retina, which shows little tendency to expand. In some cases differentation from peripheral retinoschisis is difficult.

Entirely different features are encountered in falciform retinal detachment, in which a raised retinal fold extends radially from the disc to the extreme periphery of the fundus. The peripheral end of the fold is usually linked by a local pale tissue mass to the pars plana or the posterior lens capsule, near the latter's equator. This anomaly was found in 7 eyes of 6 patients with evident DEVR in our study (V-24 A, VI-3 D, IV-16 D, IV-1 F, III-4F and II-2 G).

In these cases the falciform fold always extended from the disc in temporal or inferior temporal direction. One consequence of this localization is that the macula is severely deformed and frequently cannot even be identified in the fold. As a result, visual acuity in eyes with a raised retinal fold is usually not much better than about 1/60. Several eyes with a falciform fold as a result of DEVR showed gross chorioretinal cicatrices or areas of chorioretinal atrophy, as a rule quite near the fold.

For a discussion of the pathogenesis of the changes and of the relation between the condition known in the literature as "ablatio falciformis congenita" or " congenital retinal fold" and DEVR, I refer to Chapter 7.

In 7 eyes without light perception, cataract and retrolental organizations made it impossible to examine the fundus. On the basis of the clinical features it may be assumed that total retinal detachment had occurred, probably mostly as a result of traction from vitreous organizations originating from retinal neovascularizations. The role of other factors in the pathogenesis of retinal detachment — e.g. retinal defects and subretinal exudates — was usually no longer traceable. The history of our patients indicates that the blindness had usually developed during the primary school years. In an occasional patient, total retinal detachment proved to have occurred within a few weeks of birth (IV-1 F).

In 3 patients, total retinal detachment and leucocoria occurred during the period of observation at our department. In V-25 A, a previously functional eye showed rapid progression of traction by about age 18, with consequent gradual detachment of the entire retina. In V-16A, VOD was already poor in primary school, and traction and subretinal exudation led to total blindness by about age 20, whereupon total leucocoria developed. The left eye of II-2 G, finally, lost light perception by about age 15 due to various complications. In this case, too, total retinal detachment probably developed, although this cannot be established with certainty.

Of the total of 174 eyes of all persons with evident or probable DEVR, 23 eyes showed non-traumatic retinal detachment (including falciform fold). This amounts to a percentage of 13.

### 4.11.b    Fluorescein-angiographic changes

Of 41 eyes of 22 patients with evident DEVR, fluorescein angiograms of the posterior pole and fundus periphery were obtained which were of sufficient quality for assessment. A few angiographic changes, and their incidence in these 41 eyes, are listed in Tables 9 and 10.

Table 9. Fluorescein-angiographic changes of the peripheral fundus in 41 eyes with evident DEVR.

| Changes | Number of eyes | % |
|---|---|---|
| Abrupt termination of retinal vasculature in the temporal equatorial zone and non-perfusion of the peripheral retina | 32 | 78 |
| V-shaped configuration of the demarcation between vascular and avascular retina | 19 | 46 |
| Fluorescein leakage from peripheral retinal vessels | 36 | 88 |
| Neovascularizations | 8 | 20 |

Fluorescein angiograms were also obtained of 12 eyes of 7 persons with a tentative diagnosis of DEVR.

*Peripheral fundus*

The fluorescein angiograms disclosed the following changes in the peripheral fundus.

Abrupt termination of the retinal vasculature in the equatorial fundus and non-perfusion of the peripheral retina.

This was found in 32 of the 41 eyes with evident DEVR (78%). The retina peripheral to this termination was avascular. If present, this phenomenon was always found in the temporal periphery of the fundus, although in some cases retinal avascularity could also be demonstrated in parts of the nasal periphery. The demarcation between vascular and avascular retina was usually localized immediately anterior to the equator in the temporal sector of the fundus. Near or immediately below the horizontal meridian, this demarcation often deviated in central direction so that the avascular retinal periphery at this site showed a wedge-shaped expansion extending central to the equator (Figure 111). This configuration was observed on 19 of the 41 fluorescein angiograms.

The shape of the demarcation of the retinal vasculature closely resembles the configuration of the demarcation of the immature vasculature of the normal foetal retina during the last months of intrauterine development. The wedge-shaped zone of avascular retina between the peripheral ramifications of the superior and inferior temporal retinal vessels was demonstrated histologically in normal foetal eyes in Foos and Kopelow (1973) (see also Chapter 1). This similarity warrants the conclusion that the primary vascular anomalies in DEVR are a result of premature arrest of the foetal development of the retinal vascular system. In other words: the development of the retinal vasculature in persons with DEVR can be compared with that in a normal foetus of about 7–8 months.

A zone of aberrant leaking vessels.

The extreme ramifications of retinal vessels which form the demarcation of the avascular periphery, present a peculiar appearance: these ramifications end in irregular buds or very delicate loops, which are sometimes slightly dilatated and from which fluorescein leakage is seen in most cases. Most of these terminal ramifications have no distinct connections with other vessels (Figure 111).

Abnormal structure of the vascular bed central to the extreme zone of demarcation.

The vasculature of the retina in the area immediately central to the above described terminal ramifications likewise usually shows unmistakable changes

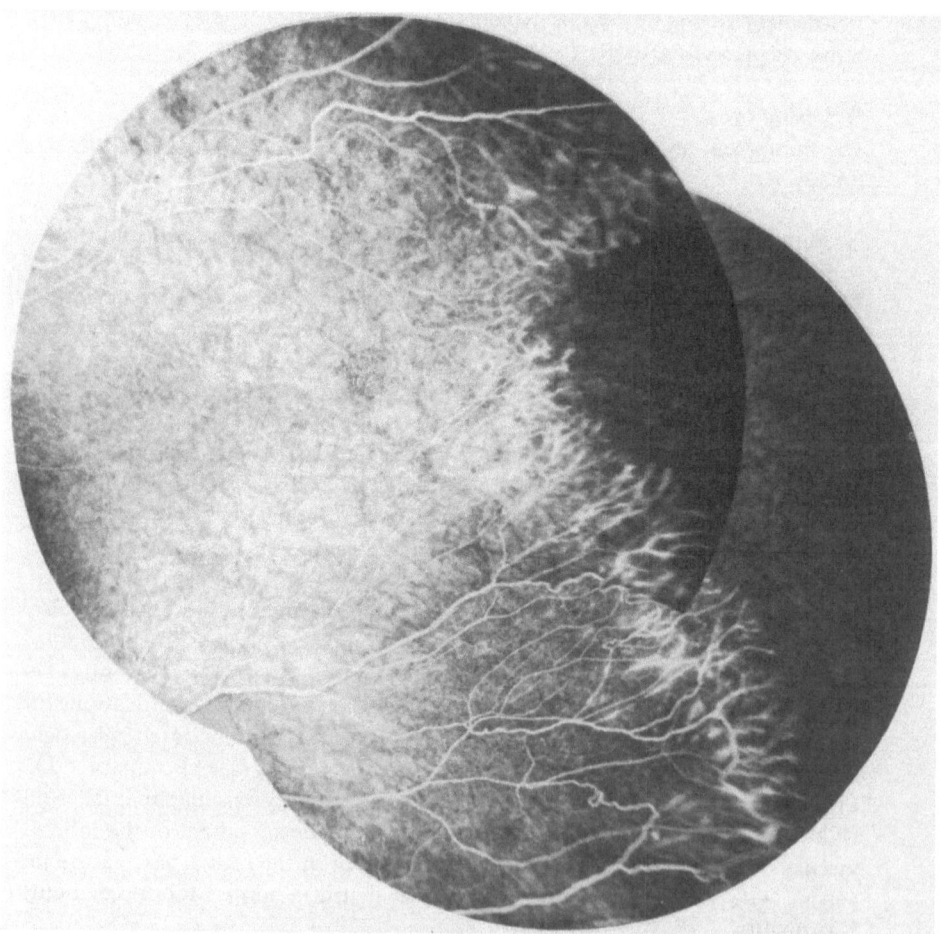

Figure 111. Fluorescein angiogram of the equatorial fundus OS near 3 o'clock. Wedge-shaped configuration of the avascular retina: the apex points to the posterior pole (V-41 A).

on the fluorescein angiogram. As previously mentioned, relatively numerous arterioles and venules are localized in this area. Fluorescein angiograms of good definition reveal that the capillary network between these vessels is irregular and poorly developed. Along many arterial as well as venous vessels, small saccular outpouchings are visible from which fluorescein leaks in the late phase (Figure 112). It looks as if these outpouchings are rudimentary developments of capillaries, but they may also be remnants of capillaries largely involuted due to retraction.

In some eyes, fluorescein leakage occurred in band-like zones localized central to the demarcation between vascular and avascular retina, and arranged more or less parallel to this demarcation (Figure 113). The retinal vessels in zones of this description sometimes showed some deformation. I have found no evidence that in such areas a vitreous membrane attached to the retina.

Fluorescein leakage from peripheral parts of the retinal vasculature was observed in a total of 36 of the 41 eyes with evident DEVR.

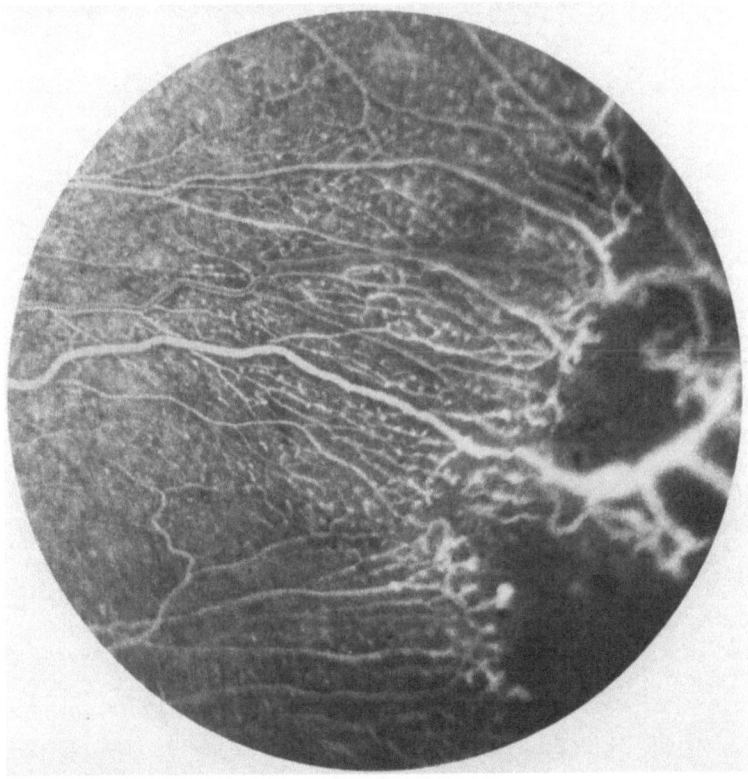

Figure 112. Small saccular outpouchings along the vascular branches in the peripheral retina (magnification of Figure 71, Chapter 3).

Arteriovenous shunts

Angiography disclosed distinct arteriovenous shunts on only a few eyes. In no case did these shunts have a large luminal width. Incidentally a shunt of this type formed a peripheral connection between the superior and the inferior temporal vessels (Chapter 3, Figure 35).

Neovascularizations

These were angiographically demonstrable in 11 of the 41 eyes with evident DEVR. In all cases they had formed at the site of the most peripheral ramifications of the retinal vessels in the zone of demarcation, and had grown into the otherwise avascular part of the retina (Figure 112). Significant fluorescein leakage from these vessels was seen in the late phase.

A large neovascularization was angiographically demonstrated in V-52 A. In this female patient the diagnosis of DEVR was not entirely certain because she had a record of neonatal oxygen administration. The clinical features in this patient with large vascular profilerations at age 15, however, are exceedingly

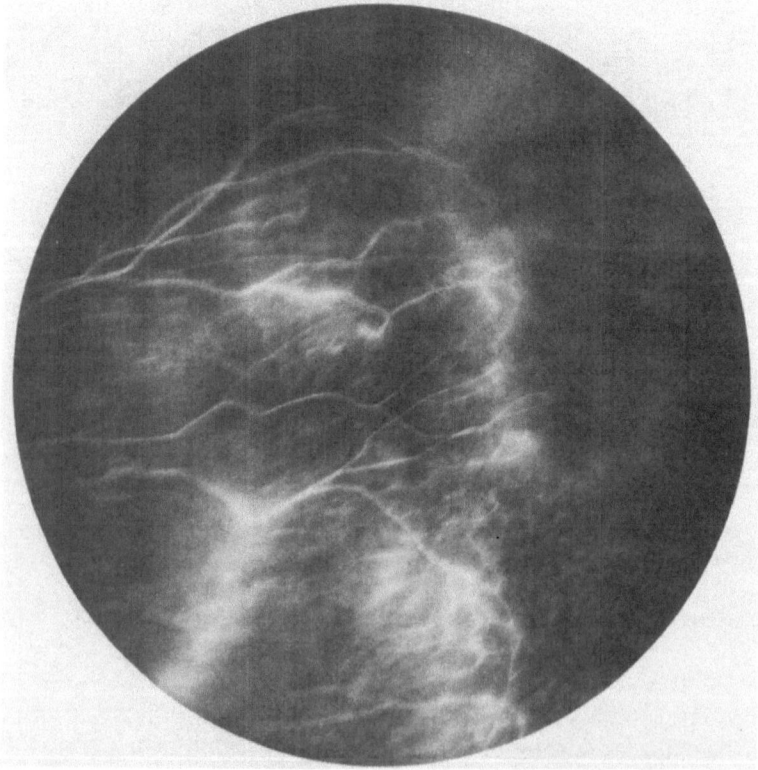

Figure 113. OS. Late phase of fluorescein angiogram shows leakage in the most peripheral zone of retinal vessels and in a band-like zone central to this (V-16 A).

rare in retrolental fibroplasia, and consequently it is highly likely that the anomalies were at least in part a result of DEVR.

The changes in the fluorescein angiogram of the peripheral fundus were as a rule confined to the retinal vasculature. In a few eyes I found strictly localized areas of atrophy of the pigmented layer of the retina in the avascular zone. Most eyes, however, showed no angiographic anomalies of the choroidal circulation. These findings corroborate the postulate that DEVR is primarily an affection of the retinal vasculature.

The above described fluorescein-angiographic changes in the peripheral retina show marked similarities to changes found in the less severe stages of cicatricial retrolental fibroplasia (RLF). These similarities were already pointed out by Canny and Oliver (1976) in their first angiographic study of DEVR. I intend to revert to these similarities in the discussion of the differential diagnosis from RLF (Chapter 8).

After Canny and Oliver (1976), Nijhuis et al. (1979) and other investigators have confirmed the disturbed perfusion of the peripheral retina in DEVR. The angiographic findings in the family described by Gitter et al. (1978), which frequently included peripheral neovascularization, also seem to be identical with the findings in DEVR.

The fluorescein-angiographic anomalies in the peripheral retina in DEVR cannot be explained by occlusions of vessels in a primordially normal vascular system. The presence of undeveloped, immature vessels in the zone of demarcation and the configuration of the demarcation of the vasculature suggest a developmental disorder of the retinal vasculature in the late phase of intra-uterine development. I intend to revert to this subject in the chapter on the pathogenesis of DEVR (Chapter 5).

Absence of leakage from peripheral retinal vessels.
The finding that a number of our patients showed no fluorescein-angiographic evidence of leakage from peripheral retinal vessels is of importance in the diagnosis of DEVR. Its consequence was that fluorographic changes in the peripheral retina could be readily overlooked. Another interesting fact is that this phenomenon was observed in its most pronounced form in members of the same family (IV-6 H, IV-10 H and IV-11 H). Only in this family was significant fluorescein leakage seen in the left eye of IV-6 H, in whom total rhegmatogenic retinal detachment existed during the angiographic examination. The peripheral retina in this eye was evidently avascular. Intensive fluorescein leakage occurred from the zone of vessels which demarcated this part of the retina. Angiography of this patient's right eye disclosed no fluorescein leakage at all (Chapter 3, Figure 98). Non-perfusion of the peripheral retina was angiographically demonstrated in a sister (IV-10 H) and a brother (IV-11 H) of this patient, but there was no peripheral zone of aberrant leaking vessels (see Chapter 3, Figures 101 and 102).

To my knowledge, none of the studies so far published on DEVR men-

Table 10. Fluorescein-angiogram changes of the posterior pole of the fundus in 41 eyes with evident DEVR.

| Changes | Number of eyes | % |
|---|---|---|
| Dilatation of macular capillaries | 10 | 24 |
| Fluorescein leakage from macular capillaries | 14 | 34 |
| Hyperfluorescent disc in the late phase | 35 | 86 |
| Leakage from the disc into the surrounding retina | 11 | 27 |

tions the absence of leakage on the fluorescein angiogram of peripheral retinal vessels.

Since the above cases occurred within one family, the question arises whether a condition other than DEVR may have been involved. I believe that this question should be answered in the negative. The configuration of the retinal vessels, the non-perfusion of the temporal retinal periphery and the pattern of hereditary transmission are all suggestive of an autosomal dominant disorder of the peripheral retinal vasculature which closely resembles DEVR.

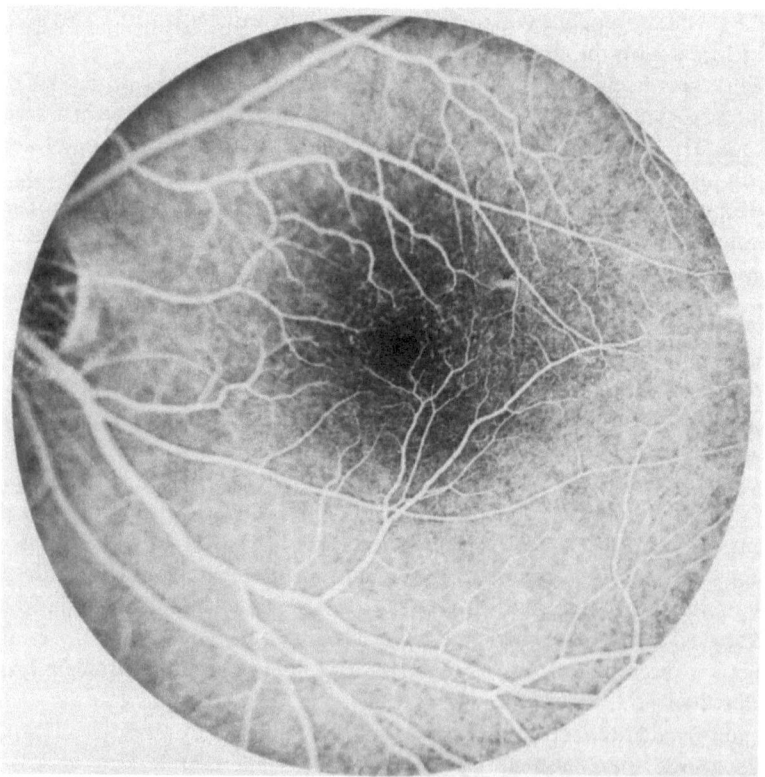

Figure 114. Slight dilatations of macular capillaries on the fluorescein angiogram (V-29 A).

It would therefore seem to me that these cases are best regarded as representing a deviant manifestation or a variant of DEVR in this family.

Similar angiographic features without peripheral leakage were found also in V-31 A.

*Posterior pole*

Fluorescein angiography revealed the following anomalies in the posterior pole of the fundus.

Dilatation of macular and perimacular retinal capillaries.
Dilatations of capillaries in the centre of the posterior pole were found in 10 of the 41 angiographically examined eyes with evident DEVR (Figure 114). Most were confined to the macula, but some were found outside it. In some cases the capillaries also showed some deformation. These changes were also

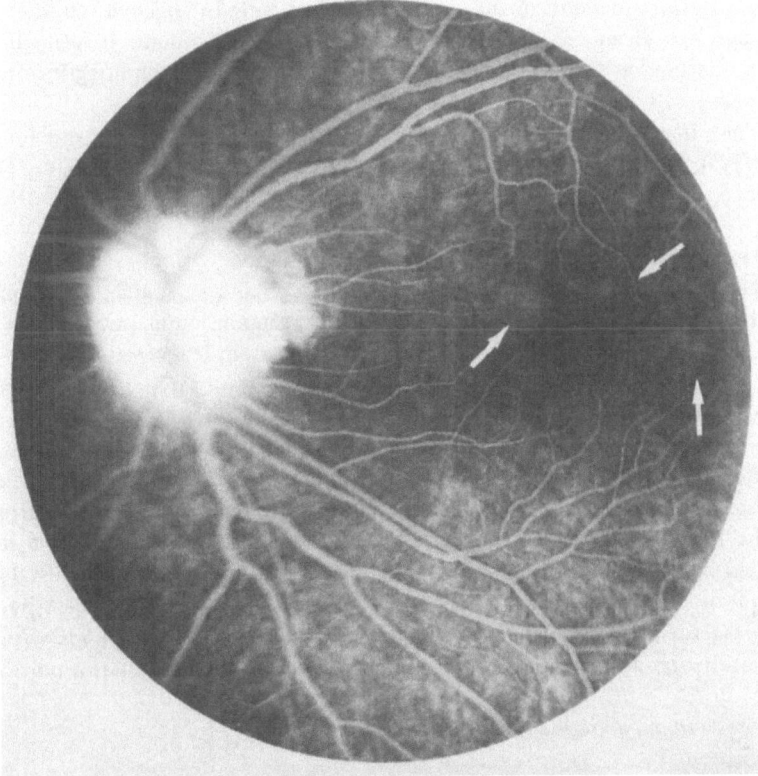

Figure 115. Late phase of fluorescein angiogram shows slight leakage from capillaries in the macular zone. Intensive hyperfluorescence of the disc (V-16 A).

found in fundi which showed no distortion of the vasculature of the posterior pole, and therefore do not seem to be caused by such distortion.

Fluorescein leakage from macular and perimacular retinal capillaries.
Fluorescein leakage from capillaries in or immediately around the macula was observed in 14 eyes (34%) (Figure 115). In most cases this leakage occurred from the abovementioned dilated capillaries in the late phase of the angiogram. In a few fundi, the late phase disclosed some leakage in the centre of the posterior pole although the early phase had shown no capillary dilatations. Not from all dilated capillaries did leakage occur.

The leakage was characterized by a not very obtrusive, spotty colouring around the fovea. In no case did the late phase angiogram reveal the features of cystoid macular oedema. In most cases the leakage in the posterior pole did not seem to be responsible for any significant diminution of visual acuity.

Extensive leakage was sometimes present in severe cases of DEVR with significant retinal deformation. The most pronounced case was the right eye of VI-3 D, in which intensive diffuse fluorescein leakage was seen throughout the posterior pole and in the retina temporal to it. In this eye the intensive leakage had given rise to flat exudative retinal detachment. It seems likely that traction on the retina had unfavourably influenced the integrity of the retinal vessels in this eye, thus intensifying the leakage.

The phenomenon of dilatation of and leakage from macular capillaries in DEVR has been previously described by Nijhuis et al. (1979) and Ober et al. (1980).

Hyperfluorescence of and leakage from the disc.
Hyperfluorescence of the disc in the late phase of the angiogram is a frequent finding in DEVR (Figure 115). I found this phenomenon in 35 of the 41 eyes (86%). It is probably caused by slight fluorescein leakage confined to the disc. In 11 eyes (27%) the late phase revealed not only hyperfluorescence of the disc but also some fluorescein leakage from the disc into the adjacent retina. In no case was colouring of the walls of the large vessels near the disc observed. It is not clear what the cause of this leakage is, nor from which vessels of the disc it comes. A possible explanation is that the leakage results from a slight lesion of the large retinal vessels at the disc. This could have been caused by their fixation within the lamina cribosa, while the more distal segments of these vessels are distorted in temporal direction. However, a hyperfluorescent disc was seen also in very mild manifestations of DEVR with no or hardly any deformation of the retinal vasculature in the posterior pole.

*Fluorescein-angiographic follow-up*

In 11 persons with evident DEVR, fluorescein angiography was repeated in an effort to demonstrate vascular changes, if any. In 9 of them (all in the A family) the interval between the two examinations was 3 years or more. The angiograms could be reliably compared because on both occasions the same fundus areas had been photographed in about the same phase.

In 20 eyes on which interpretable angiograms were available, no changes in structure of or leakage from retinal vessels was found to have occured during the follow-up period.


## Visual fields

With few exceptions, the members of the various families had no complaints which could be ascribed to visual field limitations. However, kinetic perimetry with the Goldmann perimeter revealed that visual field anomalies were not rare in DEVR.

Visual fields were measured in a total of about 20 eyes of 10 persons with evident DEVR. Normal visual fields ODS were found in 3 persons. Six eyes showed slight-to-moderate absolute limitation of the nasal visual field. Near the horizontal meridian the III-4 isopter deviated to within $50°$ in the nasal visual field, but did not come within $40°$.

Marked absolute limitation of the nasal visual field to within $40°$ was found in 6 eyes, in 4 of which the retina was entirely attached and had not been previously detached. Figure 116 shows the visual fields in a few patients with absolute nasal limitation.

The limitation of the nasal visual field in DEVR has two causes:
— The avascular part of the retina has no light perception due to non-oxygenation of the inner layers of the neuroretina. It may be assumed that only the well-vascularized parts of the retina function, and that the boundary of the nasal visual field is determined by the demarcation of the vascular part of the temporal retina (Figure 117a, 117b). That this assumption is correct is confirmed by the visual field OS in V-29 A, which shows significant absolute limitation of a large part of the superior nasal quadrant (Figure 116a). In the fundus of this eye, the inferior temporal quadrant of the retina which corresponds with this part of the visual field is most incompletely vascularized. Here, the retinal vasculature terminates more centrally than in the superior temporal quadrant of the fundus.

— The second cause of the limitation of the nasal visual field in DEVR is the temporal ectopia of the foveola. The more pronounced this ectopia, the narrower the part of the functional retina on the temporal side of the fovea, and the corresponding nasal visual field (Figure 117c).

It is evident that the two causes contribute cumulatively to the nasal visual field limitation in DEVR. The most pronounced limitation is therefore likely

210

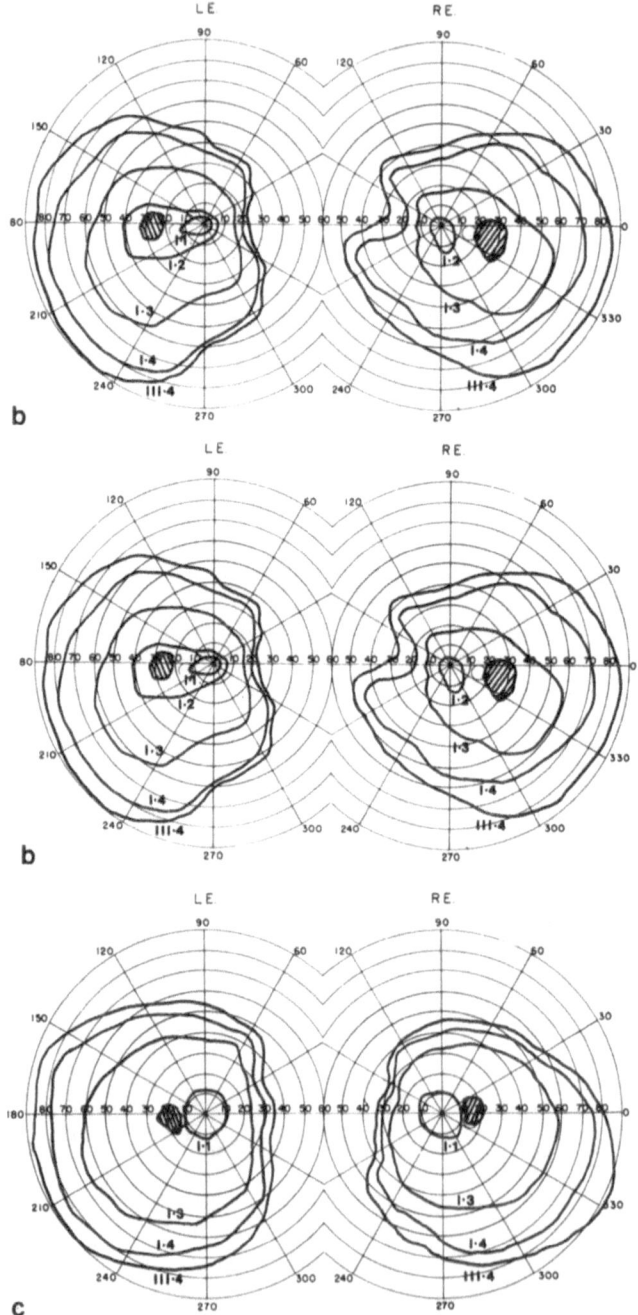

Figure 116. Absolute limitation of nasal visual field in V-29 A (a), V-12 D (b) and III-1 I (c).

to occur in eyes in which a broad zone of the temporal retinal periphery is avascular and which show significant temporal ectopia of the foveola. Temporal ectopia of the blind spot was demonstrated at perimetry of a few eyes. This phenomenon is a result of the foveolar ectopia (Figure 116b). A fact of clinical significance is that the abovementioned visual field defects can occur in asymptomatic DEVR patients. Since in such cases fundus changes are likewise often minimal, and easily overlooked, misinterpretation of visual field findings is not inconceivable. Particularly ascription of these (bi)nasal visual field anomalies to glaucoma simplex, or even to a tumour localized near the chiasm, might have serious consequences.

Visual field anomalies in DEVR has so far not been mentioned in the literature.

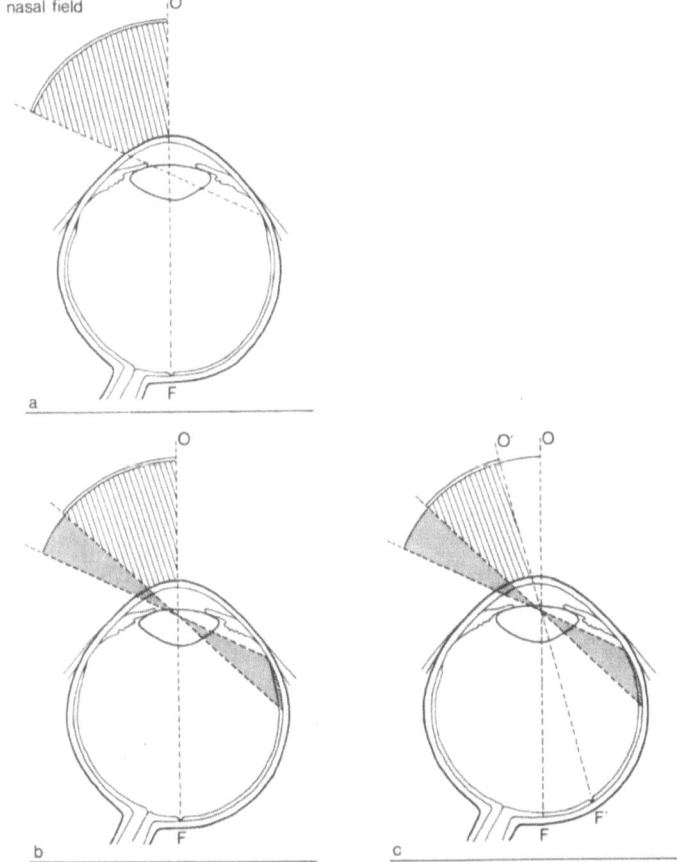

Figure 17. Origin of nasal visual field limitation in DEVR. a) Nasal visual field of a normal eye. b) Limitation of the nasal visual field in DEVR as a result of non-functioning of the avascular retina in the temporal fundus periphery. c) Further limitation of the visual field as a result of temporal ectopia of the foveola (F').

### 4.13 Ultrasonography

Ultrasonography (A-scan and B-scan) was performed on 18 eyes of 9 patients. The purpose was usually to gain an impression of morphological changes in the posterior segment of eyes with marked media opacities.

In blind eyes, the vitreous space was usually filled by opacities. Ultrasonographic localization of the retina was usually impossible in such eyes. The sclera of the posterior segment was often deformed and showed calcifications. The axis length of such atrophic eyeballs was usually no more than 20—21 mm, and in one case even as little as 14 mm (OS of IV-18 D).

An interesting finding was that ultrasonography revealed some deformation of the sclera on the posterior segment even in a few eyes without extensive vitreous organizations or retinal detachment. This phenomenon was most pronounced in ODS of IV-10 A. The A-scan revealed that the eye axis length, measured at different sites of the posterior poles, ranged from 21.5 to 23 mm. In both eyes the curvature of the sclera in the vertical plane exceeded that in the horizontal plane; this was especially evident in the B-scan (Figure 118). Moreover, the sclera of the posterior segment ODS proved not to be constant in horizontal section: the curvature was slightly more pronounced nasally than temporally in OD, while in OS the reverse was found.

This observation justifies ultrasonographic examination of DEVR patients on a larger scale than was done in this study, particularly in persons without vitreous anomalies. In combination with cycloplegic refraction and keratometry, ultrasonographic measurements might well give more information on the morphological abnormalities of the eyeball and the refracting media in DEVR, and their effect on refractive power.

### 4.14 Electroretinography and electro-oculography

An ERG was recorded of 24 eyes of 12 patients with evident DEVR and of 6 eyes of persons with probable DEVR. As expected, 9 eyes with partial or total retinal detachment all showed markedly reduced or absent photopic and scotopic responses.

The ERG of 9 eyes was quite normal. An interesting finding was that one of the eyes with a normal ERG showed a congenital retinal fold (V-24 A), whereas in another patient with similar fundus features photopic and scotopic responses were markedly reduced (OS of VI-3 D).

Minimal-to-slight ERG changes were found in 6 eyes with an attached retina. In one person (V-39 A) the photopic and scotopic responses were within normal limits but both eyes showed a slightly subnormal B-wave under mesopic conditions (about $50 \mu V$, white light stimulus of 0.2 Joule).

In OS of IV-10 A, the B-wave — both under mesopic conditions and at stimulation with a frequency of 30 Hz — was found to be distinctly lower than that in OD, which showed a normal ERG. OS differed from OD in significantly lower visual acuity, retinal pigmented layer changes temporal to the disc, preretinal vitreous membranes and fairly diffuse leakage in the posterior pole in the late phase of the angiogram. Some traction exerted on the retina by vitreous membranes was probably responsible for the ERG changes in OS in this patient.

Slightly subnormal B-wave values at stimulus frequencies between 20 and 40 Hz, and some decrease in flicker fusion frequency (about 46 Hz) suggestive of slightly diminished cone function, were found in V-40 A (ODS) and IV-16 (OS).

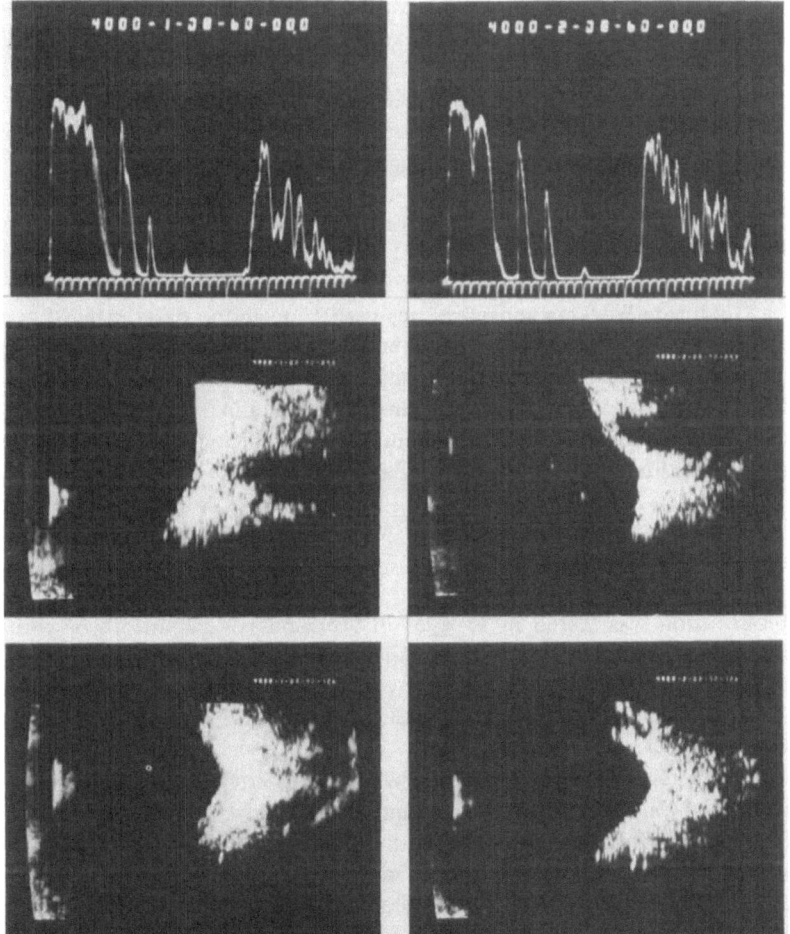

Figure 118. Ultrasonogram of OD (on the left) and OS (on the right) of IV-10 A. a) A-scan (anteroposterior). b) B-scan. Horizontal section through the posterior poles (OD: temporal side up, nasal side down. OS: nasal side up, temporal side down). c) B-scan (vertical section through the posterior poles). See also letterpress.

The literature on DEVR makes hardly any mention of ERG findings. Laqua (1980) reported that, in one eye of a DEVR patient, normal photopic and scotopic responses were found but that the flicker ERG and the oscillatory potentials were diminished. The other eye in this case showed total retinal detachment.

Our results indicate that the ERG is usually normal or virtually normal in DEVR, unless the retina is damaged or detached.

So far as possible, electro-oculography was performed in the same persons in whom electroretinography had been carried out. An EOG was recorded in 14 eyes with non-detached retinas. In 10 of these eyes, a normal ratio was found; in the remaining 4 eyes the ratio was less than 180 and had to be regarded as subnormal. One of these eyes (OS of IV-10 A) showed evidence of mechanical retinal damage.

I have been unable to find any EOG results in the literature on DEVR.

Our ERG and EOG results indicate that electrical testing of retinal function makes no contribution to the diagnosis of uncomplicated DEVR.


### 4.15  Dark adaptation

The Goldmann-Weekers apparatus was used to examine dark adaptation in 9 persons. The examination was made binocularly, but a few of these patients had only one functional eye. Dark adaptation was entirely normal in 5 persons. An increased cone threshold value was found in V-25 A. The rod threshold value, determined after 25 minutes of adaptation, was dubious in one patient and subnormal in two (IV-8 A and IV-10 A).


### 4.16  Colour vision

Colour vision was tested in 15 eyes of 9 persons, and found to be entirely normal in 7 eyes. Marked disorders of colour vision were found in IV-10 A (OS) and V-24 A (OS). In both cases visual acuity was very poor, and the disorders could be ascribed to damage of the posterior pole of the retina caused by traction.

Subtle anomalies of colour vision were found in 6 eyes of 5 patients: two patients showed a slightly excessive number of errors (for their age) in the FM 100 Hue test without specific axis direction, in combination with a slight shift on the Nagel anomaloscope to red (OS of V-25 A and V-16 A). One patient (V-29 A) showed slight anomalies ODS, which tended to a blue-yellow defect. One eye (OS of IV-16 A) showed a slight protan defect in the FM 100 Hue test and one (OD of IV-8 A) showed a bipolar deutan axis in the same test.

The causes of the abovementioned slight disorders of colour visions are far from clear to me. Some correlation with fluorescein leakage in the macular zone might be expected but was not established. ODS of V-39 A had good visual acuity and showed only minimal fluorescein-angiographic changes in the posterior pole, but nevertheless colour vision in these eyes was unmistakably defective. On the other hand, OD of IV-10 A showed significant fluorescein leakage in the macular zone in the late phase, but colour vision in this eye was found to be normal.

### 4.17  Histology

In only one of the DEVR patients I examined had an eye been enucleated (IV-1 F). This had been done six weeks after birth because retinoblastoma could not at that time be excluded on the basis of clinical findings. The original specimens of this eye, partly with haematoxylin-eosin and partly with Van Gieson staining, were available for further study. The uncut part of the eyeball, which had been embedded in celloidin, was unfortunately no longer traceable.

Although it was no longer possible to determine the exact dimensions of the eye from the available sections, there had evidently been no severe deformation or phthisis of the eyeball (Figure 119). Our findings confirmed the original pathological observations.

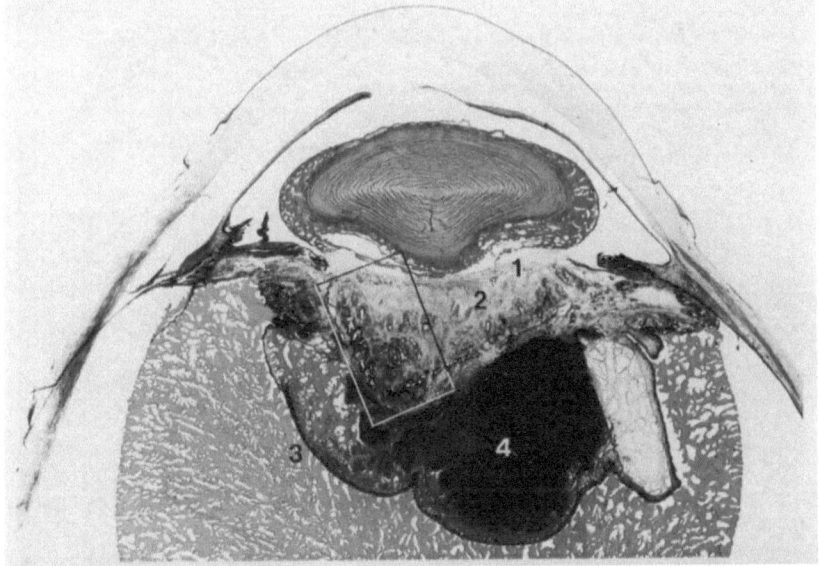

Figure 119. Sagittal section through OD of IV-1 F. 1) Retrolental fibrous tissue layer. 2) Glious tissue mass with remnants of neuroretina. 3) Posterior part of neuroretina. 4) Haemorrhage (Van Gieson, × 6).

The cornea shows artifical detachment of the endothelium but is otherwise intact. The anterior chamber is shallow due to anterior displacement of the lens and iris. The root of the iris, however, shows a normal configuration in relation to the anterior part of the ciliary body. There are no anomalies in the area of the iridocorneal angle.

The lens shows numerous vacoules, mostly localized equatorially and on the posterior side of the cortex. On the anterior side the lens capsule carries a few clumps of pigment, evidently originating from the pigment epithelium of the iris. The subcapsular epithelium is normal. On the posterior side of the lens, the capsule shows marked swelling and at some sites there are folds.

Immediately posterior to the lens capsule, a thick plaque of connective tissue colours red upon Van Gieson staining; its collagen fibres extend more or less parallel to the lens capsule (Figure 120). This layer comprises a few blood vessels. On the anterior side, this tissue is firmly attached to the posterior lens capsule at several sites, at which the lens capsule is much thinner and sometimes indistinguishable from the connective tissue layer.

The retrolental fibrous plaque is connected on either side with the ciliary processes, which are stretched in central direction due to traction exterted by the connective tissue membrane. On the posterior side the connective tissue membrane is connected with a tissue mass of mainly glia cells. Between these glia cells, several strands of connective tissue enter from the retrolental connective tissue plaque. It is evident that the tissue mass originates from the

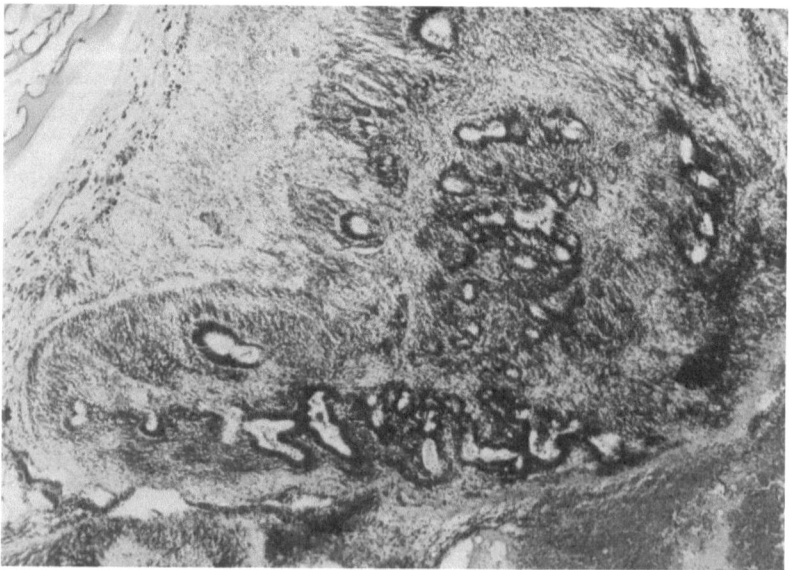

Figure 120. Magnification of the part of the section marked in Figure 119. Pseudorosettes between extensive proliferations of glia cells (Van Gieson, × 36).

totally detached neuroretina, which is hardly recognizable any longer due to glia proliferations. Some structural features of the original retinal layers are vaguely discernible at a few sites. Among the glia proliferations there are several dysplastic rosettes, varying widely in dimensions and for the most part showing what appears to be a multi-stratified structure (Figure 120).

The part of the neuroretina which is deformed by glia tissue extends on either side in the retrolental vitreous space to the pars plana, to which it is attached. At these sites the tissue mass emerges into a thin, atrophic posterior part of the neuroretina, which is likewise totally detached from the pigmented layer. The latter part of the neuroretina, which shows hardly any recognizable stratification, forms the posterior boundary of a large haemorrhage. This haemorrhage is therefore completely surrounded by retinal remnants (Figure 119). In the other sections, which include the optic nerve, the neuroretina extends from the disc in anterior direction in the shape of a funnel.

The pigmented layer of the retina has remained in touch with the choroid throughout. The largest part of the eyeball is therefore made up of subretinal space. This space comprises an eosinophilic transudate in which no cells are discernible. The choroid is thin throughout and shows little development of choriocapillaris and larger vessels.

The disc is severely deformed due to traction from the neuroretina. In the segment of optic nerve localized just outside the lamina cribosa, a relatively large amount of vascularized connective tissue is present among the axons. At no site are inflammatory changes seen.

*Discussion*

The histological changes described correspond with those found in serious manifestations of neonatal proliferative retinopathies, e.g. retrolental fibroplasia. Immediately posterior to the lens, a fibrous plaque is present which most likely originates from fibrovascular proliferations in the peripheral retina. This fibrous tissue is firmly attached on the posterior side to a totally detached neuroretina which shows rosettes of widely diverse shape and size and for the most part showing a multistratified structure. Such rosettes do not indicate primary neuroretinal dysplasia but can be found in any condition in which the neuroretina has become detached from the pigmented layer. The presence of these rosettes, therefore, does not contradict the postulate that DEVR is a developmental disorder which occurs during the final months of intra-uterine development (see Chapter 5).

Striking features of the specimen described were large haemorrhages separated from the pigmented layer by the neuroretina. This means that these haemorrhages originally developed in the preretinal vitreous space. It seems virtually certain that they came from (pre) retinal neovascularizations.

Retinal or vitreous haemorrhages were a rare complication in our clinically examined DEVR patients. I should add to this that the intravitreous haemorrhage in the above described eye had not been noticed prior to enucleation, undoubtedly due to retrolental opacities. It may therefore well be that DEVR patients who show leucocoria may have significant vitreous haemorrhages concealed behind the retrolental membrane.

Evidently the severe retinal deformation in the above specimen makes it impossible to obtain information on the structure of the retinal blood vessels. This is why histological examination of this eyeball makes no contribution what ever to our knowledge of the nature of the primary lesions underlying the above described proliferative changes.

In my opinion, the light-microscopic changes in the eyeball described seem to be indistinguishable from those in severe retrolental fibroplasia.

Recently the histopathologic findings in DEVR were reported by Brock-hurst et al. (1981), who studied two eyes enucleated from two identical twin-brothers. No family members of this twin could be examined clinically in order to give more support to the diagnosis. The neural retina in both eyes was completely detached and gliotic and was thrown into large folds by a pre-retinal membrane.

### 4.18 General physical examination

In all the families studied, specific questions were asked about the occurrence of congenital anomalies. In IV-3 H (in whose case the diagnosis of DEVR was not entirely certain), low implantation of the ears was a conspicuous finding. At the same time there was unmistakable mental retardation. No general physical examination was made. This patient's brother (IV-12 H), in whose fundi no anomalies were found, was likewise mentally underendowed.

Apart from a rather gracile habitus of a few members of the A family and a slightly elevated palate in the female proband of this family (V-25 A), no congenital anomalies or unusual physical characteristics were encountered in any of the families.

Extensive physical examination and laboratory studies were performed in 7 patients with evident DEVR. They yielded no findings of particular importance. In 7 patients a haematological study (including a coagulation study) was performed, which revealed no distinct anomalies in any of them. An oxygen dissociation curve was determined in one female patient (V-25 A). This, too, was normal.

To summarize: in the families studied I failed to find any indication that DEVR can be accompanied by general symptoms. Most publications likewise make no mention of general physical or laboratory abnormalities associated with DEVR.

Very recently Chaudhuri et al.(1982) reported abnormal platelet aggregation in a DEVR family. All five affected members of this family showed platelet aggregation tests non-responsive to administration of 15 mmol arachidonate. Abnormal responses to adrenaline and low dose (1 microgram) collagen were seen in two of their patients. These findings suggest an inherent defect in the platelet prostaglandine synthesis.

Our haematological examinations did not include the above platelet aggregation tests. Therefore, similar tests are being performed in several affected members of our DEVR families. I intend to report the results of these studies in a separate paper.

## 4.19 Stages and course

Gow and Oliver (1971) divided DEVR into three stages on the basis of the clinical features in their patients. They held that stage 1 was characterized by vitreous changes and traction on the peripheral retina, which showed white with pressure and white without pressure. Only in stage 2, they maintained, did retinal vascular changes develop. Stage 3 was described as characterized by extensive vitreous changes and retinal detachment. This classification was corrected by Laqua (1980), who pointed out that vascular anomalies and non-perfusion of the peripheral retina were general symptoms of DEVR and therefore had to be included in stage 1.

The results of a study by Nijhuis et al. (1979) and our results confirm that peripheral retinal vascular changes are a primary feature of DEVR. The pleomorphism of DEVR impedes a classification in stages. For this reason I have refrained from classifying the changes found in my patients in stages.

The natural history of DEVR poses an important question. Criswick and Schepens (1969) observed unmistakable progression in several of their patients, and therefore described the chance of complete arrest of the condition as poor. Laqua (1980) maintained that the condition is slowly progressive, but that few patients ever attain the most severe stage.

The histories and the findings obtained in the affected members of the various families in our study indicate that progression of DEVR is relatively rare, and mainly confined to juvenile patients who show fairly severe symptoms. Like Ober et al. (1980), I have been unable to demonstrate gradual progression of the condition in persons over 20 years of age. The only complication I observed in a few patients aged over 20, was rhegmatogenic retinal detachment. I found no indications that gradual diminution of visual acuity can occur in DEVR without retinal detachment or increasing traction on the posterior pole of the retina.

I found no fluorescein-angiographic changes in the peripheral retina in the course of a follow-up over a period of three years. Even small neovascularizations at the demarcation between vascular and avascular retina seemed to be entirely stationary.

As already pointed out, progression is to be expected mainly in children who show fibrovascular proliferations, intraretinal or subretinal exudates or distinct preretinal vitreous structures in the peripheral fundus. The patients examined by Criswick and Schepens (1969) were all in this category, and this selection explains why they frequently observed progression.

CHAPTER 5

# GENETIC ASPECTS AND PATHOGENESIS OF DOMINANT EXUDATIVE VITREORETINOPATHY

GENETIC ASPECTS

## 5.1 Mode of transmission

Gow and Oliver (1971) were the first to find, in a family with DEVR, a pattern of inheritance which in their opinion was consistent with autosomal dominant transmission. In most of the subsequently reported families with DEVR, too, autosomal dominant transmission was likely, even though another mode of transmission could sometimes not be excluded with certainty in smaller pedigrees (Slusher and Hutton, 1979; Dudgeon, 1980; Ober et al., 1980: pedigree 1). Since the basis of our knowledge of the hereditary transmission of DEVR is rather narrow due to the limited number of published cases (only 60 instances of DEVR have been published as such), it may be useful to consider the pattern of inheritance in our pedigrees in some detail, and to test it against the hypothesis of automal dominant transmission.

Another reason to do this is that it cannot be excluded in advance that several conditions exist which show the phenotype of DEVR, but with different hereditary characteristics.

In all families except the small E and G families, both sexes were affected. Recessive X-chromosal transmission is therefore highly unlikely. Transmission from father to son was found in three families. this entirely excludes X-chromosal transmission and indicates that autosomal recessive transmission is exceedingly improbable. In two families (D and I) the affection was diagnosed in three successive generations, and father-to-son transmission was also involved in these families. Such a combination can only result from autosomal dominant transmission.

In all families except E and G, the condition was found at least in one instance in one of the parents of an affected person. This finding argues against autosomal recessive or X-chromosomal transmission.

The combinations of the various characteristics in the A, B, C, D, F, H and I families were not consistent with autosomal recessive or X-chromosomal transmission.

If the hypothesis of autosomal dominant transmission is correct and gene penetrance is complete, then the ratio between the number of affected and the number of unaffected children of parents of whom one had evident DEVR should, at the large numbers, approximate 1:1. It was useless to calculate this ratio in the separate families because the numbers of persons examined were too small. Even for determination of the ratio in the nine families taken collectively, the numbers were still small (e.g. because only families in which all children were examined could be used for this calculation).

Another problem lay in the persons with an uncertain diagnosis of DEVR. In calculating the abovementioned ratio, members of the various families with an uncertain diagnosis of DEVR could be regarded as affected or as unaffected, or entirely excluded. The ratio calculated by each of these three methods never differed significantly from the 1:1 ratio to be expected.

The sex distribution of the affected members of the various families taken collectively has been discussed in Chapter 4 (Table 2). As was to be expected with an autosomal gene, no predominance of either of the sexes was found.

## 5.2 Gene penetrance

Determination of the gene penetrance of DEVR is of more than merely scientific importance. An approximate notion of the degree of gene penetrance is of great value for physicians asked to give genetic counselling. For practical applications I refer to section 5.5.

The literature supplies no data which could be used in even a gross approximation of the gene penetrance of DEVR. Gow and Oliver (1971) mention an "uncertain degree of penetrance", which they suspect of being "reduced". Ober et al. (1980) suspected close to 100% penetrance on the basis of the observation that three of six descendants with a 50% chance of developing the symptoms of DEVR, did in fact show these symptoms. Evidently, however, such small numbers of cases warrant no conclusion, however cautiously formulated.

### Determination of penetrance

There is a simple method to determine the penetrance of an autosomal dominant gene. It is based on the fact that the genotype of the condition must be present in the parents of children of whom one or several suffer from the condition in question. By determining in which percentage of such parent couples symptoms of the condition can be found, one obtains the percentage of persons with the phenotype of the condition in relation to the total number of persons with the genotype. This percentage corresponds with the gene penetrance. In this determination, errors can be introduced by selection of families in which one of the parents shows changes versus families in which one of the parents has the genotype without showing symptoms of the condition. The various causes of these errors need not be discussed in detail here.

The influence of most of these errors on calculated penetrance is such that the calculated value exceeds the true value. It is impossible to determine the influence of these errors exactly, but it is not likely to be significant in the calculation of penetrance in our families.

Table 11. Approximation of the penetrance of the DEVR gene.

| Family | Parent couples with one or several children with evident DEVR | |
| | Total number of couples examined | Number of couples in whom abnormalities were found |
| --- | --- | --- |
| A | 5 | 5 |
| B | 1 | 1 |
| C | 5 | 5 |
| D | 4 | 4 |
| E | 1 | 0 |
| F | 1 | 1 |
| G | 1 | 0 |
| H | 2 | 2 |
| I | 3 | 3 |
| Total | 23 | 21 |

Penetrance: $\frac{21}{23} \times 100\% = 91\%$

Our calculation of the penetrance of the DEVR gene is shown in Table 11.

The first column lists the number of parent couples examined in the various pedigrees, of whom one or several children had evident DEVR. The second column separately lists the number of these parent couples in whom symptoms of DEVR were found. The table shows only two instances in which no anomalies were found in the parents of affected patients (E and G families). It is evident that gene penetrance is high. The calculated degree of gene penetrance is:

$$21/23 \times 100\% = 91\%.$$

As in any autosomal dominant condition, the calculated gene penetrance is based on clinical observations. Whether symptoms are or are not found depends on the method of investigation used and on the investigator's experience with the condition in question. The abovementioned degree of penetrance was calculated mainly on the basis of observations made with the aid of the slit-lamp and the three-mirror contact lens.

I am convinced that, if examination of the fundi had been limited to indirect ophthalmoscopy, many cases of DEVR with minimal lesions would not have been identified as such. Evidently, such a procedure would have yielded a lower degree of penetrance.

## 5.3 Gene expression

The severity of the ophthalmological changes found in patients with DEVR ranges from hardly perceptible symptoms in the peripheral fundus without any diminution of visual acuity, to fibrovascular organizations throughout the vitreous space with resulting total retinal detachment. Most publications on

DEVR describe such variations in the severity of symptoms. Our study does not confirm the view of some authors (Criswick and Schepens, 1969; Gow and Oliver, 1971; Laqua, 1980) that DEVR probably has a gradual progressive course in most cases (Chapter 4). Since few patients show any evidence of progression, especially after childhood years, the difference in severity of symptoms between these patients can hardly (if at all) be interpreted as indicating different stages of the disease. The interindividual difference in severity of symptoms should be regarded mainly as a result of the widely variable expression of the DEVR gene.

The significance of complications such as neovascularizations and rhegmatogenic retinal detachment has been discussed in Chapter 4. The occurrence or non-occurrence of these complications is largely decisive for the ultimate function of the eye involved.

### 5.3.a Genetic factors

The question may arise whether genetic factors could exert an influence on gene expression. In principle, they very well may because several genes undoubtedly play a role in the embryonic development of the retina. The difference in composition of such a group of genes, which can be expected in different individuals, might be a cause of the difference in expression of the DEVR gene.

This influence of the genetic background on the gene expression in DEVR can certainly not be excluded. The marked variation in gene expression in the two eyes of the same individual which is frequently observed in DEVR, can of course not be explained by genetic factors. I regard this important clinical observation as a strong argument in favour of the postulate that genetic factors can only partly be responsible for the variability of DEVR gene expression.

### 5.3.b Influence of the "environment"

It seems a logical premise that external influences may be of some significance in the aetiology of symptoms of DEVR. Different external conditions could lead to differences in gene expression. Since the primary disorder of vascular development in DEVR occurs in the course of the final months of pregnancy, different conditions of the foetus in utero during this period may influence the severity of the symptoms. It is virtually impossible to demonstrate the influence of such "external" factors. I have been unable to find a correlation between birth weight and severity of fundus changes. A very interesting question is whether prematurely born children with DEVR have been especially sensitive to neonatal oxygen administration. This subject is discussed in some detail in Chapter 8.

To environmental factors which might influence the embryo or the infant, the same applies as to the abovementioned genetic factors: it is inconceivable that these factors as such could cause the marked differences in gene expression between OD and OS in a given individual.

## 5.4 Incidence and distribution of the gene

At this time it is impossible to estimate the incidence of the gene. A large group of persons who possess the gene have no visual complaints, and no readily discernible fundus changes; the clinically working ophthalmologist will consequently tend to underestimate the incidence of the DEVR gene.

Our study has shown that even severe cases of the conditions are often not correctly diagnosed. This is not surprising because, until a few years ago, DEVR was still a virtually unknown condition. It is therefore also understandable that the diagnosis is not included in recent statistics on causes of blindness and diminished visual acuity in children, e.g. those compiled by the International Association for Prevention of Blindness (Schappert-Kimmeyser, 1975).

In my opinion, DEVR is not rare in The Netherlands. Instances of DEVR are encountered relatively often if one is specifically looking for its symptoms.

Recent observations in Great Britain suggest that there, too, the condition is not rare (Bird, 1981).

### 5.4.a Ethnic and geographical distribution

All the DEVR families described in this study are caucasian and, so far as I know, originate from Dutch ancestors. Although some of the publications on DEVR supply no information on the racial constitution of the family or families studied, yet most cases have been observed in caucasians. It is certain, however, that the condition is not found exclusively in whites.

Ober et al. (1980) described DEVR in a brother and sister in a Chinese family. In a family of Iranian origin described by the same authors, DEVR was diagnosed in a father and three daughters.

The fluorescein angiograms which Minoda and Kanagami (1976) published as obtained in various Japanese patients referred to their department for rhegmatogenic retinal detachment are highly suggestive of DEVR. The history of most of these patients was unfortunately uncertain, and consequently it is possible that the changes found in some of them were based on retrolental fibroplasia. It is likewise unfortunate that no family data are presented in their study.

The syndrome described by Kimura and Uemura (1977) is probably also identical to DEVR, but I have no certainty that this is true.

Van Manen (1944) published a case of bilateral congenital retinal fold in a native inhabitant of Nias, a small island near Sumatra in the Indonesian Archipelago. Despite the negative family history, the detailed description of the fundus changes found in this patient is quite consistent with a diagnosis of DEVR, although of course it is impossible to establish this diagnosis in retrospect. According to Van Manen, the population of Nias is probably of Mongoloid origin.

## 5.5 Genetic counselling

Genetic counselling is an important component of the care to be extended to DEVR patients or their family. A more detailed discussion of this subject is not superfluous, because the literature provides but little information on this aspect of DEVR.

This section intends to give some information on the risks of certain DEVR manifestations in the offspring of members of families in which the condition occurs. It should be emphasized that these risks as a rule cannot be calculated with any exactness; we must accept approximations based on the available knowledge.

If we are to provide genetic counselling, we should have some knowledge of the following three characteristics of the DEVR gene:
— mode of transmission
— penetrance
— expression.
As previously explained, we may assume autosomal dominant transmission of DEVR; and we may assume that gene penetrance, as calculated in the families studied, is about 90%.

Gene expression is somewhat less easily determined. It is evident that the severity of symptoms in a given person is determined by the diminution of his binocular visual acuity. This is why it is important for the ophthalmologist or geneticist to know how large the risk is that persons who possess the gene have visual acuity values below a particular level. To calculate this risk, we would have to know the binocular visual acuity of a large group of persons with the DEVR gene.

Table 5 of Chapter 4 presents the distribution of visual acuity in the better eye in our DEVR patients. This distribution reflects the degree of visual handicap in DEVR patients and thus gives some indication of the risk of a certain diminution of visual acuity in persons who possess the DEVR gene. It is postulated in this context that visual acuity in the persons on whom the table is based, undergoes no changes as a result of the condition. This postulate certainly seems plausible for most of these persons because, as we have seen, DEVR is rarely progressive after adolescence.

The number of persons with a visual acuity in the better eye of 0.5 or less was 13 (18%) in this table. In providing genetic counselling, therefore, a risk of 18% can be used as roughly approximating the risk of such a visual handicap in persons with the gene in whom fundus changes are found.

The risk of severe diminution of visual acuity, at least binocularly, is relatively small for children of parents of whom one has the DEVR gene.

In genetic counselling it is therefore not sufficient to calculate the risk that a child will possess the gene or show the changes of DEVR. It is of importance to point out that most persons affected have good or fair visual acuity, and that only a minority of them are visually handicapped. This information is the more important as the category of parents or parents-to-be who ask for advice, is largely confined to those who know of severe cases of DEVR in near relatives or who themselves suffer from severe DEVR.

PATHOGENESIS

## 5.6 DEVR as a vascular developmental disorder

On the basis of recent studies (Canny and Oliver, 1976; Nijhuis et al., 1979; Laqua, 1980; Ober et al., 1980) and our own observations, it has become evident that DEVR is primarily an affection of peripheral retinal vessels. The other fundus and vitreous changes are most likely secondary to the vascular disorder.

Although the peripheral retinal changes have often been interpreted as capillary closure, they evidently cannot have been caused by occlusion in a primordially normal vascular system. The finding of aberrant, irregular terminal ramifications adjacent to the avascular retinal periphery indicates a vascular developmental disorder.

In view of the fact that in most eyes with DEVR the nasal retinal periphery shows complete vascularization, while the vascularization of the temporal retinal periphery extends to about the equator or slightly peripheral to it, it is plausible that the disorder of vascular development has occurred between the 7th and the 9th month of intra-uterine development. This postulate proceeds from the hypothesis that the rate of vascular development had been more or less normal before the disorder developed.

The question arises how abrupt the disturbance in vasculogenesis may have occurred in DEVR patients. The knowledge now available is not sufficient to answer this question. In many cases, fluorescein angiography of the equatorial retina of DEVR patients reveals not only structural changes of and leakage from the most peripheral vessels, but similar changes in slightly more central parts of the vascular system. This suggests that the disturbance has not developed abruptly but has exerted its influence for some time before leading to complete arrest of vasculogenesis.

The process underlying the disorder of vasculogenesis in DEVR has so far remained obscure. Some of several theoretical possibilities are listed and criticized below.

1. The DEVR gene causes structural anomalies in the peripheral retina which prevent vascular development in this part of the fundus.

*Criticism.* In most patients, clinical examination has failed to reveal distinct anomalies of the avascular retinal periphery. The changes found in this part of the fundus in more severe cases seem to be a result rather than a cause of the disturbed retinal vascularization. The above hypothesis is therefore not supported by clinical observations.

2. The disturbed vascular development results from abnormal development or involution of the foetal hyaloid system.

*Criticism.* Before it develops its own vascularization, the neuroretina is partly oxygenated from the hyaloidal vasa propria. It is therefore conceivable that changes of the hyaloidal system may have consequences for the vascularization of the retina. The finding of cases of congenital retinal fold (a malformation regarded by some as a result of a developmental disorder of the primary vitreous and the foetal hyaloidal system) in DEVR families prompted Dudgeon (1979) to launch this suggestion. I have found no remnants which might indicate abnormal regression of the hyaloidal system. Moreover, a more plausible explanation of a congenital retinal fold in DEVR presents itself (Chapter 8). To summarize: there is no sufficient clinical evidence to support this hypothesis.

3. Vascular development becomes disturbed by anomalous oxygen transport in the foetal blood.

*Criticism.* This hypothesis is based on the similarity in clinical symptoms between DEVR and retrolental fibroplasia (RLF). The vascular anomalies in RLF as a rule develop in response to a significant increase in the oxygen pressure of the arterial blood. It is quite inconceivable that the presence of foetal blood with an abnormal oxygen affinity (e.g. due to an abnormal haemoglobin or abnormal replacement of foetal haemoglobin by normal adult haemoglobin or abnormal concentrations of co-factors such as 2, 3-diphosphoglycerate) could lead to any significant increase in arterial oxygen pressure in utero (Lorijn, 1980, 1981).

Another argument against the above hypothesis is that, so far as I know, there has been no report on a human foetal haemoglobinopathy manifested exclusively by ocular changes.

Although I had no occasion to study oxygen dissociation in neonates with DEVR, examination of older children and adults revealed no anomaly in the morphology of the blood, and no indications suggesting the presence of abnormal haemoglobins. An oxygen dissociation curve was determined in one young female patient, and found to be quite normal (V-25 A).

4. The disorder of vascular development results from a local metabolic disorder which is limited to the complex of vasoformative tissue in the foetal neuroretina, and which occurs in response to the anomalous gene present in the cells of this tissue.

*Criticism.* According to this hypothesis the disorder is confined to the zone of production of immature blood vessels in the foetal retina, and extraretinal anomalies play no role in its pathogenesis. The local metabolic disorder may be based on or associated with an increased sensitivity to oxygen, so that vasculogenesis is disturbed even at normal oxygen pressure (this, of course, is uncertain).

In my opinion few (if any) objections can at this time be made to this hypothesis. However, as long as the pathogenesis of DEVR has not been elucidated, the search for extraretinal anomalies which may play a role in this pathogenesis must not be discontinued.

## 5.7 Deformation of the foetal network of retinal vessels as direct consequence of disturbed vascular development. A hypothesis.

A striking feature of DEVR is the abnormal configuration of retinal vessels in and around the posterior pole. As mentioned in Chapter 4, this was found in 60% of the eyes examined. In severe cases of DEVR this deformation of the vascular network can be ascribed to traction exerted by preretinal membranes in the temporal periphery of the fundus. However, many eyes with an abnormal retinal vascular pattern in the posterior fundus, show no discernible structure in the preretinal vitreous space which might have caused such deformation. This absence of a tractional cause in a fair number of eyes with DEVR suggests that other factors play a role in the deformation of the retinal vascular system.

It has been previously explained in this chapter that DEVR is based on premature termination of vasculogenesis of peripheral retinal vessels, probably in the final months of the intra-uterine period. It seems likely that this disturbance not only leads to incomplete peripheral retinal vascularization but also plays a direct role in the deformation of more central, primordially earlier parts of the vascular system.

That such a disturbance could influence a primordially earlier and therefore normal part of the vascular bed would hardly be conceivable if the latter would have attained its definitive configuration prior to the period in which the developmental disorder occurs. However, this is not the case. As outlined in Chapter 1, the normal human retinal vasculature has not yet assumed its adult configuration even at the time of birth, but growth, maturation and remodelling of the immature vascular network continue after birth (Cogan, 1963). In my opinion the latter process is inevitably influenced by a late foetal disorder of vasculogenesis of the type involved in DEVR. It is probably by this influence on the otherwise physiological process of remodelling that an abnormal arrangement of primordially normal parts of the retinal vasculature is caused.

A fact of importance in this conception is that the disturbance in peripheral retinal vasculogenesis occurs in a vascular system which in its totality is still immature. Consequently the disturbance not only has its consequences for the peripheral vasculature but leads to some deformation of the entire vascular network.

In DEVR it is in particular the development of the peripheral ramifications of the temporal retinal vessels that is disturbed and finally arrested completely. Since growth and maturation of the primordially established parts of the retinal vascular bed in the posterior pole and nasal periphery continue normally, it is conceivable that some displacement occurs in the direction of the areas in which vascular development lags behind. This is why displacement from the nasal to the temporal periphery occurs. However, the fixation of retinal vessels at the site of the disc turns this displacement into a slight rotation round the posterior pole (Figure 121).

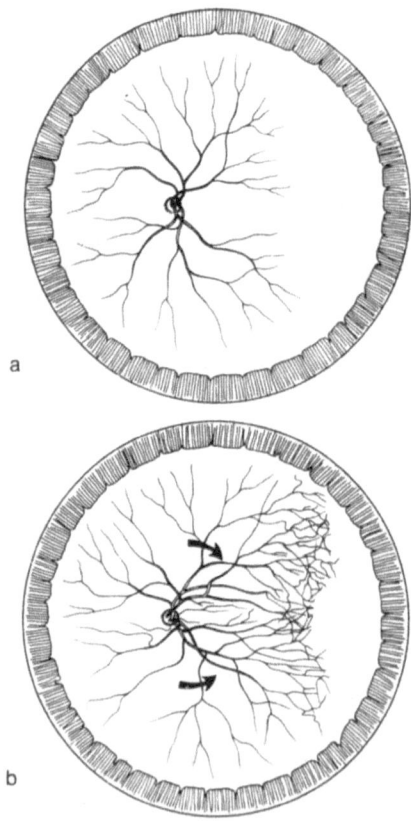

Figure 121. Schematic representation of the late foetal deformation of the retinal vascular system in DEVR. a) About the 7th month: normal development; unlike the temporal half of the retina, the nasal half shows virtually normal vascularization. b) About the 8th–9th month: late disturbance in vasculogenesis manifesting itself in the temporal half of the fundus. Deformation of the other parts of the vascular network with displacement in temporal direction (arrows).

The above hypothesis affords an explanation of the abnormal configuration of vessels and the macular ectopia in eyes with DEVR which show no signs of traction. Nor can traction explain the aberrant structure of the retinal vasculature between posterior pole and temporal equator, which is characterized by an increased number of parallel vascular ramifications (Figure 122). As demonstrated angiographically in Chapter 4, the capillary network between such vessels is often poorly developed. The hypothesis that such vascular ramifications have pushed together as a result of the vascular development disorder is more consistent with the clinical observation than the hypothesis of a tractional course. The role of traction exerted by epiretinal membranes in the pathogenesis of the deformation of the retina and its vasculature seems significant only in the severe forms of DEVR.

The hypothesis that disorders in the development of the peripheral retinal vasculature may have consequences for the configuration of vessels in the posterior pole, is supported by observations made in some cases of Wagner's disease (see Chapter 10).

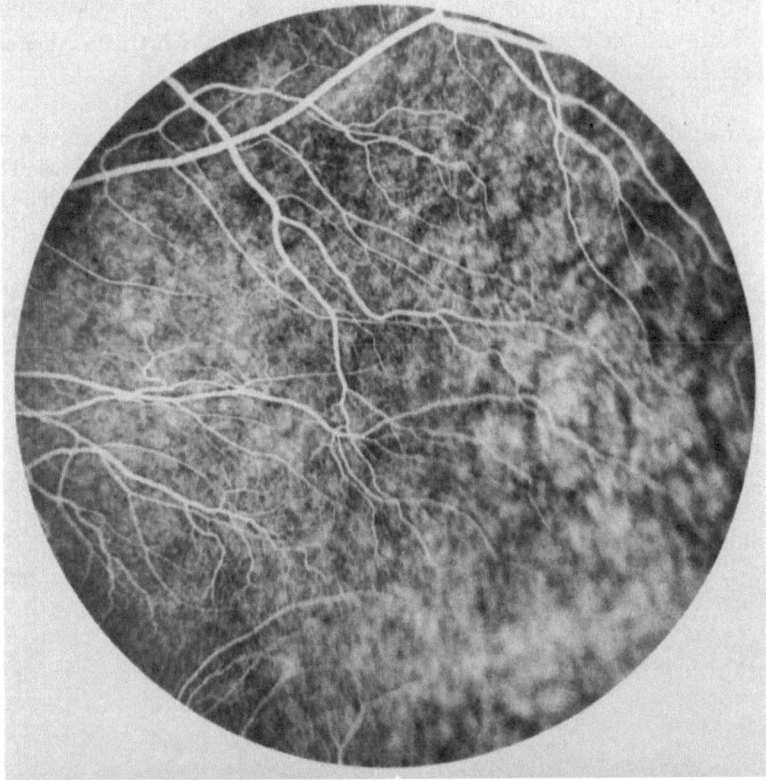

Figure 122. Increased number of vascular ramifications in retinal areas temporal to the posterior pole OS. This phenomenon can apparently not be explained by traction, but is probably a direct consequence of disturbed vascular development.

### 5.8 Objections to qualification of DEVR as "vitreoretinal dystrophy"

Several ophthalmological studies published in recent years classify DEVR among the vitreoretinal degenerations (Tolentino et al., 1976), vitreoretinal dystrophies (Deutman, 1977; Naumann, 1980) or "hérédodégénérescences vitréo-rétiniennes". (Bec et al., 1980). To my mind, these designations are not consistent with the nature of DEVR.

The degeneration concept has found wide acceptance especially as a pathological anatomical term, used with reference to disorders of tissue metabolism which become manifest in characteristic morphological changes (Hogan and Zimmerman, 1962).

The term dystrophy is likewise used to refer to conditions associated with premature cellular changes and cell death. Of importance is that both degeneration and dystrophy concern (fully developed) mature tissues (Apple and Naumann, 1980).

Dysplasia, however, involves disturbed tissue development, although Waardenburg (1963) maintains that dystrophy can occur on the basis of a dysplastic disorder, whereupon apparently normal cells or tissues gradually degenerate and are destroyed.

As we have seen, DEVR is a condition characterized by a late foetal developmental disorder of the retinal vascular system. It does not involve a process of gradual degeneration of initially normal cells during (extra-uterine) life, and the terms dystrophy and degeneration therefore do not apply. Clinically, this is evident from the absence of slowly progressive morphological and functional changes in DEVR, which in this respect differs from, say, the hereditary retinal dystrophies. The fact that in a minority of eyes with DEVR signs of progression of the changes may be observed in a particular period of life (e.g. due to increasing exudates or vitreous organizations) does not imply that the condition may be qualified as degeneration or dystrophy.

A second critical note on the designation vitreoretinal degeneration or vitreoretinal dystrophy concerns the adjective "vitreoretinal", which suggests that the vitreous is always affected. Absence of vitreous changes in more than 50% of the eyes with DEVR has already been mentioned in Chapter 4. In my opinion, DEVR is a retinopathy rather than a vitreoretinopathy. The vitreous anomalies in DEVR should be regarded as a consequence of the retinal vascular anomalies.

CHAPTER 6

# PREVENTION AND TREATMENT OF COMPLICATIONS OF DOMINANT EXUDATIVE VITREORETINOPATHY

## 6.1 Early diagnosis and selection of high-risk patients

Unlike many other hereditary affections of the retina, DEVR is not characterized by slowly progressive degeneration. Visual function is determined largely
by the occurrence or non-occurrence of complications, some of which can be
treated or even prevented.

These facts justify attempts to reduce the incidence of visual loss as a result
of DEVR.

Unlike retrolental fibroplasia (RLF), there is no tainted neonatal history
in DEVR; consequently the condition is usually not identified until visual loss
is evident in one or both eyes. Early diagnosis of DEVR, before symptoms
develop, is possible in young children in families in which the condition is
known to occur. Parents who show symptoms of DEVR should be instructed
about the importance of examination of their children and future children. It
is of importance to point out that the condition as a rule takes a benign
course, and that treatment is required only in a minority of cases.

It is difficult to decide at which age young children are best examined. Because DEVR can cause marked anomalies even shortly after birth, the examination ought to be made in the neonatal period. This, however, poses practical problems in most cases. Examination at the age of 2–4 months seems
more acceptable. When fundus examination in mydriasis reveals no lesions, it
is advisable to re-examine the infant in early childhood, because such an
examination probably cannot exclude minimal manifestations of DEVR with
certainty.

Follow-ups on children with minimal lesions should probably be made
periodically before school age is reached. Older children and adults with minimal lesions need not, in my opinion, be examined more frequently than once
every 1–2 years.

It is of great importance to ensure that, in families with DEVR, children
with an increased risk of complications are selected at the earliest possible age.
The presence of the following symptoms in young children most likely indicates an increased risk of complications:
− traction on the peripheral retina, exerted by vitreous membranes
− significant deformation of the retina in the posterior pole
− vascular proliferations

— retinal and subretinal exudates
— retinal defects
— anisometropia.
Children in whom these symptoms are found, need frequent follow-up examinations.


## 6.2 Treatment

*Amblyopia*

In children with DEVR who show subnormal visual acuity in one eye, efforts should be made to establish whether this is (partly) a result of amblyopia. Whenever amblyopia is considered possible on the basis of orthoptic and ophthalmoscopic examination, it should be treated as soon as possible. Anisometropia, if present, should be corrected. It is important to ensure that treatment by occlusion is not unnecessarily intensive and prolonged: very often it is impossible to restore normal visual acuity when there are structural retinal changes in the posterior pole as well.

*Strabismus*

When an operation to correct strabismus is contemplated, the frequently enlarged positive kappa angle due to temporal macular ectopia should be taken into account. It is therefore important to ascertain, before intervention, to which extent the abnormal kappa angle contributes to the visible eye position. The worst error that could be committed is to mistake a pseudodivergent eye position for divergent strabismus, and to make an attempt at surgical correction.

*Neovascularization*

The most serious complications of DEVR are a result of neovascularization, and it is logical to attempt to treat this by cryocoagulation or photocoagulation. Some therapeutic effect can be expected only if this treatment is instituted at a time when the vascular proliferations have not yet led to extensive vitreous organizations.

Unfortunately, severe cases which would require coagulation have so far nearly always been overlooked until marked visual loss has occurred. It is therefore a sine qua non that children with DEVR be ophthalmologically examined before visual loss occurs. As already pointed out, this can be ensured only if DEVR families are recognized and registered as such, and if affected family members are instructed about the importance of an examination of their children (if any) at an early age.

It is far more difficult to trace cases of DEVR in infants than it is to trace RLF: in the latter case it is reasonably possible on the basis of the history to establish which children are running a grave risk of developing severe lesions.

There are only two publications which supply data on the results of coagulation therapy in DEVR: Criswick and Schepens (1969) treated five patients with peripheral neovascularizations by photocoagulation or cryocoagulation (three were treated bilaterally). Some time after treatment two eyes showed rhegmatogenous retinal detachment, which in one case was successfully treated while in the other case the features of massive periretinal proliferation (MPP) were found. A few eyes responded favourably to coagulation, but in some cases the neovascularizations persisted or even expanded. The average age of the patients treated was about 12 years.

Gow and Oliver (1971) treated four patients with fibrovascular proliferations in the fundus periphery by cryocoagulation, and one patient by photocoagulation. The last patient showed no signs of progression during a follow-up over 12 months; the four patients treated by cryocoagulation all showed atrophy of the fibrovascular cicatrix. The average age of these five patients was about 9 years.

Only three of our patients were treated by photocoagulation in view of neovascularizations. In V-25 A the fundus OD was treated with the Argon laser (only slight active vascular proliferations were present). No signs of progression were observed in the fundus, and visual acuity remained unchanged, during a follow-up over 5 years.

In III-2 B the avascular zone of the temporal fundus periphery OD was elsewhere treated with the Argon laser on several occasions. This patient only had a small neovascularization which seemed not very threatening and disappeared completely as a result of the coagulations.

Larger neovascularizations (V-52 A) were treated by photocoagulation. In this female patient a fan-shaped preretinal neovascularization was treated by direct Xenon coagulation; it was found to be markedly reduced after a few weeks. A few leaking remnants of this proliferation were subsequently treated with the Argon laser. During a follow-up over 5 years this patient developed no symptoms of traction or neovascularization, and her visual acuity remained unchanged (1.0). In none of these three patients were complications observed after coagulation.

Progressive vascular proliferation in young patients with DEVR would seem to be the principal indication for coagulation. Adults with DEVR have small neovascularizations which seem to be stationary and need no treatment (V-2 D).

*Leakage from retinal vessels*

In eyes in which leakage from retinal vessels leads to progression of oedema and intraretinal and subretinal exudates, attempts may be made to exert a favourable influence on this process by photocoagulation or cryocoagulation of the retinal areas involved. I have only incidentally resorted to such treatment (VI-3 D).

## Retinal defects and retinal detachment

Small circular atrophic defects are the type of retinal defect most commonly found in DEVR. The question whether this type of defect in an attached retina requires treatment, is not readily answerable. General studies have shown that the risk of a complicating detachment of the retina when there are asymptomatic defects of this type is very small (Byer, 1974), but it is uncertain whether this applies also to DEVR. Prophylactic coagulation of such small defects seems to carry no undue risk, and is certainly indicated in DEVR patients with a history of rhegmatogenous retinal detachment in the other eye, or with a history of this complication in the immediate family.

The type of treatment of horseshoe ruptures — in DEVR as in other patients — depends on several factors. Generally, the therapist confronted with such ruptures has a choice between coagulation therapy or a scleral buckling procedure combined with coagulation.

Retinal detachment in DEVR is a serious complication, and its treatment may pose grave problems. As in RLF, the prognosis of this complication seems to depend largely on the patient's age: the earlier in life the retina becomes detached, the less favourable the prognosis. As in RLF, rhegmatogenic retinal detachment in DEVR seems to occur mostly after age 10, and can be treated by a classical scleral buckling procedure. Successful treatment of rhegmatogenous retinal detachment in DEVR by this technique was reported by Criswick and Schepens (1969) and by Dudgeon (1980). In two of our patients the retina was re-attached in this way (VI-3 B and III-3 H).

A problem often encountered in the treatment of retinal detachment due to cicatricial RLF is the difficult localization of small peripheral defects, which in some cases are probably concealed behind preretinal glious membranes (Tasman, 1975). The same problem is unlikely to pose itself in DEVR, and probably also existed in some of our patients (VI-3 D, IV-6 H and IV-33 C).

A grave problem in the operative treatment of retinal detachment — both in DEVR and in RLF — is that its pathogenesis is often tractional as well as rhegmatogenous and exudative. This forces the surgeon to select a combination of techniques most likely to do justice to the various factors which have led to the detachment.

In the case of retinal detachment with severe traction from the vitreous space, scleral buckling alone is often inadequate. In these cases this procedure can be combined with vitrectomy via the pars plana. Such a combined operation was performed on III-5 B, IV-6 H and IV-33 C.

There are only incidental reports on pars plana vitrectomy in DEVR (Laqua, 1980). Treister and Machemer (1971) described this procedure in the

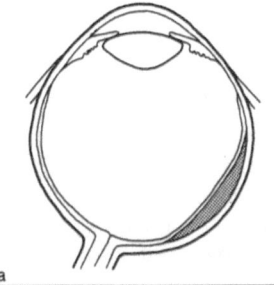 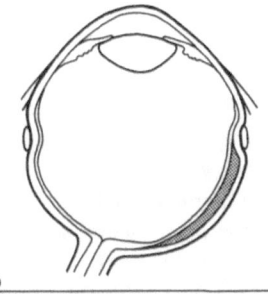

Figure 123. a) Retinal detachment with contraction of the retina due to epiretinal membranes. b) Insufficient effect of scleral buckling procedure.

treatment of a 16-year-old female with no history of neonatal oxygen administration, who showed the typical fundus anomalies of DEVR. They successfully treated a total retinal detachment in the posterior pole by removing vitreous adhesions to the retina.

Another problem in severe DEVR is that contraction of epiretinal membranes shortens the detached retina. Whether an episcleral or intrascleral buckle is an adequate therapeutic technique in these circumstances, is questionable: this method does not abolish the incongruence of sclera and neuroretina (Figure 123). In patients with a severely shortened retina it seems more

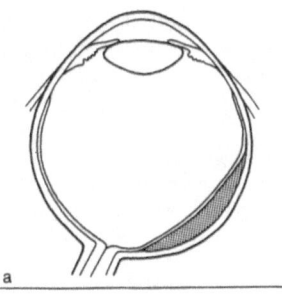

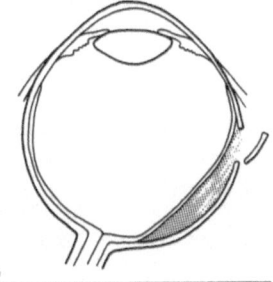 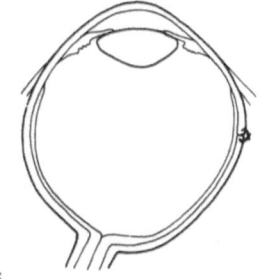

Figure 124. Treatment of a detached and contracted retina (a) by scleral excision (b, c).

effective to use the old technique of scleral excision as introduced by Müller in 1903, which if necessary can be combined with pars plana vitrectomy as recently suggested by Hanscom and Machemer (1980) (Figure 124).

So far there have been no reports on operative treatment of retinal detachment in very young children with DEVR. In view of experience gained with operative treatment of RLF, the chance of successful re-attachment surgery at a very early age seems limited. However, some investigators have demonstrated that re-attachment surgery can have hopeful results in very young children with RLF, although long-term follow-up data on such patients have not been published (McPherson and Hittner, 1979).

The technique of injecting silicone oil into the preretinal vitreous space seems to be justified in selected cases in which extensive vitreous membranes have fixed the retina in rigid folds, or in which other operative techniques have failed. Although data on long-term results are still rather scanty, injection of silicone oil can effect adequate unfolding of the retina (VI-6 H: Figure 125). In patients with large retinal defects this procedure is risky because oil can flow through the defect into the subretinal space (III-5 B).

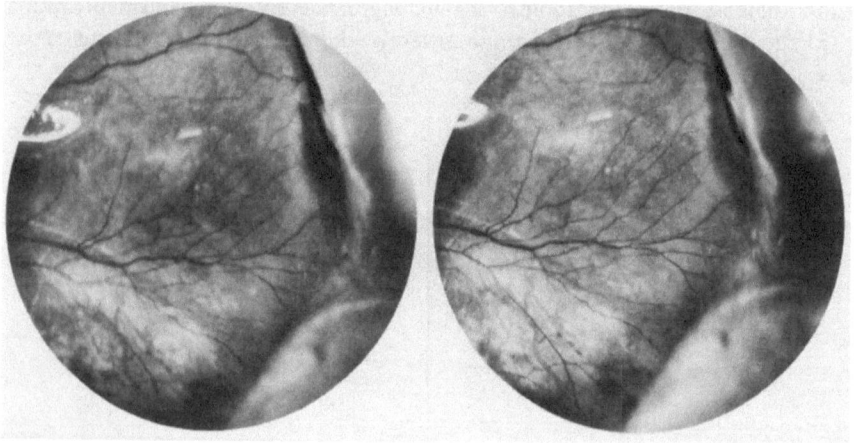

Figure 125. OS. Stereo-photograph. Re-attachment of the retina by means of silicone oil injection after a former unsuccessful scleral buckling procedure (VI-6 H).

CHAPTER 7

# CONGENITAL RETINAL FOLD (ABLATIO FALCIFORMIS CONGENITA)

The term congenital retinal fold (ablatio falciformis congenita) refers to an allegedly congenital malformation which is characterized by the presence of a raised retinal fold extending radially from the posterior pole to the fundus periphery. Since the end of the 19th century this condition has been the subject of a considerable number of ophthalmological publications. Of several hypotheses on its pathogenesis, that advanced by Ida Mann (1935) is the most widely known.

It is now generally accepted that congenital retinal fold is not a clinical entity but can be a manifestation of a diversity of conditions. The literature on congenital retinal fold is full of contradictions. So far, the relation between DEVR and congenital retinal fold has hardly been studied. This chapter focuses mostly on this relation.

## 7.1 The clinical features of congenital retinal fold

Weve (1935) described the anomaly as a duplicature of the retina, which was stretched like a sail between the disc of the optic nerve and the area between lens and ciliary body. He nearly always observed this anomaly in the inferior temporal quadrant of the fundus, and described it as "ablatio falciformis congenita".

The patients described by Mann (1935) likewise showed a retinal fold extending from the disc to the extreme periphery of the fundus, or even to the equator of the lens; in most cases, several radially arranged blood vessels were distinguishable in this fold. However, the folds observed by Ida Mann were not always localized in the inferior temporal quadrant of the fundus.

The reports published by Weve (1935) and Mann (1935) were not the first on this condition. Pflüger (1885) had already described bilateral changes in the temporal fundus periphery in a microcephalic child which he interpreted as coloboma but which in all likelihood were based on falciform retinal detachment, i.e. congenital retinal fold.

A patient described by Sulzer (1888) showed a congenital retinal fold in the inferior temporal quadrant of one eye, whereas the other eye was entirely normal.

Heine (1904) found bilateral changes in a 9-year-old girl which he described as congenital cystic retina; these changes also seem to correspond with the clinical features of congenital retinal fold, but in this case the diagnosis in not entirely certain.

Salffner (1902) published a detailed description of the histopathological changes in the eye of a 10-month-old infant, which had been enucleated because a "glioma" had been suspected. In the inferior part of the vitreous space, a retinal duplicature extended from the disc to the posterior side of the lens.

In 1904, De Vries described a 5-year-old boy with a posterior pole cataract OD and, in OS, a strand extending in anterior temporal direction from the disc; the strand contained vessels, some of which extended into the retina. The retina outside this strand, however, was virtually avascular. This patient died at age 11 as a result of multiple tumours interpreted as endotheliomas and neurofibromas. The histological findings were published by Ancona (1935). Her description and illustrations clearly show that in this patient, too, there had been a falciform retinal detachment in the inferior temporal quadrant of the fundus.

Many other publications clearly showed the predilection of congenital retinal fold for the inferior temporal quadrant of the fundus. Apart from Weve's patients (1935, 1938) and the abovementioned cases, congenital retinal folds were reported in this quadrant by numerous other authors (Hoffman, 1926; Stübel, 1927, 1928; Tillema, 1937; Gartner, 1941; Theodore and Ziporkes, 1940; Poulsen, 1947; Van Manen, 1944; Von Winning, 1952; Badtke, 1954, 1960; Heydenreich, 1959; Joannidés and Protonotarios, 1965; Thiel, 1968).

*Terminology*

In this text I use "congenital retinal fold" and "ablatio falciformis congenita" as synonyms. In section 7.5 it will be explained that the anomaly is usually based on a late developmental disorder of the retinal vasculature, and that in most cases it is impossible to establish whether the changes developed shortly before or after birth. Although in the latter case the anomaly is not, strictly speaking, congenital, I nevertheless generally use the term congenital retinal fold because this is the generally accepted term for this condition. In my opinion, retinal folds which lack the characteristic features described by Weve and Mann, should not be referred to by the above terms even though the changes are already present at birth.

## 7.2 Conditions which may be associated with congenital retinal fold

Table 12 lists the conditions in which the features of congenital retinal fold can sometimes be found (in retrolental fibroplasia it is of course beyond doubt that the symptoms are of postnatal origin).

Table 12. Conditions associated with a congenital (or neonatal) retinal fold.

Dominant exudative vitreoretinopathy
Retrolental fibroplasia
Incontinentia pigmenti (Bloch-Sulzberger syndrome)
Norrie's disease
Reese-Blodi-Straatsma syndrome (including trisomy 13)
Microcephaly; Hydrocephaly (congenital encephalo-ophthalmic dysplasia).
Congenital toxoplasmosis
Posterior persistent hyperplastic primary vitreous
Meckel's syndrome

The relationship between DEVR and congenital retinal fold has only recently been studied (Van Nouhuys, 1981a) and will subsequently be discussed in detail.

Incontinentia pigmenti, Norrie's disease, the Reese-Blodi-Straatsma syndrome and RLF are discussed in the relevant chapters.

Persistent hyperplastic primary vitreous – a rather controversial cause of congenital retinal fold – is discussed in detail in Chapter 13.

Congenital retinal fold in combination with microcephaly is discussed in section 7.4.

Congenital retinal fold in association with Meckel's syndrome is a rarity. This syndrome, which is associated with severe systemic anomalies, is not within the scope of this study.

## 7.3 Congenital retinal fold as a manifestation of DEVR

A comparison between the often detailed descriptions of fundus features in cases of congenital retinal fold and the changes we found in several of our DEVR patients with a raised retinal fold from the disc to the peripheral fundus, reveals the close similarity of these two conditions.

When Criswick and Schepens (1969) introduced familial exudative vitreoretinopathy as a separate clinical entity, they already suggested a possible aetiological relationship between this condition and congenital retinal fold, Gow and Oliver (1971), however, maintained that idiopathic congenital retinal fold shows but little similarity to the features found in the DEVR family they studied.

It seems to me that the prevalent uncertainty and confusion with regard to congenital retinal fold and its relationship to DEVR has two causes:
1. congenital retinal fold is a descriptive term with multiple aetiological connotations;
2. DEVR can manifest itself in widely diverse ways; owing to the relatively small number of cases so far described, few investigators have had occasion to familiarize themselves with the condition in its various forms.

I am firmly convinced that many of the cases of congenital retinal fold described in the literature represent manifestations of DEVR (Van Nouhuys, 1981b).

This conviction is supported by the following similarities between the fundus features in many published cases of congenital retinal fold and those found in patients in the families we studied:

Localization of the retinal fold in the inferior temporal quadrant has already been discussed. It is likely, however, that a falciform fold can in exceptional cases be found on the nasal side in DEVR also. I observed a nasal localization near the horizontal equator on fundus photographs of one eye of a patient who was very likely a member of a DEVR family. I was shown these photographs by Professor Bird at the Moorfields Eye Institute in London.

Attachment of the peripheral end of the retinal fold to the ciliary body or the posterior lens capsule via white glious tissue. Most publications on congenital retinal fold describe a usually white tissue mass at the end of the retinal fold which, as in our DEVR patients, is often connected with the posterior lens capsule near the temporal equator of the lens (Chapter 4, Figure 105).

Gross retinal pigmentations. Such pigment deposits have been very frequently described in congenital retinal fold. As in our cases, these pigmentations are usually localized in the attached part of the retina on either side of the insertion of the falciform fold (Chapter 3, Figure 76).

Atrophy of the choroid. There are frequent reports on pale yellow areas in which large choroidal vessels are clearly visible as a result of atrophy of the choriocapillaris and possibly also of the pigmented layer of the retina. These descriptions tally with observations made in some of our cases. Sharply defined atrophic scars, through which the white sclera is clearly visible, are another observation made in both conditions. Such cicatrices have often been erroneously qualified as colobomas (Chapter 3, Figure 77).

Aberrant retinal vascular pattern is a finding frequently mentioned in case reports on congenital retinal fold. Many authors express their surprise at the scantiness of retinal vessels in the attached parts of the neuroretina. On the other hand, mention is usually made of a substantial number of blood vessels which extend from the disc in anterior direction in the retinal fold, or at some distance from the disc extend from the fold into the attached part of the neuroretina. These findings are likewise consistent with our observations on falciform folds in DEVR (Chapter 3, Figure 77).

Apart from the fundus features, other characteristics of congenital retinal fold also correspond with findings obtained in DEVR: numerous patients with congenital retinal fold prove to show fundus changes in the contralateral eye, or even to show bilateral ablatio falciformis. Apart from the presence of bilateral symptoms, familial occurrence is not a rarity; nor is the combined presence of cases of ablatio falciformis and total retinal detachment (so-called pseudoglioma) in one family.

Such familial cases of congenital retinal fold with localization in the inferior temporal quadrant and often with bilateral fundus changes without a history of premature birth or neonatal oxygen administraion, and without systemic congenital anomalies, very likely represent manifestations of DEVR.

Cases of congenital retinal fold which meet all the above criteria have been described by Hoffman (1926), Weve (1935, 1938), Theodore and Ziporkes (1940), Von Winning (1952), Scialdone and Artifoni (1962), Joannidés and Protonotarios (1965) and Ohba et al. (1981).

In most of the abovementioned familial cases of congenital retinal fold, the mode of transmission could not be established with certainty. In the various families the condition was found in male as well as in female members; and this excludes X-chromosomal transmission.

Autosomal dominant transmission, however, has only incidentally been demonstrated (Scialdone and Artifoni, 1962). In my opinion, this is no argument against the diagnosis of DEVR in these families.

As demonstrated in most of our families with DEVR, gene expression is extremely variable. Should such families be examined solely by indirect ophthalmoscopy, then many (if not most) members with minimal symptoms

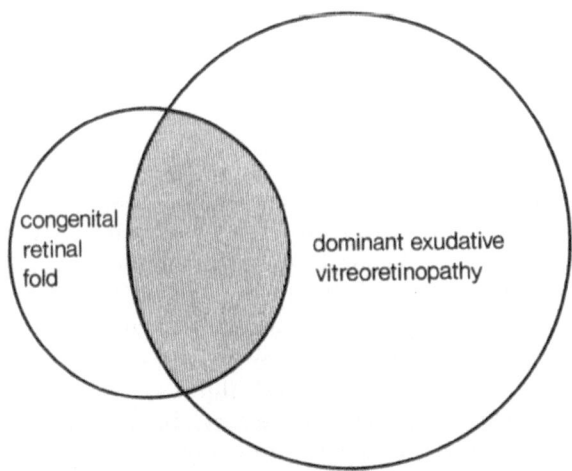

Figure 126. Relation between congenital retinal fold and DEVR.

would not be identified, and the chance of demonstrating a distinct autosomal dominant pattern of transmission would be small.

Most reports on congenital retinal fold, however, make no mention of
examination of patients' relatives. In view of the clinical symptoms described,
however, it seems likely that a number of these sporadic cases are based on
DEVR.

The relationship between DEVR and congenital retinal fold is schematically represented in Figure 126: the area within the small circle indicates cases
of retinal fold; many of these cases involve DEVR (hatched part). This group
represents only a small fraction of the total number of cases of DEVR. The
total area within the DEVR circle was therefore made substantially larger than
that within the congenital retinal fold circle. It is to be noted that the propor-
tional dimensions of the circles and the area of overlapping are based on a
general impression of the incidence of these conditions, and were not produced
on the basis of any epidemiological research.

## 7.4 Congenital retinal fold and microcephaly

Several reports on patients with bilateral congenital retinal fold mention the
presence of microcephaly (Pflüger, 1885; Stübel, 1927; Von Pelláthy, 1931;
Gartner, 1941; Mackensen, 1953; Masuda, 1962; Von Barsewisch, 1968;
Warburg, 1976; Jarmas et al., 1981).

One female patient with this combination was known at our department,
and I had occasion personally to examine her and her immediate relatives. Of
the numerous ophthalmological, paediatric and neurological examinations
made in this case in the course of the years, only the more important results
are presented below.

*Case history IV-7 (16-12-65)*

*History*

At the time of my examination this 15-year-old, mentally underendowed girl
showed unmistakable microcephaly. At the age of 1 year she had been referred
to an ophthalmologist by a paediatrician who had noticed a convergent position of the left eye. Our department found horizontal nystagmus when the
girl was 2 years old, as well as ablatio falciformis in the temporal fundus ODS.
Correcting spectacles were prescribed in view of bilateral mixed astigmatism
of about 6 diopters. Since a serious visual handicap obviously existed, the
patient was referred to a home for visually handicapped children.

There was a record of premature birth (birth weight 2300 g), but the neonate had been in fair condition and no oxygen administration had taken place.
The pregnancy had been of normal duration (40 weeks) but had been complicated by an ovarian cyst which assumed very large dimensions and had to
be surgically removed soon after parturition.

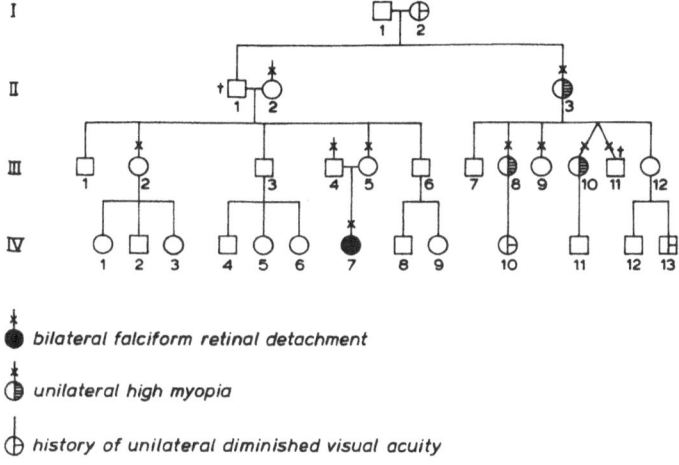

Figure 127. Pedigree of the family of patient IV-7 (16-12-65).

The ophthalmological family history revealed nothing abnormal in the parents, but maternal relatives included several persons with unilateral visual loss.

*Ophthalmological examination*

| | |
|---|---|
| Visual acuity | VOD: Cyl. − 6.0 axis 160° 4/60. |
| | VOS: S + 2.0/Cyl. − 6.0 axis 10° 1/60. |
| Eye position | Convergent strabismus OS; pronounced horizontal nystagmus. |
| Anterior segments | ODS: Entirely normal cornea, iris and anterior chamber. No marked microphthalmia. Some opacities of the posterior lens capsule on the temporal side; lenses otherwise clear. |
| Vitreous | ODS: Syneresis with optically empty lacunae and liquefaction. A fragile preretinal vitreous membrane in the temporal fundus periphery. |
| Fundi | OD: Marked deformation of the retinal vessels on the disc. A narrow, increasingly prominent retinal fold extends from the disc in inferior temporal direction to the extreme fundus periphery, where it ends in a local mass of white glious tissue attached to the pars plana. The macula is not visible. Several vessels extend |

radially from the disc in the retinal fold (Figure 128). The central segments of the nasal vascular branches are distorted in the direction of the fold. In the posterior pole, a number of retinal vessels are visible outside the fold, but they soon end in terminal ramifications, mostly in the superior nasal quadrant. The retinal mid-periphery presents a whitish appearance and seems avascular. Nowhere are remnants of hyaloid vessels seen.

OS: As in OD, a falciform fold extends from the disc to the temporal fundus periphery, where it disappears near 3 o'clock in a white tissue mass attached to the lens equator and

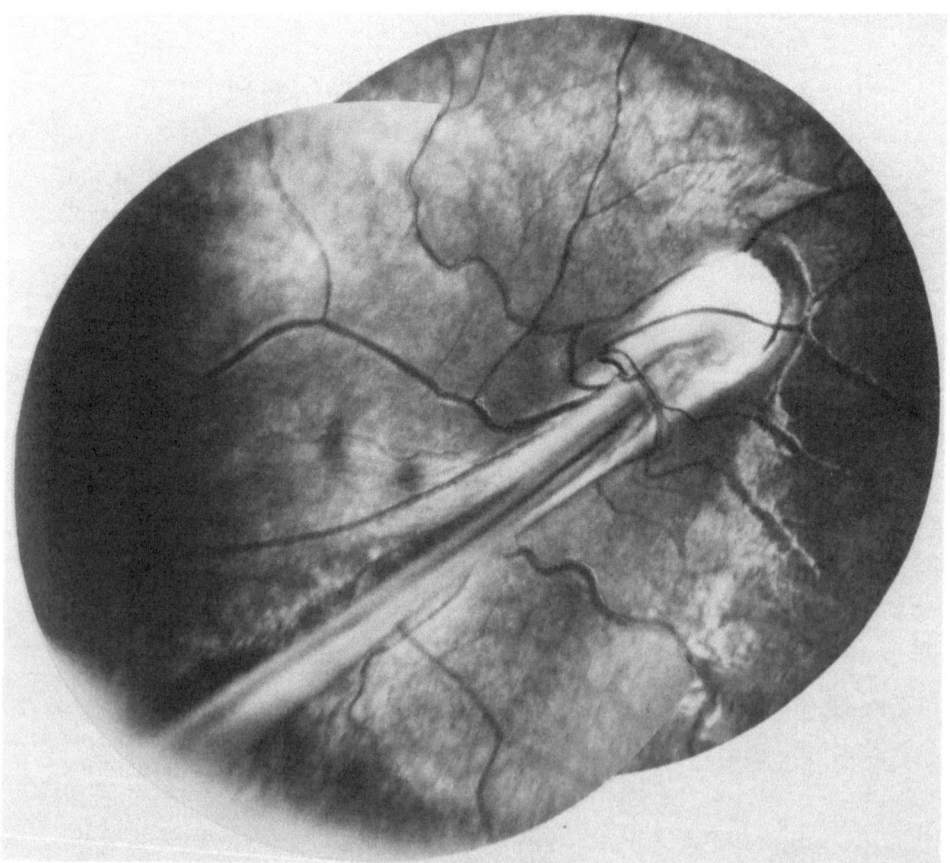

Figure 128. Falciform retinal fold extending from the disc to the inferior temporal quadrant of the fundus.

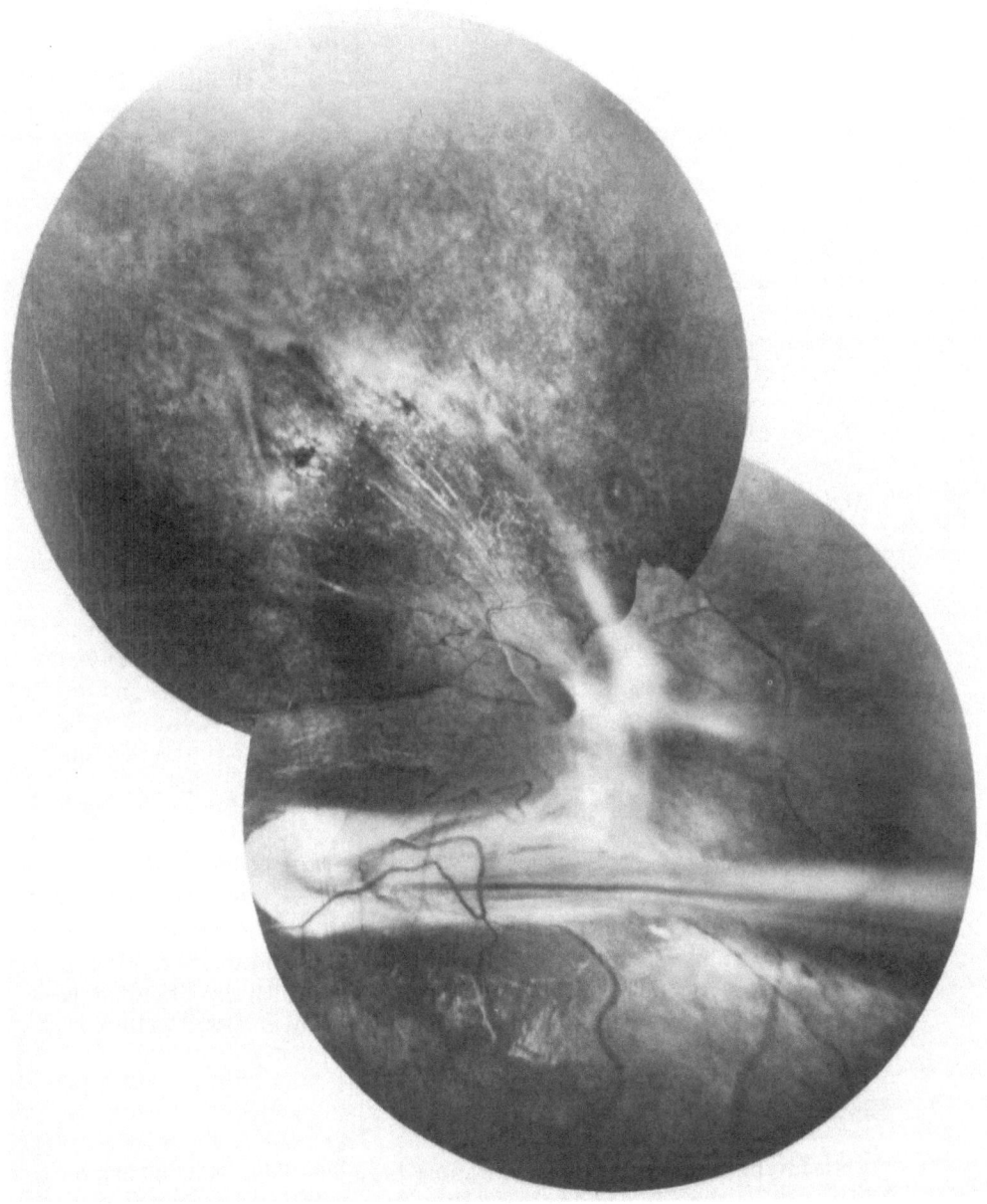

Figure 129. OS. Posterior pole. Falciform retinal fold extending from the disc in temporal direction. The retina superior to the posterior pole is avascular.

the pars plana. The retina shows several gross pigmentations on either side of the fold. The pattern of the retinal vasculature closely resembles that in the fundus OD: the vessels outside the fold again seem to end not far outside the posterior pole, leaving the major part of the retina avascular (Figure 129).

### General anomalies

In view of the microcephaly and epileptic manifestations, the patient was submitted to extensive neurological and paediatric examinations at several different ages. The cranial circumference was only 29 cm at birth, and always remained far below the P 10 curve on several subsequent occasions. Six café-au-lait spots were found scattered over the body surface. Other changes which might be consistent with Von Recklinghausen's disease were not found. The girl showed unmistakable mental and motor retardation. General internal and laboratory studies revealed no anomalies. A chromosome study disclosed a normal female karyotype.

### Family study

Contact lens examination of the fundus periphery in the mother (III-5) revealed a few whitish areas anterior to the equator in both fundi, and a small defect in the temporal fundus OS. In view of this, fluorescein angiography of the peripheral fundus was carried out, which failed to demonstrate any distinct retinal vascular anomalies. The fundi of the father (III-4) proved to be normal. Ophthalmological examination of II-3, III-9 and III-10 revealed unilateral high myopia without vascular anomalies in the retinal periphery.

### Summary and conclusions

This mentally deficient girl combined a bilateral ablatio falciformis in the inferior temporal quadrant with marked microcephaly. In view of the café-au-lait spots on the skin and some orthodontic problems, the diagnosis incontinentia pigmenti was considered; however, the neonatal history was not very suggestive of this condition. The hereditary unilateral high myopia found in several persons in the family study seemed to be totally unrelated to the condition of this patient.

### Discussion

As already pointed out, several publications have described the combination of congenital retinal fold and microcephaly. As in our case, nearly all patients described showed a bilateral falciform fold extending from the disc to the inferior temporal quadrant of the fundus periphery. This similarity of clinical features of ocular anomalies in this group of microcephalic patients is suggestive of a clinical entity.

Most instances of this syndrome were sporadic cases. The parents of the patients described by Gartner (1941) and Masuda (1962) were consanguineous, which might indicate autosomal recessive transmission. In our case, the possibility of intra-uterine damage as a result of pregnancy complications in the mother is to be considered. Very recently, Jarmas et al. (1981) observed the combination of falciform retinal folds, microphthalmia and microcephaly in two brothers, whose mother was decidely microcephalic but showed no ocular anomalies. The mother of the girl described by Pflüger (1885) likewise showed a degree of microcephaly without ocular anomalies. The observations of Jarmas et al. (1981) and Pflüger (1885) are compatible with autosomal dominant transmission with variable expression. However, there is as yet no certainty about the heredity of this condition.

Incontinentia pigmenti and the Reese-Blodi-Straatsma syndrome are the principal possibilities in differential diagnosis.

Incontinentia pigmenti (Bloch-Sulzberger syndrome) is characterized not only by anomalies of the eyes and the central nervous system but also by anomalies of the skin, teeth and nails — which of course are not necessarily all present in the individual patient (see also Chapter 9). Unlike incontinentia pigmenti, which is virtually limited to females, the combination of microcephaly and falciform retinal fold has been found in both sexes.

The syndrome described by Reese and Blodi (1950) and Reese and Straatsma (1958), which as a rule is probably based on trisomy 13, is characterized by malformations of organs other than only the eyes and the central nervous system, and thus differs from the above discussed syndrome.

RLF-like ocular anomalies in combination with congenital cranial changes such as hydrocephalus and microcephaly have been described by Krause (1946), and subsequently by others. This combination of ocular and cranial anomalies is interpreted by some investigators as "congenital encephalo-ophthalmic dysplasia", and is discussed in Chapter 9. The ocular anomalies of this syndrome are in my opinion based on a primary developmental disorder of the retinal vasculature (Chapter 9).

The next section of this chapter discusses the pathogenesis of congenital retinal fold. The formation of a falciform retinal fold in microcephaly as well as in several other conditions, is probably a result of disturbed foetal development of retinal vessels. It is therefore highly likely that the syndrome characterized by microcephaly and congenital retinal fold has the same pathogenesis as congenital encephalo-ophthalmic dysplasia, and can be regarded as a specific manifestation of the latter.

In view of the clinical features of the above described case of microcephaly combined with bilateral congenital retinal folds, I have included this patient's history in this chapter rather than in Chapter 9, section 4.

Falciform retinal fold has been observed also in patients with hydrocephalus (Warburg, 1978). In these cases, too, the pathogenesis of the ocular anomalies seems identical to that of other manifestations of "congenital encephalo-ophthalmic dysplasia" (Chapter 9, section 4).

## 7.5 Pathogenesis of congenital retinal fold

Several hypotheses have been advanced regarding the pathogenesis of congenital retinal fold. Pflüger (1885), who described bilateral falciform retinal folds in the inferior temporal quadrant of the fundus in a girl with some degree of microcephaly, ascribed these changes to contraction of cicatricial tissue in the vicinity of a coloboma. The atypical localization of the structures he described as coloboma could, he believed, be explained by some rotation of the eyeball in the course of foetal development.

The view that a falciform retinal fold might result from persistence of hyaloid vessels is not of recent date either. Sulzer (1888) already thought that the anomaly found in his patient was based on a developmental anomaly of the foetal vascular system of vitreous and retina. He based this view on the presence of a few structures on the posterior side of the lens, which he regarded as remnants of the lens capsule.

The most widely known hypothesis on the pathogenesis of congenital retinal fold is that advanced by Mann (1935). She held that the anomaly is a result of an abnormal "adhesion of the primary vitreous and its contents to one portion of the inner layer of the optic cup". The secondary vitreous which forms between these two structures later in the course of development, is absent at the site of the abnormal adhesion of the primary vitreous to the inner layer of the optic cup. Due to the production of secondary vitreous, the two structures are displaced near the site of the adhesion, the "inner layer of the optic cup being detached and raised up in a ridge, and the contents of the primary vitreous becoming displaced from the optic axis towards the side of the adhesion". This theory was based mainly on the observation (made by Mann and a few other investigators) of vascularized tissue attached to the neuroretina at the site of the "ridge of the fold". This tissue was believed to originate from the primary vitreous and the hyaloid vessels, and to have raised the neuroretina from its pigmented layer at the site of the adhesion.

Another microscopical observation which supported Mann's theory that a congenital retinal fold is formed early in the course of foetal development, was the presence of atypical rosettes and signs of hypoplasia in the neuroretina at the site of the falciform fold. Mann maintained that these changes were to be expected because the fold was probably formed before retinal differentiation was far advanced.

As early as 1902, Salffner described his histopathological findings in an eye with a congenital retinal fold. This author, too, found a tissue strand connected with the apex of the retinal duplicature, in which he found blood

vessels which he regarded as hyaloid vessels. The tissue strand, however, consisted mainly of (ectodermal) glia cells which, he thought, originated mainly
from the optic nerve and had grown in anterior direction along the hyaloid
artery.

So far, the view that the formation of a congenital retinal fold is a result of
or related to a disturbance in the development of the primary vitreous has
been fairly generally accepted. Some authors even go so far as to regard the
congenital retinal fold as synonymous with "posterior persistent hyperplastic
primary vitreous" (Michaelson, 1965; Pruett and Schepens, 1970; Pruett,
1975).

Badtke (1954, 1960) pointed out that in several cases of congenital retinal
fold it was impossible to find remnants of hyaloidal vessels or other elements
of the primary vitreous. Persistence of these structures can therefore not be
regarded as of primary significance in the formation of a falciform retinal fold.
In Badtke's opinion, and that of Palich-Szántó (1954), the disorder affects
the development of the ectodermal optic cup in the region of the foetal
ocular fissure. Like the previously discussed theories, this hypothesis postulates that a congenital retinal fold is a disturbance which occurs early in the
course of foetal development.

In my opinion, there are clear indications that, in most cases, a congenital
retinal fold results from a disturbance which occurs during the final months
of intra-uterine development and that in fact the complete picture of the anomaly does not develop until after birth. Before discussing the pathogenesis as
I envisage it, it should be pointed out that (as already mentioned previously)
a congenital retinal fold is decidedly not a clinical entity. It is therefore
possible that a pathogenesis other than the one I envisage may be involved in
some cases (see also the final subsection of this chapter).

An important argument against the postulate that congenital retinal folds
are usually a result of a developmental disorder (more specifically: persistence)
of the primary vitreous lies in the fact that in many cases there are no discernible hyaloid remnants. This fact has been established, not only by Badtke
(1954) but also by Weve (1935) and Joannidés and Protonotarios (1965) in
clinical observations, and by Ancona (1935) and Tillema (1937) in histopathological studies. Our DEVR patients with clinical symptoms of a congenital retinal fold, likewise showed no remnants of hyaloidal vessels or other elements of the primary vitreous. In several cases, however, I did find one or
several blood vessels localized very superficially near the ridge of the fold, and
more or less parallel to it. Both at ophthalmoscopy and at histological examination, such blood vessels are only too easily confused with persistent hyaloidal vessels. The fact that, in the fold, the retinal vessels continue to the
posterior side of the lens further increases the confusion.

A persistent hyaloid artery is nearly always connected with the posterior
pole of the lens or a point slightly nasal to it. In this respect it differs from
retinal vessels in the falciform fold, which are usually connected with the

posterior lens capsule in the inferior temporal quadrant near the equator of the lens.

That a congenital retinal fold can also develop after birth is demonstrated by observations on this anomaly in retrolental fibroplasia. Many publications on RLF describe this manifestation (Owens, 1955; Tasman, 1970). It is evident that persistence of the primary vitreous is of no significance in the pathogenesis of RLF, as several investigators (Terry, 1942; Reese, 1949) used to believe.

Undoubtedly, some published instances of congenital retinal fold can be ascribed to RLF. For example, probably, the patient described by Van Wien and Sullivan (1955). Weve (1953), too, was convinced — years after his first publications — that RLF was the cause of the anomalies found in some of the patients he described.

The formation of a falciform retinal fold in RLF is regarded as a result of local proliferations of fibrovascular tissue and contraction of these structures to a local mass of cicatricial tissue. It is not difficult to envisage that this tissue often constitutes a connection with the posterior lens capsule, for neovascularizations often grow from the retinal periphery in anterior direction, extending into the vitreous space where they establish contact with the posterior side of the lens (Kingham, 1977). The predilection of local masses of cicatricial tissue and of the falciform fold caused by these structures for the inferior temporal quadrant, corresponds with the predilection of neovascularizations for this part of the fundus. This pathogenesis is schematically represented in Figure 130.

To my mind it is certain that the pathogenesis of congenital retinal folds in DEVR is the same as that of these folds in RLF. Both conditions are characterized by disturbed vascularization of the peripheral retina, manifested especially in the inferior temporal quadrant of the fundus. In both conditions, secondary neovascularizations can occur in this part of the retina. The white tissue masses observed at the peripheral end of the raised radial folds in all our DEVR patients undoubtedly originate from neovascularizations and, in my opinion, cannot possibly be regarded as remnants of embryonic tissue, as Dudgeon (1980) postulates. The period of development of a falciform fold is less readily determinable in DEVR than in RLF, where of course the changes always develop postnatally. It is evident that, in DEVR, the anomaly cannot occur before the final two months of intra-uterine development, because it is only at about this time that the primary developmental disorder of the peripheral retinal vasculature occurs.

It is certainly possible that the secondary neovascularizations and the contraction of fibrovascular tissue do not lead to the formation of a radial fold until after a few months, and that consequently the clinical features of congenital retinal fold are not observed until some time after birth in DEVR. That the anomaly can be observed shortly after birth is demonstrated by the finding of a congenital retinal fold in OS of IV-1 F at the age of one month.

Congenital retinal folds which result from DEVR (whether or not it is diagnosed as such) therefore have a late foetal or even, possibly, a neonatal pathogenesis. The adjective "congenital" is therefore possibly wrong in some cases.

Falciform retinal folds have been observed shortly after birth, not only in DEVR and RLF but also in incontinentia pigmenti (Bloch-Sulzberger syndrome). Reports have been published by Findlay (1952), Grüneberg (1955) and Fried and Meyer-Schwickerath (1980). I agree with Best and Rensch (1974) that there are no clear indications of a role of anomalies in the development of the hyaloid system in the pathogenesis of this condition, as some investigators maintain.

For a more detailed description of the manifestations of this condition I refer to Chapter 9. At this time it is sufficient to point out that the primary lesion of the ocular fundus would seem to be occlusion and probably also disturbed development of the peripheral retinal vessels which, as in DEVR

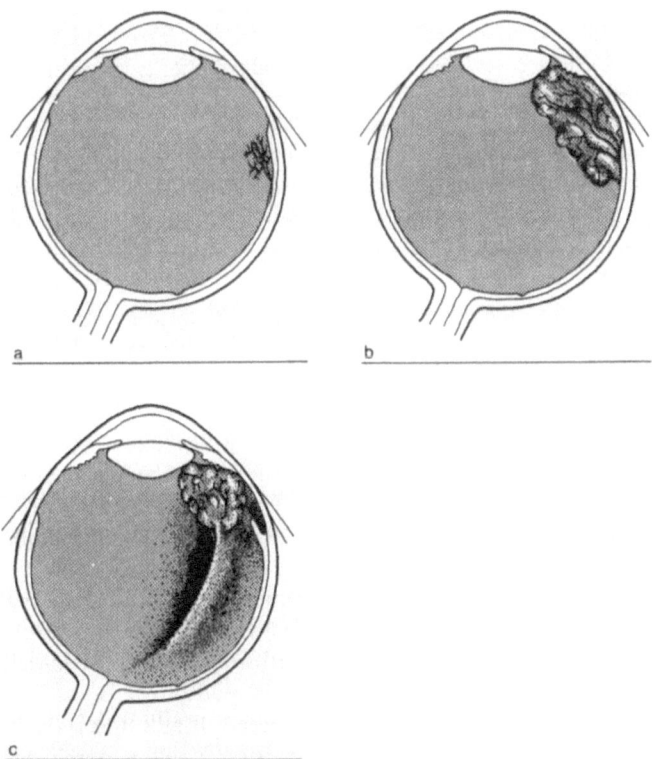

Figure 130. Pathogenesis of a falciform retinal fold. Neovascularizations develop in the temporal retinal periphery (a) and extend anteriorly into the vitreous space as far as the posterior side of the lens (b). Contraction of fibrovascular tissue causes formation of a retinal fold (c).

and RLF, leads to non-perfusion of the temporal retinal periphery at a neonatal age.

I am therefore convinced that the pathogenesis of a falciform retinal fold
in incontinentia pigmenti is mainly a result of secondary retinal neovascularizations, as in DEVR and RLF, and likewise occurs only during or after the
phase of development of peripheral retinal vessels. The fact that the acute
phase of incontinentia pigmenti is usually observed within a few days of birth
or, in the case of congenital symptoms, has probably occurred shortly before
birth, is entirely consistent with the abovementioned hypothesis.

Like patients with DEVR, RLF and incontinentia pigmenti, our female
patient with bilateral falciform retinal folds and microcephaly showed no evidence of a disturbance in early embryonic development, nor any discernible
remnants of persistent hyaloidal vessels. The incomplete vascularization of
the retina outside the posterior pole in both eyes demonstrated that – in this
case, too – disturbed vascularization had led to the retinal deformation. The
identical fundus features with bilateral retinal folds in the inferior temporal
quadrant which Pflüger (1885), Stübel (1927), Gartner (1941) and Von
Barsewisch (1968) described in microcephalic patients, suggest an identical
pathogenesis.

I would summarize my conclusions from the above observations as follows:
a falciform retinal fold of the type found in DEVR, incontinentia pigmenti,
and also in combination with microcephaly, is the result of a disorder of the
peripheral retinal vascularization which occurs late in the course of development, and its pathogenesis is similar to that of the falciform retinal fold
found in RLF.

In all these conditions, total retinal detachment with massive organizations
throughout the vitreous space can develop at an early age if the vascular proliferation is more severe. Such manifestations have been described in the literature, usually as "pseudoglioma".

There are also reports on several not exactly diagnosed cases of the combination of falciform retinal fold and total retinal detachment with vitreous
organizations, either in a single patient (Weve, 1935; Otuki, 1939; Poulsen,
1947; Von Winning, 1952; Heydenreich, 1959) or in several members of the
same family (Weve, 1935; Babel, 1966).

Norrie's disease (see also Chapter 9) is manifested in the vast majority of
cases by congenital or immediately postnatal leucocoria as a result of total
retinal detachment (Warburg, 1966). Falciform retinal folds have been observed in a few cases of this condition (Jacklin, 1980).

Although the pathogenesis of Norrie's disease is still uncertain, the histopathological findings obtained in this condition would certainly seem to be
compatible with a proliferative retinopathy secondary to disturbed retinal
vascularization. Fluorescein-angiographic findings recently obtained in a neonate (Fujita et al., 1980) support this postulate. Although it is yet to be
proven, it seems plausible that the falciform retinal fold (and of course also

the much more frequently observed total retinal detachment) in Norrie's disease – as in the other conditions discussed above – results from neovascularizations which occur late in the course of development.

The Japanese investigator Nishimura (1980) recently pointed out the absence of peripheral retinal vasculature in a number of patients with falciform retinal folds who had been born at term. The author described these cases as "retinopathy of prematurity in term infants". I would attach paramount importance to examination of relatives of such patients, because the manifestations described are strongly suggestive of DEVR.

### 7.5.a. Early versus late hypothesis

It has been attempted above to demonstrate that a falciform retinal fold is a complication to be found in several conditions, usually as a result of late foetal or even neonatal developmental disorders.

The question arises whether – apart from the pathogenesis outlined above – there are cases which involve an early developmental disorder, as assumed by Mann and other authors. Remnants of the hyaloid system and other primary vitreous elements have been ophthalmoscopically observed near the falciform fold in many cases. The ascription of preretinal membranes and superficially localized blood vessels in the fold to elements of the hyaloid system on the basis of a clinical observation seems rather questionable. In most cases a histological diagnosis cannot be made, because enucleation of eyes with a falciform retinal fold is fortunately a rare procedure nowadays.

For a critical review of the literature on congenital retinal fold as a manifestation of so-called posterior persistent hyperplastic primary vitreous (PHPV) I refer to section 13.1.

Finally, the postulate that a falciform retinal fold results from an anomaly in the region of the embryonic ocular fissure (Pflüger, 1885; Badtke, 1954, 1960; Palich-Szántó, 1954) strikes me as hardly acceptable, because it is extremely rare to find the anomaly in the area where the embryonic optic cup closes, i.e. the inferior aspect of the eyeball, or even in the sector localized slightly nasal to it. Reports on well-documented cases of falciform retinal fold in this region are rare (Eisenberg, 1948).

### 7.5.b Additional pathogenic mechanisms

In the discussion of the presumably late pathogenesis of falciform retinal folds, local neovascularizations arising from retinal vessels in the peripheral fundus were regarded as the primary cause of the lesion. It is highly unlikely that these proliferations (and local vitreous haemorrhages from these vessels, as observed in the active phase of RLF: King, 1950; Foos, 1975) are the principal basis of the cicatricial tissue found at the peripheral end of a falciform retinal fold. However, it cannot be excluded that the stimulus to form cicatricial tissue can also arise from other peripheral structures, e.g. the avascular retinal periphery, as Flynn et al. (1979) assumed to be the case in RLF.

That simple traction exerted by peripheral cicatricial tissue does not seem to be the only prerequisite for falciform fold formation, is apparent from the fact that proliferative retinopathies which develop later than the neonatal age – e.g. diabetic retinopathy, sickle cell retinopathy, Eales' disease, etc. – never show the features of a typical falciform fold. Retinal folds of the type previously described in some of our DEVR patients are never found in the above conditions, even though these are not infrequently accompanied by local fibrovascular proliferations in the fundus periphery. The odd pattern of the retinal vessels in the posterior pole in eyes with a congenital retinal fold is wellknown. Most clinical studies on this condition mentioned the peculiar accumulation of parallel vascular branches in the attached parts of the neuroretina. This phenomenon can only be explained by marked temporal displacement of retinal vessels and their rotation on their point of fixation at the site of the disc.

In Chapter 5 I have advanced a hypothesis to explain this phenomenon of displacement of retinal vessels in DEVR. According to this hypothesis, an aberrant configuration of retinal vessels in DEVR does not result exclusively from traction exerted by secondary preretinal vitreous organization, but some deformation of the vascular bed occurs in direct response to the vascular development per se.

The resulting deformation of retinal vessels is illustrated in Figure 121 of Chapter 5, which shows temporal displacement of all retinal vessels and rotation of the superior branches of the central artery and vein in a direction opposed to the rotation of the inferior branches of these vessels. The superficial retinal layers are deformed due to displacement from two different directions towards one meridian: the horizontal meridian or the one slightly inferior to it. It is quite conceivable that, as a result, the neuroretina at this site tends to detach itself from the pigmented layer in a radial fold. Whether this displacement of retinal vessels and inner retinal layers as a result of the mechanism postulated is as such able to create the duplicature, remains uncertain.

The fact that falciform retinal folds are generally found only in severe forms of RLF and DEVR, in which signs of old fibrovascular proliferations are present, suggests that this is not the case. The mechanism outlined above can only be assigned an additional role in the pathogenesis of a congenital retinal fold.

### 7.5.c  *Unilateral congenital retinal fold of obscure pathogenesis*

The patient whose case history follows, showed the features of unilateral congenital retinal fold. Unlike previously described patients, this boy showed no evidence of a developmental disorder of the retinal vasculature.

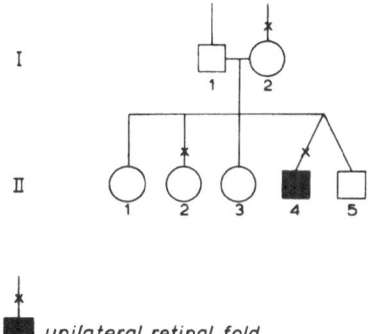

unilateral retinal fold

Figure 131. Pedigree of the family of patient II-4 (11-05-73).

*Case history of patient II-4 (11-05-73) (Figure 131)*

*History*

This boy was referred to our department at age 3 with a recently detected divergent position of OD. He had been born as one of a pair of apparently not identical twins. Pregnancy and parturition had been uneventful. The boy's birth weight was 2500 g. His postnatal condition was good. He was placed in an incubator for a few days but received hardly any oxygen. His twin brother (II-5) was in moderate condition and remained in the incubator for a few weeks. No ocular or visual complaints in members of the boy's family.

*Ophthlamological examination (age 3)*

| | |
|---|---|
| Visual acuity | VOD: 1/60. |
| | VOS: 0.6, uncorrected. |
| Eye position | Divergent strabismus OD; no nystagmus. |
| Intraocular pressure | OD: 14 mm Hg. |
| | OS: 15 mm Hg. |
| Anterior segments | ODS: Normal. |
| Vitreous | OD: Minute particles; normal structure. |
| | OS: Normal. |
| Fundi | OD: A whitish, somewhat transparent tissue strand extends from the disc to the inferior temporal sector. Immediate inferior and temporal to the disc, this strand seems connected with a raised fold of the neuroretina. About three disc diameters away from the disc, there is a distinct swelling in the retinal fold, which at this site shows a striking yellow colour. This colour and the localization near the centre of the posterior pole suggest that the yellow spot is included in the retinal fold. |

258

Fluorescein angiogram

Outside the posterior pole the radial fold detaches from the retina and continues as a preretinal tissue strand to the extreme fundus periphery, where it attaches with a wide, not very prominent plaque of white glious tissue.

OS: Entirely normal posterior pole and periphery.

OD: The early phase of the disc shows more or less normal filling of the central retinal artery, although this is slightly deformed in the direction of the fold. The superior temporal artery extends in the upper margin of the retinal fold over a small distance, but slightly temporal to the disc enters the attached part of the retina, where it ramifies. Immediately superior to the fold, near the disc, the retinal pigment epithelium shows a fair-sized atrophic scar. The venous phase clearly reveals retinal vessels in the falciform fold immediately temporal and inferior to the posterior pole; the fold is wrinkled at this site (Figure 132). The late phase shows diffuse hyperfluorescence of the entire retinal fold with leakage into the vitreous (Figure 133). No remnants of hyaloid vessels are visible anywhere. The vascularization of the peripheral retina outside the fold is normally developed throughout.

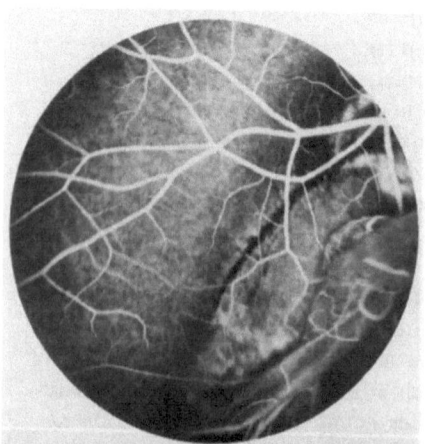 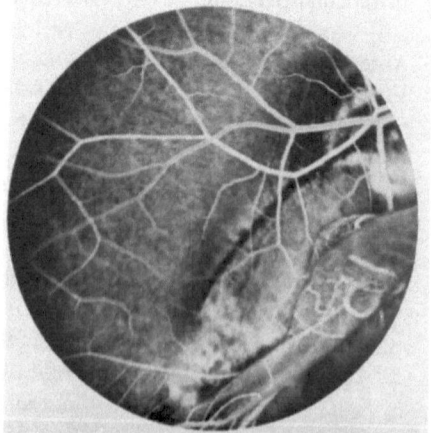

Figure 132. OD. Stereoscopic fluorescein angiogram of the posterior pole. Several retinal blood vessels are visible in the falciform fold.

*Family study*
The mother (I-2) and a sister (II-2) showed no fundus changes in mydriasis. The other members of the family could not be examined.

*Laboratory findings*

| | |
|---|---|
| Toxoplasmosis | Negative immunofluorescence; negative complement fixation test. |
| Toxocara | Negative complement fixation test. |
| Ascaris | Negative complement fixation test. |

*Course*
At age 8, visual acuity is unchanged after correction of slight myopia. The features of the media and fundi are likewise unchanged.

*Summary and conclusions*
The fundus anomaly described above evidently has the character of a congenital retinal fold, as the presence of retinal blood vessels in the fold demonstrates. However, there are a few differences from the retinal folds normally observed in DEVR and RLF: the fold does not as such completely traverse the fundus periphery, but outside the posterior pole continues as a tissue strand, extending to the pars plana. Another difference is the absence of symptoms indicating disturbed development of the retinal peripheral vasculature. Moreover, the features of the central part of the fold differ slightly from those observed in most cases of congenital retinal fold. The unusual swelling near the centre of the posterior pole was not observed in my other cases, nor is it mentioned in the literature.

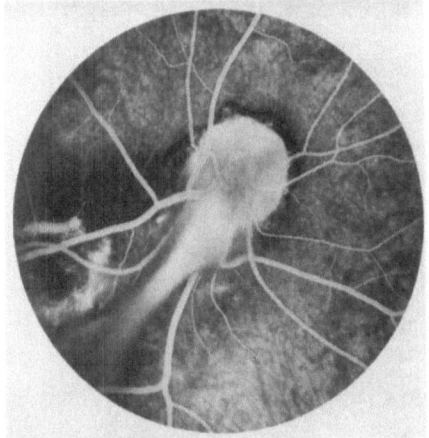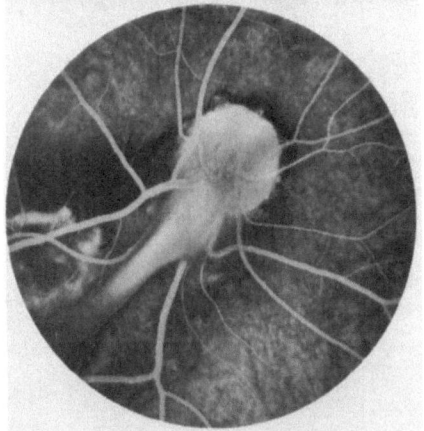

Figure 133. Stereoscopic fluorescein angiogram. Late phase shows hyperfluorescence of the fold near the disc.

The question may arise whether the pathogenesis of the falciform fold in this case might be consistent with one of the classical hypotheses, e.g. that advanced by Mann (1935) or by Badtke (1960). The localization of the lesion, however, is not suggestive of a developmental disorder in the region of the embryonic ocular fissure. The presence of a preretinal tissue strand in the fundus periphery might be interpreted as indicating a remnant of the primary vitreous; however, the absence of hyaloid vessels renders this interpretation speculative.

It seems better to admit my inability to reconstruct the pathogenesis of the anomaly in this patient. The principal conclusion to be drawn from the findings obtained is that not every (congenital) retinal fold results from a late embryonic developmental disorder of the retinal vasculature, but that the anomaly can in some cases have a different cause.

CHAPTER 8

# RETROLENTAL FIBROPLASIA

Retrolental fibroplasia is a condition based on a lesion of the developing retinal vascular system caused by neonatal oxygen administration to prematurely born infants. The symptoms of this condition were first described by Terry in 1942, but it was not until 1951 that oxygen administration was identified as the cause of these symptoms (Campbell, 1951). Controlled studies (Patz et al., 1952; Kinsey and Hemphill, 1955; Kinsey, 1956) confirmed the hypothesis that oxygen administration played an important role in the pathogenesis of RLF.

## 8.1 Clinical symptoms

### 8.1.a Active retrolental fibroplasia

The retinal vascular lesions which develop in response to neonatal oxygen administration, are qualified as acute or active RLF. Involution of these vascular changes usually occurs after a few months, and this is associated with fibrosis or the development of other residual symptoms. From this phase on, the term cicatricial RLF applies.

Classification of active RLF in various stages has been suggested by several authors (Reese et al., 1953; Schaffer et al., 1979).

The most pronounced symptoms of active RLF are usually found in the temporal fundus periphery which, as already explained, is the last part of the retina to be vascularized in normal embyronic development. The presence of a rather pale avascular retina peripheral to the temporal equator in a premature infant, therefore, does not indicate the presence of slight RLF but is an expression of the incomplete vascularization which is physiological in such children. In my opinion this feature of the peripheral retina in premature infants is often erroneously regarded as a symptom of RLF.

The transition from vascular to avascular retina is rather abrupt in premature infants who have received no oxygen administration. An early symptom of active RLF, however, is the development at the site of this transition of a slightly raised, pale structure in which abnormally dilatated arterioles and veins terminate on the central side (Flynn et al., 1977; Flynn et al., 1979). The fluorescein angiogram of this area shows filling of this transitional structure between vascular and avascular retina, but fails to visualize a vascular pattern. The late phase discloses marked leakage from this structure. Flynn et al. (1977, 1979) described this structure as an arteriovenous shunt or mesenchymal shunt. In this stage, the large retinal vessels in the posterior pole often show some dilatation and tortuosity. In a more advanced stage of RLF, neovascularizations arise from the retinal vessels posterior to the mesenchymal shunt and enter the vitreous space through the internal limiting membrane. In other cases the neovascularizations arise from the mesenchymal shunt itself (Kingham, 1977). Intraretinal haemorrhages are not rare in this stage, and sometimes haemorrhages in the vitreous space are observed. In severe cases the peripheral neovascularizations grow deep into the vitreous space. They often also grow anteriorly until they touch the posterior lens capsule.

Any RLF associated with extraretinal neovascularizations entails a risk of total or partial tractional retinal detachment.

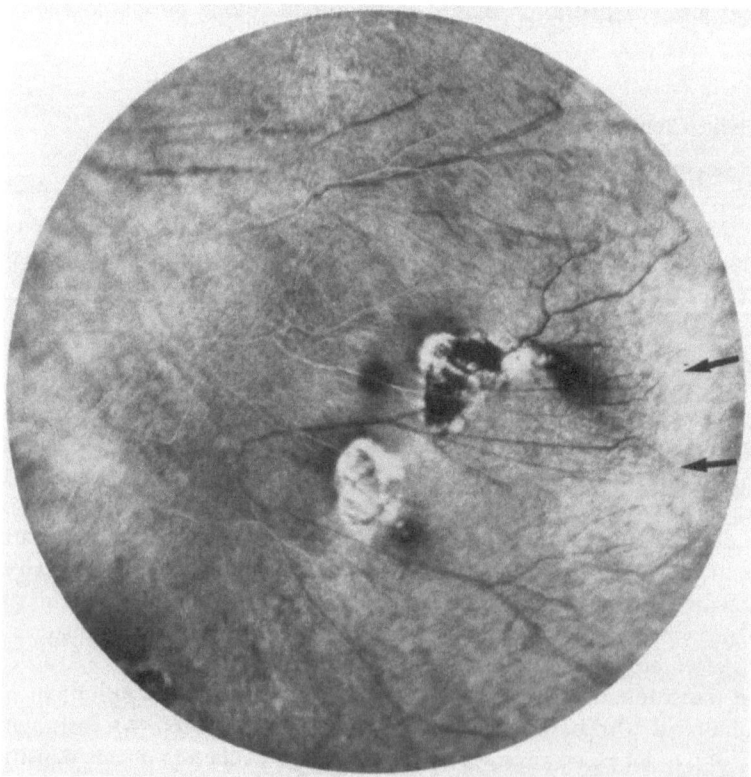

Figure 134. OS. Fluorescein angiogram of the temporal fundus periphery in a patient with RLF. The venous vascular ramifications of the retina have not yet filled. The retinal vasculature terminates immediately anterior to the equator (arrows).

### 8.1.b  Cicatricial retrolental fibroplasia

The changes which persist after the acute phase are collectively known as cicatricial RLF. As for active RLF, systems have been advanced to classify cicatricial RLF according to severity (Reese et al., 1953; McCormick, 1977; Patz, 1975; Schaffer et al., 1979). In mild cases of cicatricial RLF, retinal pigmentations are found, as a rule in the temporal fundus periphery. Moreover, thin veils are sometimes visible in the vitreous space, as a rule localized preretinally in the temporal periphery.

Surprisingly, none of the classifications of cicatricial RLF makes mention of the absence of retinal vessels in the temporal fundus periphery, although this is readily visible at slit-lamp biomicroscopy or fluorescein angiography (Figure 134). This incomplete vascularization of the peripheral fundus is a basic characteristic of RLF, and one that is rarely absent. Moderate or high myopia is not uncommon in RLF (Hittner et al., 1978), and is often associated with atrophic lesions of the choroid and pigmented layer in the posterior pole (Figure 135).

In many cases there is a significant difference in refraction between the two eyes, which can lead to amblyopia. Another phenomenon often observed even in mild cases of RLF is the wide positive kappa angle associated with a pseudo-divergent eye position. This is caused by temporal or inferior temporal ectopia of the macula, accompanied by some deformation of the retinal vessels in the posterior pole (Figure 136).

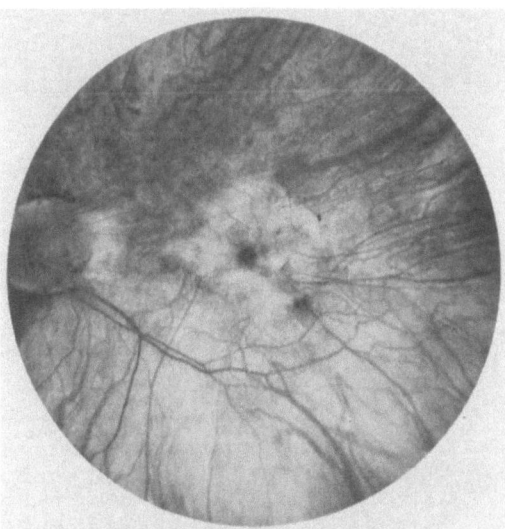

Figure 135. The posterior pole of the same eye as in Figure 134 shows extensive atrophic changes of the choroid and pigment epithelium.

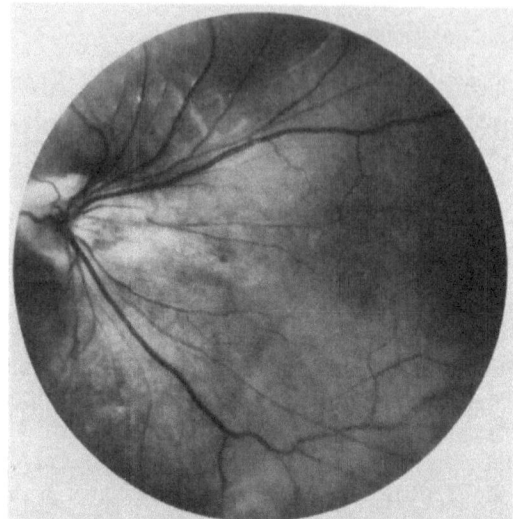

Figure 136. Abnormal vascular configuration and ectopia of the macula in cicatricial RLF. The features are identical to those of DEVR.

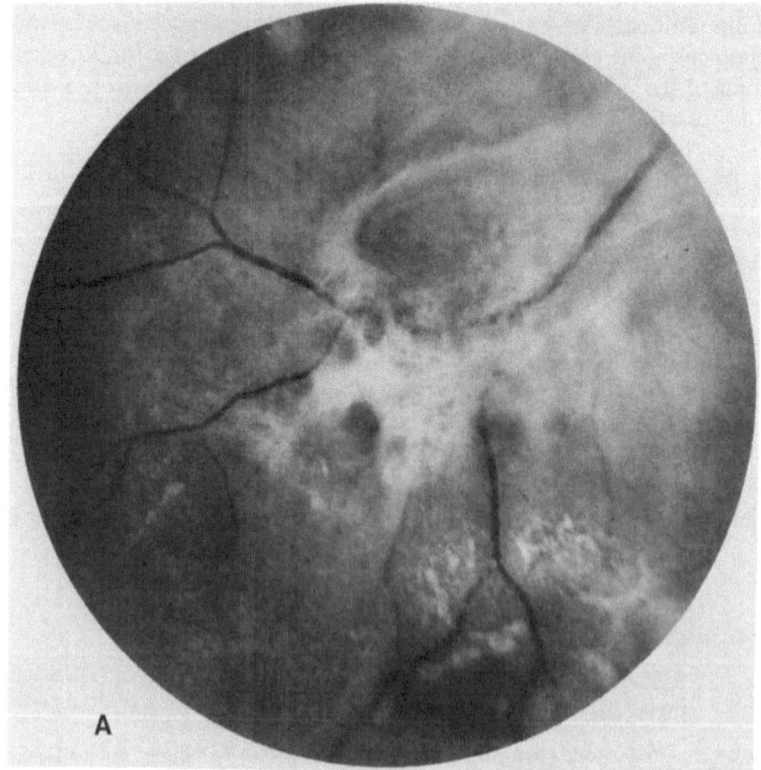

Figure 137. A) OD. Preretinal vitreous organizations near the inferior temporal vessels.

More severe cases of cicatricial RLF are characterized by fibrovascular pro-liferations, usually localized anterior to the temporal fundus periphery. Con-traction of this fibrotic tissue has often led to traction on the retina in tem-poral direction.

A wellknown complication is a falciform retinal fold, which in RLF usually extends from the disc through the centre of the posterior pole to the tem-poral fundus periphery, where it is usually connected with the posterior lens capsule via cicatricial tissue (Reese and Stepanik, 1954).

In some cases traction has given rise to a peripheral retinal detachment which can be fairly stable. An eye thus affected can have fair visual acuity as long as no duplicature has formed in the posterior pole.

In severe cases of cicatricial RLF, significant organizations of glial tissues can occur in the posterior cortex of the vitreous, with strong adhesions to the

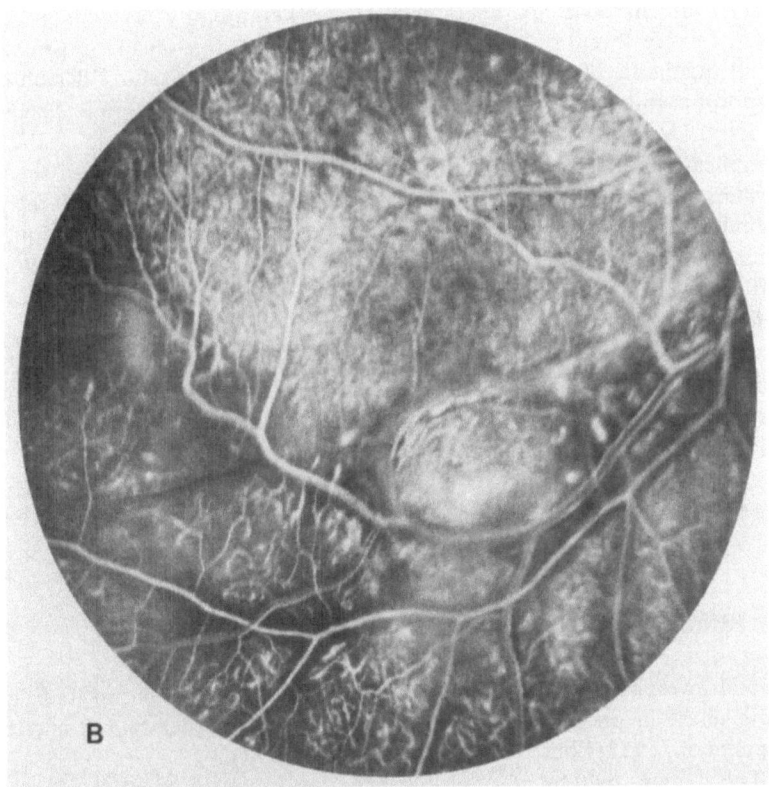

Figure 137. B) Fluorescein angiogram of the same area. Abnormal structure of the capillary network, broadened periarterial capillary-free zones and constriction of the arterioles near their origin at the inferior temporal artery.

retina, both in the periphery and in the posterior pole (Figure 137A). The fluorescein angiogram of such structures shows that they are often avascular, and need not originate from retinal vascular proliferations (Figure 137B).

Another interesting angiographic feature in cicatricial RLF is likewise demonstrated in Figure 137B: significant broadening of the periarterial capillary-free zone and apparent stenosis of the smaller ramifications of the temporal artery, especially near their origin. Few clinical studies on RLF have so far mentioned this phenomenon, and further investigation would seem to be desirable.

Anomalies of the anterior segment are not uncommon (Cohen et al., 1964; Hittner et al., 1979). In many cases there is a shallow, sometimes even a collapsed anterior chamber which can lead to glaucoma as a result of occlusion of the iridocorneal angle. A less common finding is an abnormally deep anterior chamber (Cohen et al., 1964). The iris often shows synechiae and loss of stroma, so that the pupil is of irregular shape. Varying degrees of lens opacity are likewise not uncommon. Band keratopathy develops in severe cases. In very severe cases of RLF there is marked fibrovascular organization in all quadrants of the vitreous space, leading to total retinal detachment. Hypotonia and shrinking of the eyeball is often seen in such terminal stages.

Exudative and rhegmatogenous retinal detachment are among the late complications of cicatricial RLF. The latter type is more common than the former, and usually develops as a result of small multiple defects in the peripheral retina. Due to their small dimensions and peripheral localization, and because of the often present preretinal vitreous opacities, it is often very difficult to detect such defects (Tasman, 1975). As in the case of DEVR, these defects are usually localized in the temporal periphery (Tasman, 1970).

A less common phenomenon is retinal detachment as a result of accumulation of subretinal exudates (Tasman, 1976). In most cases, such exudates form in or temporal to the posterior pole and cause retinal detachment which it is difficult to treat by operation.

## 8.2 Histology

Several investigators have studied the histopathological lesions of RLF in the acute phase in premature neonates given oxygen (Friedenwald et al., 1951; Reese et al., 1952; Foos, 1975; Kushner et al., 1977).

The earliest light-microscopic changes occur in the inner layers of the neuroretina at the site of the most peripheral zone, where primitive vessels develop centrifugally. This zone, which on the central side merges into newly formed primitive capillaries and on the peripheral side is adjacent to the not yet vascularized part of the retina, consists of conglomerates of mesenchymal cells with PAS-positive inclusions in the cytoplasm, localized in the most superficial layers of the neuroretina.

In response to neonatal oxygen administration, abnormal proliferations of these mesenchymal cells develop which cause thickening of the retina. Transverse sections through the retina reveal irregular vascular canals, mostly localized on the central side of the conglomerates of mesenchymal cells. These microscopic structures correspond with the structure interpreted ophthalmoscopically and fluorographically as arteriovenous shunt and, in view of the cell type involved, are also known as mesenchymal shunt (Flynn et al., 1977; Kushner et al., 1977). In trypsin-digest specimens, the retinal vascular bed posterior to this shunt shows peculiar dilatations and small outpouchings of some capillaries (Kushner et al., 1977), which can also be observed on some fluorescein angiograms of active RLF.

In a subsequent stage of RLF, the microscopic specimen is found to contain primitive capillaries which, from the posterior aspect of the mesenchymal tissue of the arteriovenous shunt in the retina, invade the vitreous (Foos, 1975). These vessels are made up of endothelial cells, a few intramural pericytes, and a delicate basement membrane (Foos, 1975). Specimens of eyes with advanced severe RLF usually show funnel-shaped retinal detachment, with a large plaque of fibrovascular tissue forming the connection with the posterior lens capsule. The detached neuroretina often shows pseudorosettes (Klein, 1949).

## 8.3 The influence of oxygen on the development of the immature retinal vasculature

*Experimental studies*

The influence of administration of increased oxygen concentrations to neonates has been studied in many animal species. The retinal vasculature in several mammals is incompletely developed at (normal) birth and develops to its adult configuration during the neonatal period. Experiments have shown that such immature vascular systems are very sensitive to administration of increased oxygen concentrations. In full-term neonates of such animals, the toxic effect of oxygen on the retina can be successfully studied.

Ashton's experiments have been of great importance for our knowledge of the pathogenesis of RLF. Oxygen administration to newborn kittens leads within about 6 hours to occlusion of the immature capillaries, soon followed by degenerative changes in the cytoplasm of the endothelial cells of these capillaries (Ashton and Pedler, 1961).

The pathogenesis of this early effect of oxygen still remains partly obscure. Vacuoles form in the endothelial cells, and these cells disintegrate soon after, so that the already stenosed lumen of the affected capillaries is filled with remnants of cellular material. Similar light-microscopic or electron-microscopic changes suggestive of primary damage caused by oxygen cannot be found either in other vessels of newborn kittens or in other neuroretinal cells. However, Uemura et al. (1977) were able to demonstrate toxic degeneration of the outer segments of the receptor cells in addition to oxygen damage of endothelial cells in newborn rabbits, which made a rapid recovery after return to a normal atmosphere. Oxygen damage of immature retinal capillaries, as found in cats and other test animals, is not confined to the endothelial cells. Pericytes of this part of the vascular bed likewise disintegrate, often leaving only a tubular basement membrane structure with or without remnants of degenerated cells, which sometimes provoke a macrophage reaction (Ashton, 1970). Return of the kittens to a normal atmosphere is followed by a phase of proliferation of endothelial cells, which form vascular buds that grow into the vitreous through the internal limiting membrane. In this phase, Ashton (1970) also observed another electron-microscopic phenomenon: the Müller cells in the innermost layers of the neuroretina form buds which protrude into the vitreous space but remain covered by the internal limiting membrane. After return of the kittens to a normal atmosphere, the retinal capillaries whose endothelial cells have not been totally destroyed by oxygen show bizarre proliferations of endothelial cells, sometimes forming several layers of these cells in the vascular wall (Patz, 1965).

Some endothelial cells still show swelling of mitochondria with loss of mitochondrial crests and vacuoles of the cytoplasm 14 days after termination of the hyperoxia (Patz, 1965).

The response of various mammals to neonatal oxygen administraion can vary widely: in mice, which at birth have a poorly developed retinal vascular system and still show an extensive network of hyaloid vessels, oxygen administration can induce marked proliferation of the hyaloid vessels and neovascularizations on the iris (Gyllenstein and Hellstrom, 1955; Patz, 1965).

To which extent the vascular lesions of human RLF are caused by diffusion of oxygen from the choroid, cannot be established with certainty at this time. It may well be that the supply of oxygen from the choriocapillaries plays a more important role in the pathogenesis of RLF than the supply of oxygen by the retinal arterioles because the latter, unlike the former, show significant constriction during hyperoxia. The effect of artificial retinal detachment on the oxygen damage to immature retinal vessels has demonstrated the influence of oxygen diffusion from the choriocapillaries in animal experiments (Ashton and Cook, 1955).

## 8.4 Treatment

Coagulation treatment of RLF is still a rather controversial subject. Some authors, particularly in Japan, are fairly optimistic about the therapeutic results of early coagulation. Good results of photocoagulation have been reported in premature infants with active RLF (grade III according to Owens) by Nagata et al. (1972), Tanabe and Ikema (1972) and Nishimura et al. (1975). Some Western investigators have also reported a few instances of a favourable response of active RLF to cryocoagulation or photocoagulation (Hindle and Leyton, 1978; Harris, 1976; Payne and Patz, 1972). Other studies describe cryocoagulation of active proliferative RLF as ineffective or even deleterious (Kingham, 1978). Harris (1976) pointed out that vitreous haemorrhages may occur, especially after photocoagulation.

One problem in evaluating the effect of coagulation is the high incidence of spontaneous regression of vascular proliferations in active RLF. It seems highly likely that, in a number of successfully treated cases, regression of the neovascularizations would also have occurred without treatment (Nagata, 1977; Kingham, 1978). A prospective controlled clinical trial might contribute to our knowledge of the importance of coagulation in active RLF. Some authors consider the possibilities to perform such a study to be rather limited (Kalina, 1980).

The problems encountered in the operative treatment of retinal detachment in cicatricial RLF are the same as those in the treatment of DEVR. Tractional and rhegmatogenous retinal detachment in RLF has been treated by conventional scleral buckling techniques, sometimes even in infants, with encouraging results (McPherson and Hittner, 1979). Vitrectomy procedures have also been used, but their efficacy in the treatment of RLF is still uncertain. Tasman (1979) reported a high incidence of retinal re-detachment in a small series of patients. This may have been due to the difficulty of adequate removal of the cortical vitreous in cicatricial RLF.

## 8.5 Differential diagnosis

As already pointed out, the clinical symptoms of RLF and DEVR are highly similar. Both conditions result from a disturbance in the late development of the retinal vasculature. The difference is that RLF is caused by exogenous factors, whereas DEVR is caused by a pathological gene. Goldschmidt (1935) described such an exogenously influenced imitation of a genetically determined condition as "phenocopy". We can therefore regard RLF as a phenocopy of DEVR. It is remarkable that the phenocopy was the first of the two conditions to be detected, especially because its history is still relatively short.

It is evident that differential diagnosis between the two conditions is based mainly on the neonatal history, and the ophthalmological history and examination of family members.

An important question is whether the ocular anomalies in the two conditions are entirely identical or whether differences may be demonstrable in some cases. In my opinion it is usually impossible in the individual patient to distinguish the anomalies of DEVR from those of cicatricial RLF. The fundus changes as well as the anomalies which may be found in refraction, anterior segment and vitreous would seem to be clinically identical. The fluorescein angiogram in mild cases of cicatricial RLF reveals non-perfusion of the temporal retinal periphery, demarcated on the central side by a zone of aberrant vascular ramifications which show delicate dilatations and fluorescein leakage (Flynn et al., 1979). These features seem hardly different (if at all) from those of the fluorescein angiogram in DEVR.

According to Brockhurst et al. (1981) it is possible to distinguish DEVR from RLF by clinical examination in the two following respects: the neovascular membrane in DEVR, unlike in RLF, is posterior to the ora serrata, and, secondly, myopia is common in RLF, whereas eyes of DEVR patients are often hyperopic. It is my opinion that the neovascular membrane in both RLF and DEVR originates from the peripheral retina and may obscure the ora serrata and pars plana in the more severe cases of both conditions. Myopia, like in RLF, is very common in DEVR (Chapter 4.4) and, therefore, plays no role in the differential diagnosis of both disorders.

It may well be that certain characteristics are more frequent or more pronounced in one condition than in the other. For example, it seems that small neovascularizations persist longer and fibrose less quickly in DEVR than in RLF. However, such minor neovascularizations are incidentally also found in adults with RLF (Jampol and Goldbaum, 1980).

### 8.5.a  *"Retrolental fibroplasia" without neonatal oxygen administration or prematurity*

In the course of the years, several publications in the paediatric and ophthalmological literature have described RLF in individuals who had received no neonatal oxygen administration. Some had been prematurely born Huggert, 1954; Seedorff, 1968; Bruckner, 1968; Brockhurst and Chishti, 1975), while others had been born at term (Brockhurst and Chishti, 1975; Adamkin et al., 1977). Other studies mentioned RLF in full-term infants who had received only a small amount of oxygen (Kraushar et al., 1975) or who had no record of neonatal oxygen administration (Reese, 1949).

Symptoms of RLF have been reported also in premature infants who, despite neonatal oxygen administration, showed a persistently decreased arterial oxygen pressure in the high-oxygen environment, due to a congenital cardiac anomaly (Kalina et al., 1972; Foos, 1975; Naiman et al., 1979).

In view of such observations, many investigators regard RLF as a condition which can develop in full-term infants as well as in prematures, and in fact need not always be a result of increased arterial oxygen pressure in the newborn.

Several hypotheses have been advanced to explain the development of RLF under these conditions. Some authors consider it possible that, at parturition, the retina of the neonate is more sensitive to the increase in arterial oxygen pressure due to preceding intra-uterine hypoxia (Bruckner, 1968).

Adamkin et al. (1977) described severe RLF in a virtually full-term infant not given neonatal oxygen administration. Icterus neonatorum had necessitated postnatal exchange transfusions in this case. The authors maintained that increased arterial oxygen pressure due to the shift in the dissociation curve during the transfusions must have been responsible for the ocular complications.

Like Stefani and Ehalt (1974) and Svedburgh (1975), I would prefer to restrict the term RLF to cases in which the ocular changes result from neonatal oxygen administration.

Alhtough neonatal oxygen sensitivity can vary, RLF is an iatrogenic condition which, in principle, can be produced by oxygen administration in any premature baby.

When symptoms of RLF develop in infants not given neonatal oxygen administration, an endogenous disorder of retinal vascular development should be the first possibility considered. Although the cause of the anomaly is obscure in such cases, it is most likely to be found primarily in the infant. The pathogenesis of such an anomaly differs decidedly from that of retinal lesions caused in normal prematures by oxygen administration, and the term RLF is therefore confusing.

Another disadvantage of the term RLF in cases with no record of neonatal oxygen administration is that one tends to hold some exogenous cause responsible for the retinopathy. Although exogenous factors cannot be excluded, their role is in my opinion often overestimated, while on the other hand genetic factors are usually disregarded (quite erroneously).

It seems unlikely that RLF might develop solely as a result of exchange transfusions in full-term infants, or solely as a result of intra-uterine asphyxia, as some publications postulate. The simple fact that ocular complications are as a rule not found after exchange transfusions and intra-uterine hypoxia, warrants the conclusions that these conditions cannot have been the sole cause of the retinopathy.

At clinical examination of the individual patient, DEVR is indistinguishable from RLF. In the absence of a history of premature birth and neonatal oxygen administration, RLF-like symptoms should be primarily interpreted as suggestive of possible DEVR. However, most publications on patients with RLF for which no aetiological factors can be found in the neonatal history, make no mention of the possibility of DEVR. This is not surprising, because DEVR has only recently been given wider attention.

In the publications mentioned in the early paragraphs of this subsection, I found no ophthalmological data obtained by examination of family members, and the family history was often not even mentioned.

As already mentioned, a negative family history is not uncommon in DEVR; the only method to demonstrate the condition in such cases is by examination of the patient's parents and, if possible, of other close relatives. Even if examination of the parents fails to reveal anomalies, however, DEVR cannot be excluded with certainty, for penetrance is incomplete. Brockhurst and Chishti (1975) did mention DEVR as possible differential diagnosis in their report on six cases of cicatricial RLF without a history of neonatal oxygen administration. On the basis of the clinical findings in their patients, however, they excluded DEVR. As already mentioned, differential diagnosis between RLF and DEVR is impossible without a family study. In my opinion, the clinical manifestations described in this article are by no means incompatible with a diagnosis of DEVR.

Schulman et al. (1980) considered the diagnosis of DEVR in a fullterm patient with RLF-like changes in both fundi, who had received no neonatal oxygen administration. They examined the patient's mother, who showed no anomalies, but examination of the father was not possible. These authors correctly described their findings, not as RLF but as "fundus changes consistent with RLF" and "peripheral proliferative retinopathy".

At this time it is not clear whether RLF-like retinopathies not resulting from neonatal oxygen administration or DEVR, and not accompanied by general symptoms, are in the same aetiological group. Some of these cases may well be caused by a gene with a different autosomal dominant transmission, or by non-hereditary factors. I have observed a few instances of the occurrence of bilateral RLF-like juvenile proliferative retinopathies in otherwise healthy children whose relatives showed no fundus changes. Such observations may indicate that DEVR is not the only imitator of RLF.

Future research into RLF-like retinopathies with no exogenous cause in the neonatal history, will have to focus on the detection of genetic factors. The aetiological importance of DEVR in such cases can only be established by family studies.

## 8.6 Consequences of oxygen administration to premature neonates with the genotype of DEVR

An important question, which cannot be answered at this time, is whether premature neonates with the genotype of DEVR are excessively sensitive to oxygen.

It is conceivable that the already disturbed angiogenesis in DEVR stagnates more readily in response to increased arterial oxygen pressure than in normal premature infants. We do not know whether vascular development merely stagnates in DEVR, or also takes a retarded course. If the latter is true, then the vascular system in a premature neonate should be in a less mature stage than might be expcted on the basis of gestational age, and sensitivity to oxygen should be relatively high.

It is very difficult to demonstratè a possibly increased sensitivity of the retina to oxygen administration in DEVR by clinical examination. The variability of expression of the condition makes it virtually impossible to establish – in the incidental DEVR patient given neonatal oxygen administration – to which extent the symptoms are of genetic origin, and to which extent they are caused by exogenous factors.

The presence of marked proliferative changes in an occasional member of our DEVR families who received neonatal oxygen administration (V-52 A) in a period in which this treatment rarely gives rise to serious complications, might indicate an additive effect of endogenous and exogenous factors.

The extent to which neonatal sensitivity to oxygen administration is genetically determined, can be established only by further research.

CHAPTER 9

# AFFECTIONS WITH CONGENITAL OR NEONATAL
# VITREOUS ORGANIZATIONS AND RETINAL DETACHMENT

## 9.1 Incontinentia pigmenti (Bloch-Sulzberger syndrome)

Incontinentia pigmenti is a rare condition which becomes clinically manifest
in female infants. It is usually characterized by erythematous skin rashes and
formation of intradermal vesicles. These lesions are often already present at
birth, but may also develop in the neonatal period. There is usually marked
eosinophilia of the blood during this active period. The inflammatory eruptions
gradually disappear, leaving pigmented scars which usually fade in the course
of a few years. The condition may be accompanied by anomalies of the central nervous system, hair, teeth, skeleton and eyes. In severe cases the ocular
anomalies can cause a grave visual handicap, thus overshadowing the other,
usually less disabling changes.

### 9.1.a  Clinical ocular symptoms

The classical fundus symptoms in incontinentia pigmenti are massive vitreous
organizations with total retinal detachment, producing the clinical picture of
a "pseudoglioma". The young patient described by Bloch (1925) already
showed this anomaly in one eye, which was enucleated because a retinoblastoma was suspected. Carney (1975) collected from the world literature
653 cases of incontinentia pigmenti. Of the 455 cases suitable for statistical
analysis, 160 showed ocular anomalies. Strabismus was the most frequently
found anomaly (83 cases). Other not uncommon symptoms were cataract
(18 cases), retinal detachment (13), microphthalmia (13), atrophy of the
optic nerve (18), pseudoglioma (16), retinal telangiectases (10) and retinal
pigmentations (18 cases).

Disease symptoms have also been observed in the anterior segment: posterior synechiae were described by Uebel et al. (1950), Scott et al. (1955),
Wollensak (1959) and Mensheha-Manhart et al. (1975).

Retinal vascular anomalies have been described by such authors as Lieb
and Guerry (1956) and Krey and Laux (1974).

Conspicuous aberrations of the peripheral retinal vasculature have been
described by Best and Rentsch (1974) and Watzke et al. (1976). The vessels
central to the temporal equator were tortuous and showed variations in
luminal width. There were ramifications on the equator, some of which showed

arteriovenous anastomoses. A striking finding was complete avascularity of the retina peripheral to these aberrant vessels. Some neovascularizations were visible at the demarcation between the vascular and the avascular retina.

Similar findings were obtained in a female patient with the Bloch-Sulzberger syndrome examined at our department. Her case history follows.

*Patient M.R.K. (13-12-65)*

*History*

This girl was referred to our department at age 3 with divergent strabismus OD. The paediatric department of our hospital was found to have admitted this patient shortly after birth with acute disease symptoms and vesicular skin eruptions on the trunk, associated with unmistakable eosinophilia. Incontinentia pigmenti had been diagnosed on the basis of these symptoms.

The birth weight was 2700 g; no record of neonatal oxygen administration. Pregnancy had been uneventful. The patient's mother was reportedly in good health and had never miscarried. A younger brother and sister of the patient were reported to be in good health, with good visual acuity. No family history of systemic or ocular anomalies.

*Ophthalmological examination (at age 3)*

| | |
|---|---|
| Visual acuity | VOD: 0.25, uncorrected. |
| | VOS: 0.8, uncorrected. |
| Cycloplegic refraction | OD: S + 2.0. |
| | OS: S + 1.5. |
| Eye position | Strabismus sursum vergens OD. |
| Anterior segments | ODS: Normal. |
| Vitreous | ODS: Normal. |
| Fundi | ODS: Pale disc, especially in OD. Otherwise normal appearance of posterior poles. |

*Treatment*

Correcting spectacles and occlusion OS to correct the strabismus. The latter was discontinued because VOD failed to improve. Strabismus correction was performed elsewhere when patient was 7 years old. Regular follow-ups at our department were resumed from age 11 on.

*Ophthalmological examination (at age 11)*

| | |
|---|---|
| Visual acuity | VOD: S + 2.5/Cyl. − 1.5 axis 15° 3/60. |
| | VOS: S + 1.5 1.0. |
| Eye position | Slight divergent strabismus OD. |
| Anterior segments | OD: Subcapsular posterior cataract (Figure 138). |
| | OS: Normal. |

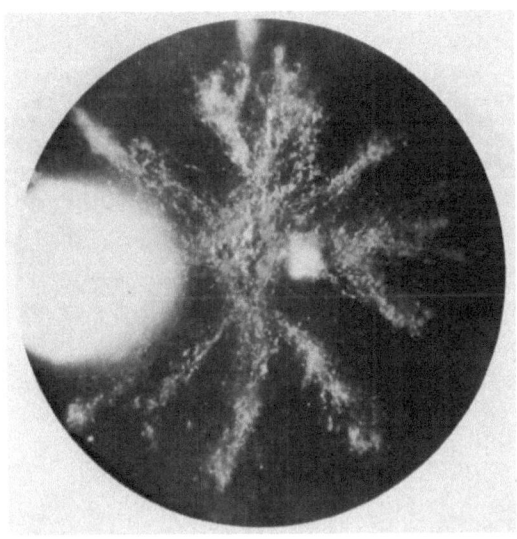

Figure 138. Subcapsular posterior cataract OD.

Vitreous

Fundi

Fluorescein angiogram

OD: Normal structure. Minute white particles.
OS: Normal.

OD: Pale atrophic disc (Figure 139). A few ramifications of the central retinal artery in posterior pole show white vascular sheaths (Figure 139). Temporal to the posterior pole, too, a few arterioles with white, degenerated walls are visible (Figure 140). Slightly more peripherally, a few venules are strikingly irregular and tortuous. The temporal retina anterior to the equator is entirely avascular. A few gross pigment deposits are seen in this non-perfused part of the retina. The nasal retinal periphery shows a normal vasculature.

OS: Disc somewhat pale. Normal vascular configuration and structure throughout the retina.

OD: The early phase of the area central to the equator in the inferior temporal quadrant shows a very-low-density network of capillaries, some of which have dilatated to form wide arteriovenous anastomoses (Figure 141). The late phase very clearly shows non-perfusion of the temporal retinal periphery as far as a level central to the equator (Figure 142). The

278

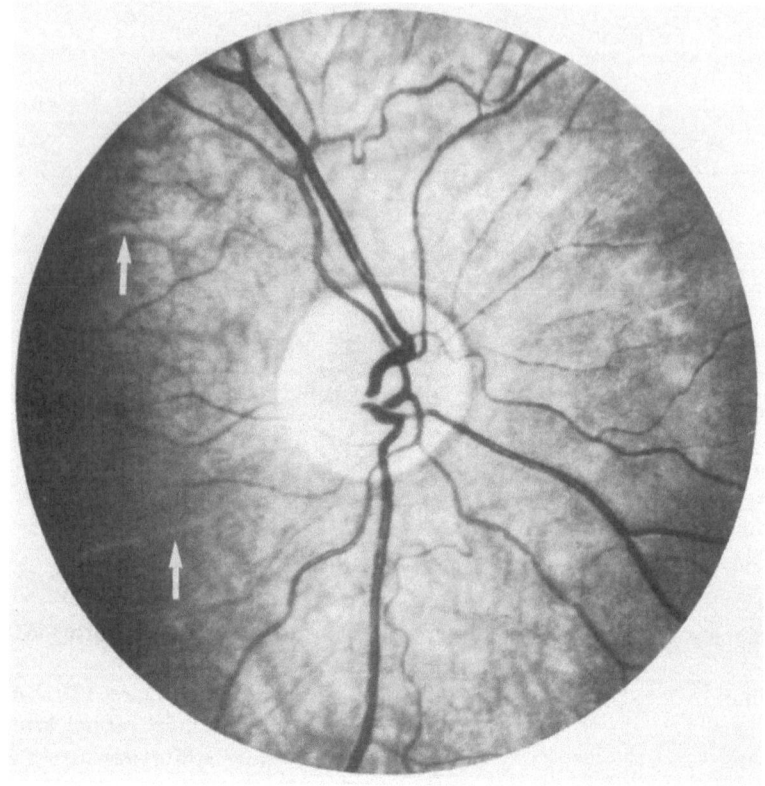

Figure 139. OD. Very pale disc and some arterial branches with white vascular sheaths (arrows).

most peripheral zone of retinal vessels shows very tortuous venous ramifications reversing in central direction.

OS: The late phase reveals normal retinal perfusion.

Visual fields      OD: Slight absolute limitation of the visual field in all quadrants, and slightly reduced general sensitivity.

OS: Normal.

ERG      ODS: The scotopic and photopic responses are within normal limits, but slightly lower in OD than in OS.

*General findings*

A few large, light-brown pigment spots, not raised, on the skin of the chest and the inguineal region (Figure 143). Trophic skin lesions. Some facial asym-

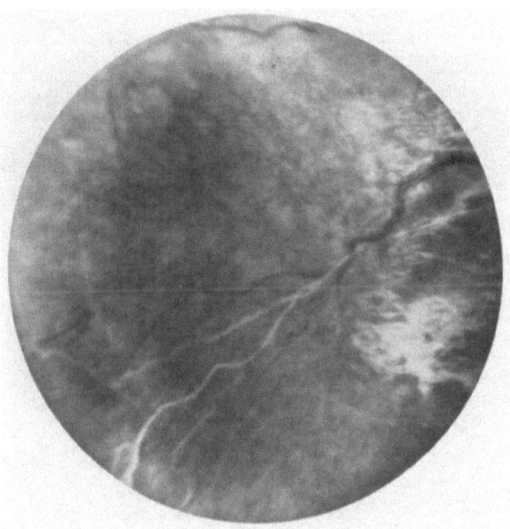

Figure 140. OD. White sclerotic arteries inferior and temporal to the posterior pole.

metry due to flattening of the right side. Scalp hair implantation thinner on the right than on the left. Marked hypoplasia of the right mandible, in which only one permanent molar has developed. The developed teeth show unmistakable morphological abnormalities. Neurological examination reveals no distinct abnormalities. The IQ is rather low.

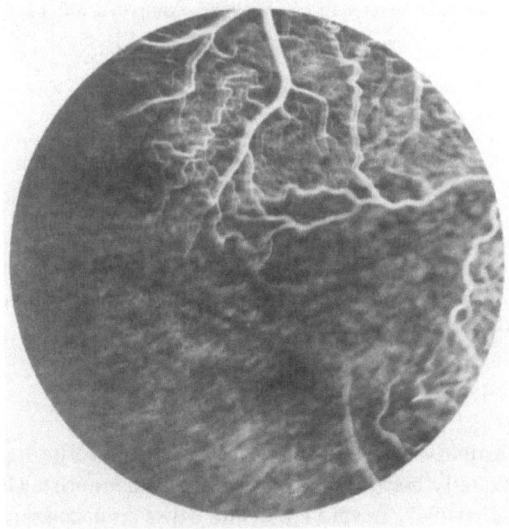

Figure 141. Fluorescein angiogram showing dilated arteriovenous shunt vessels.

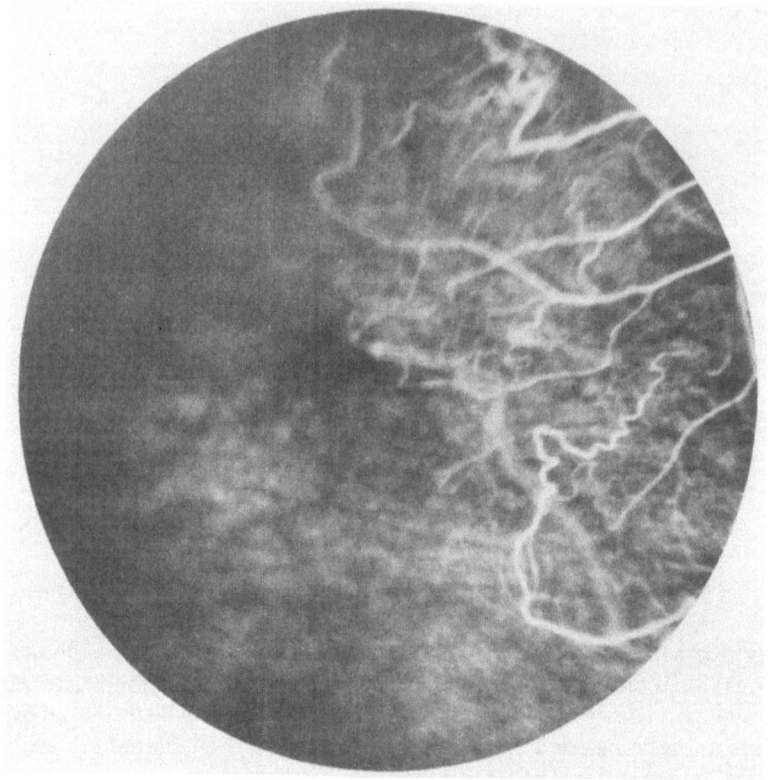

Figure 142. Late phase of the angiogram showing non-perfusion of the temporal retinal periphery.

*Family study*
Ophthalmological examination of the patient's mother revealed nothing abnormal.

*Summary*
A girl with incontinentia pigmenti and visual loss and strabismus OD. Fundi ODS show pale discs, and OD constricted retinal vessels with non-perfusion of the temporal retinal periphery.

### 9.1.b  Genetic aspects

Incontinentia pigmenti is encountered almost exclusively in females. Carney found a positive family history in 55.4% of the cases reported in the literature. Male embryos are virtually never viable, and cause spontaneous abortion.

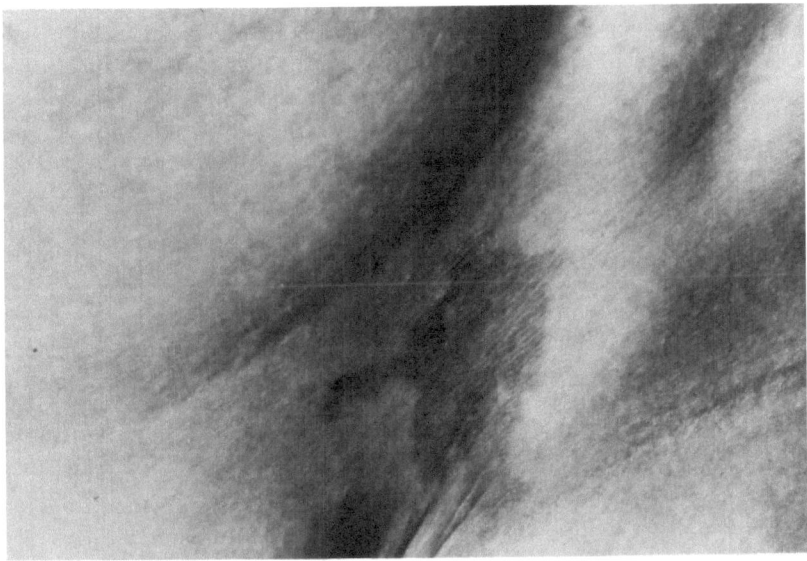

Figure 143. Irregularly shaped but not raised pigmented lesion in the inguinal region.

Transmission of the condition may be X-chromosomal as well as autosomal. It is beyond doubt that the aberrant chromosome originates from the mother. However, the fact that the male heterozygote is not viable is suggestive of X-chromosomal dominant transmission.

### 9.1.c *Histology and pathogenesis*

In the past few decades, several hypotheses have been advanced on the pathogenesis of the ocular anomalies in incontinentia pigmenti. Some authors ascribed the ocular changes to an inflammatory process, e.g. foetal iridocyclitis (Wollensak, 1959). The inflammatory skin changes in the acute phase and the development of posterior synechiae supported this hypothesis.

Other investigators regarded fibrovascular structures found in the vitreous at histological examination as persistent elements of the primary vitreous (Krümmel and Rausch, 1955; Benedikt and Ehalt, 1970). The pigment deposits in the skin lesions in the early phase of the disease focused the attention of several investigators on the retinal pigment epithelium as a possible site of the primary disorder in the eye. Histological examination of the skin revealed deposition of melanin in the dermis by epidermal melanocytes and an abnormal population of melanocytes in the epidermis (Guerrier and Wong, 1974).

Mensheha-Manhart et al. (1975) described light-microscopic and electron-microscopic findings in the enucleated eye of a young patient with incontinentia pigmenti. The pigment epithelium posterior to the totally detached retina showed nodular proliferations with macrophages which contained much melanin and lipofuscin. On the basis of these findings they considered it possible that a primary disturbance of the pigment epithelium is followed by secondary lesions of the neuroretina.

Best and Rentsch (1974) reported clinical findings obtained in the eye of an infant which a few months later could be microscopically examined. On both occasions they observed that the vascular system on the temporal side of the retina had failed to develop: the peripheral retina was avascular. A study of the histological specimen revealed that the ophthalmoscopically observed neovascularizations had developed into a thick fibrovascular membrane which had totally detached the retina. They regarded the hypoplasia of the retinal vasculature as the primary ocular anomaly in incontinentia pigmenti, which can lead to secondary neovascularization. In severe cases the latter can give rise to massive fibrovascular proliferations in the vitreous, and total retinal detachment.

Watzke et al. (1976) confirmed the clinical observations of Best and Rentsch in seven patients they examined. Our patient, too, showed an avascular temporal retinal periphery, but complicating neovascularization had not occurred.

The retinal vascular changes in incontinentia pigmenti closely resemble those of RLF and DEVR. The three conditions are all characterized by a developmental disorder of the retinal vasculature which mainly involves the temporal fundus periphery. It is therefore likely that incontinentia pigmenti, too, involves damage to the retinal vasculature which occurs late in the course of foetal development. This conclusion is consistent with the fact that the acute skin symptoms develop either in the neonate or (probably) in utero shortly before birth. It seems plausible that the developmental disorder of the retinal vessels is as much more serious as the acute phase of the disease occurs earlier. If this hypothesis is correct, then the patients with a postnatal acute phase are likely to show less marked fundus changes than those with congenital skin eruptions. I have been unable to find data in the literature on incontinentia pigmenti which could be used to test thus hypothesis.

There are no longer any clinical or microscopic indications for interpretation of the vitreous organizations as a consequence of metastatic ophthalmia. The postulate that persistence of the primary vitreous and the hyaloid system plays a role in the pathogenesis, is probably based on misinterpretation of the presence of preretinal fibrovascular tissue in microscopic specimens. Best and Rentsch (1974) already discussed this mistake. They maintained that larger retinal vessels which lead to neovascularizations can easily be mistaken for persistent hyaloid vessels.

The theory that the neuroretinal changes in incontinentia pigmenti result from primary affection of the pigment epithelium seems no longer tenable. It is true that extensive pigment deposits have been found in severely affected eyes (Benedikt and Ehalt, 1970; Mensheha-Manhart et al., 1975), but these deposits are not a rare finding in eyes with retinal detachment of longer standing. Distinct changes of the pigment epithelium are usually absent in milder cases of incontinentia pigmenti with ocular anomalies described in the literature.

The presence of posterior synechiae, as observed in incontinentia pigmenti with serious ocular complications, is certainly not suggestive of primary uveitis. In milder cases (as in our patient) they can be completely absent. Posterior synechiae also frequently develop in a late stage of other serious infantile proliferative retinopathies, e.g. RLF and DEVR.

### 9.1.d Differential diagnosis

The frequently present skin changes facilitate differentiation of incontinentia pigmenti from other juvenile cause of leucocoria. In less severe cases the fundus changes cannot be detected until the child is a few years old, when skin pigmentations have faded. In these cases the diagnosis can usually be established on the basis of historical data on the neonatal period and examination of the skin, teeth and hair. Non-raised pigmented spots on the skin of especially the trunk and extremities, malformations or absence of teeth, or alopecia, are important findings in support of the diagnosis. Central nervous system symptoms such as convulsions, spastic paralysis and mental retardation likewise are not uncommon (Carney, 1976).

It is important to examine mothers of patients with incontinentia pigmenti because, as already pointed out, transmission of the anomalous gene is possible only from mother to daughter (not in the paternal line). Nevertheless, general and ophthalmological examination of mothers of patients often reveals no indication of the disease; it did not in the mother of the above described patient. In these cases, a mutation in the maternal gametes may have occurred. Another possible explanation is that the mother does possess an abnormal X-chromosome, but that it does not become manifest in her. This could be due to inactivation of the X-chromosome with the anomalous gene, as postulated in the hypothesis advanced by Lyon (1961).

It is interesting to compare the fundus changes in incontinentia pigmenti with those in DEVR. However closely the fundus changes in the two conditions resemble each other, they are not identical. In my opinion an essential difference lies in the presence of white vascular sheaths and sometimes occlusion of medium-size arterioles in incontinentia pigmenti. I have never observed this phenomemon in DEVR. In most cases of incontinentia pigmenti, moreover, the pattern of the retinal vasculature along the central demarcation from the avascular periphery seems more pronounced and more irregular than in DEVR and RLF. A third difference lies in the fact that optic nerve atrophy is not encountered in DEVR and RLF, but is not an uncommon finding in incontinentia pigmenti. In the latter condition it may be that occlusion of retinal arterioles leads to hypoxia of the innermost layers of the more peripheral retina, thus arresting the further development of foetal retinal vessels.

In incontinentia pigmenti, as in DEVR and RLF, neovascularizations need not cause total vitreous organizations but may be restricted to the temporal retinal periphery and sometimes cause a falciform retinal fold (Fried and Meyer-Schwickerath, 1980).

### 9.1.e    Treatment

In particular photocoagulation may be indicated for the treatment of neovascularizations. This seems especially the case when there is progression of vascular proliferations. There are only a few reports on patients thus treated (Best and Rentsch, 1974; Watzke et al., 1976), and consequently the value of coagulation in incontinentia pigmenti is still uncertain.

## 9.2 Norrie's disease

### 9.2.a    Clinical symptoms

Norrie's disease is characterized by severe bilateral ocular changes and, in some cases, by hearing defects and disorders of cerebral function. The condition is found exclusively in males, and X-chromosomal transmission has been demonstrated in several families (Warburg, 1966; Blodi and Hunter, 1969; Holmes, 1971). The most conspicuous ocular anomaly is leucocoria due to the presence of a whitish-grey or yellowish retrolental tissue mass which usually shows some vessels at slit-lamp examination.

The leucocoria is usually detected shortly after birth. In a few instances the parents do not notice their child's visual handicap until the end of the second year of life (Warburg, 1966). The anterior chamber is sometimes shallow, and in several cases the aqueous humour shows a positive Tyndall phenomenon. Anterior and posterior synechiae are often present.

Most patients become blind in the course of the first few months of life as a result of shrinking and detachment of the retina. Older children and adults with this disease show atrophy of both eyeballs, and band keratopathy of the cornea.

Adult patients are often of subnormal intelligence, and sometimes show other evidence of cerebral lesions, e.g. epileptic seizures or psychotic symptoms. Neither the incidence nor the cause of hearing defects in Norrie's disease is known (Warburg, 1966).

Although the disease is rare, several affected families have been described in negroes as well as in caucasians (Hansen, 1968), and also in North American indians (Wilson, 1949).

Hamburg (1970) observed the disease in three brothers in The Netherlands. Von Winning (1952) described a family in which two brothers and a maternal cousin were virtually blind as a result of bilateral "pseudoglioma". Although it is unknown whether these patients showed other ocular anomalies as well, Warburg (1966) considered the clinical picture of the ocular anomalies and the presumably X-chromosomal transmission in this family to be typical of Norrie's disease.

### 9.2.b  Histology

Several eyes of patients with Norrie's disease have been enucleated, and the microscopic features of the condition are therefore wellknown. Unfortunately, most of the enucleated eyes were severely deformed by fibrotic and glial tissue, so that early histological changes could not be studied.

The specimen of an atrophic eyeball described by Andersen and Warburg (1961) showed a hypoplastic iris with synechiae in the iridocorneal angle. The anterior surface of the iris was covered by a fibrovascular membrane. The lens had shrunken and was cataractous, with duplicatures in the capsule. The deformed vitreous space was full of fibrovascular cicatricial tissue with gross collagen fibres and proliferations of retinal pigment epithelium cells. Immediately posterior to the lens, a plaque of hyalinized vascular tissue was seen which, according to the authors, was suggestive of persistent hyperplastic primary vitreous. In this specimen the neuroretina could not be traced anywhere but, possibly, in a haemorrhagic and necrotic area. In the optic nerve, both myelin sheaths and axons showed virtually complete aplasia.

In a less atrophic eyeball, Apple et al. (1974) likewise found haemorrhages and fibrovascular proliferations in the vitreous space. The detached neuroretina showed proliferation of glial tissue and dysplastic rosettes. No gross deformation of retinal vessels was observed. In microscopic specimens of both eyes of a patient with Norrie's disease, Townes and Roca (1973) found extensive fibrovascular cicatricial tissue in the vitreous space. In one eye, the retina formed a funnel-shaped strand extending from the disc to a retrolental mass of fibrotic tissue; in the other specimen the neuroretina was no longer identifiable. Extensive fibrovascular vitreous organizations were described also by Wilson (1949) and Stefani and Ehalt (1974), but in the latter case the diagnosis was not entirely certain.

I had occasion to study the histological changes in the eyes of two patients with Norrie's disease. The first boy was a member of the family described by Hamburg (1970). Like his two brothers, this boy became blind shortly after birth.

The sagittal sections of the eye enucleated shortly after birth revealed total retinal detachment. The retina formed a funnel-shaped strand extending from the disc to a thin membrane of fibrotic tissue which attached to the posterior side of the lens and the ciliary processes. The posterior part of the detached neuroretina showed proliferation of glial tissue. The anterior part of the retina immediately behind the fibrovascular membrane was necrotic and showed hardly any recognizable structure.

The second specimen came from a boy who developed bilateral leucocoria shortly after birth. This child also showed central nervous system symptoms such as convulsions and psychomotor retardation. Family studies had been made at the ophthalmological and paediatric departments of the Utrecht University Hospital. It had been found that, in the maternal family, several boys had been blind or virtually blind shortly after birth, and that some had died within the first year of life. Norrie's disease had been diagnosed on the basis of the clinical manifestations and the pattern of transmission, which was consistent with X-chromosomal transmission. Figure 144A shows a section through the eye enucleated two months after birth. Funnel-shaped detachment of the retina is visible. Proliferation of glia cells renders the retinal structure virtually unrecognizable. There are no distinct dysplastic rosettes, but several remnants of retinal layers are visible which show deformation due to duplicatures (Figure 144B). Several small blood vessels among the glial proliferations are surrounded by some fibrotic tissue. On the anterior side, the neuroretina is attached to the posterior lens capsule via fibrovascular tissue, which also attaches to the ciliary processes. The retinal pigment epithelium is still completely in contact with the choroid. Most of the space between neuroretina and pigmented layer is filled with blood.

### 9.2.c Pathogenesis

The severity of the changes in the vitreous space greatly impedes efforts to establish the pathogenesis of the changes in Norrie's disease. Unlike, say, DEVR, Norrie's disease shows but little variability in gene expression, and the disease leads to the terminal stage of phthisis bulbi during infancy in nearly all cases. This greatly limits the changes of clinical fundus examination.

According to Warburg (1966) the disease may well be based on a developmental disorder of the neuro-ectoderm. Apart from the ocular anomalies and the microscopic changes in optic nerve and optic tract, the dysplasia of the cerebral cortex she found, and possibly also the hearing defect, might be ascribed to this. She maintained that the ocular anomalies could result from disturbed differentiation of the inner layer of the optic cup, leading to disturbed production of secondary vitreous. The latter could lead to persistence of the primary vitreous. She interpreted the fibrovascular organizations in the vitreous space as persistent hyperplastic primary vitreous.

Apple et al. (1974) postulated a similar pathogenesis, although in addition

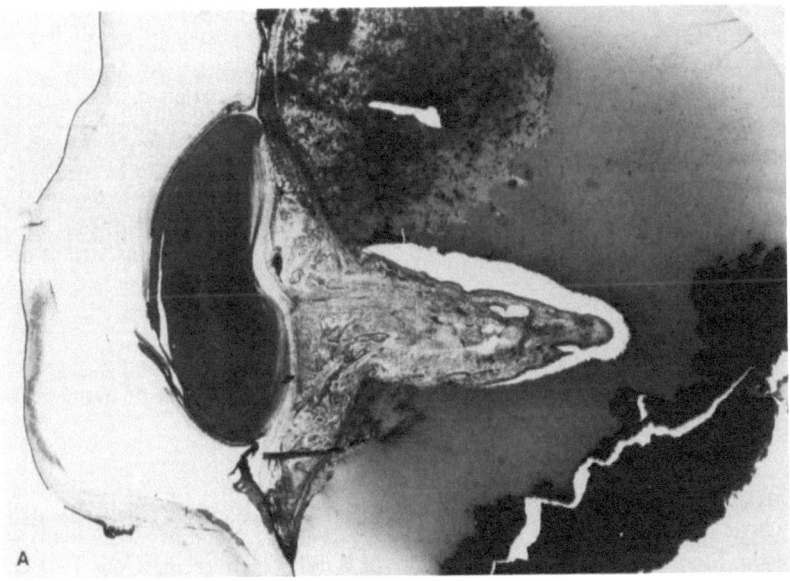

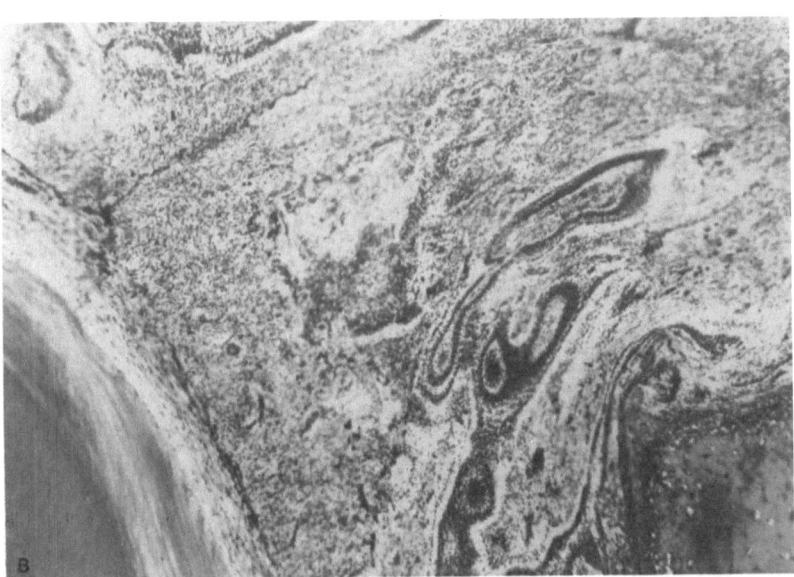

Figure 144. Norrie's disease. Anteroposterior section of the globe. A) The retina is totally detached and has become a funnel-shaped mass attached to the posterior lens surface. The eyeball is almost entirely filled with blood (× 6). B) Higher magnification of the same section as in Figure 144A. The retrolental mass consists mostly of glia cells. Deformed layers of the neuroretina are distinguishable at some sites (× 36).

to persistence of primary vitreous they did not exclude the possibility that the fibrotic tissue masses may result from fibrovascular proliferations.

It seems plausible that the primary disorder in Norrie's disease occurs in the embryonic neuroretina, for in most cases the sclera, choroid and retinal pigment epithelium showed no signs of abnormal primordial development. It seems less likely to me that the retrolental fibrotic tissue structures could originate from hyperplastic remnants of the primary vitreous. The postulate that these structures originate from neuroretinal neovascularizations strikes me as more plausible. The following observations support this theory:

The histological features of eyes of patients with Norrie's disease do not differ from those in terminal stages of other congenital or neonatal proliferative retinopathies such as DEVR or RLF.

Rapid postnatal progression of vitreous organizations has been observed in several cases of Norrie's disease. Jacklin (1980) examined a neonate with this disease and found progression of a falciform retinal fold to a total retrolental tissue mass in which the retina was included. Such progression is more suggestive of active vascular proliferation than of persistence of hyaloid elements.

Persistent hyperplastic primary vitreous of hereditary origin is not known in man, but hereditary proliferative retinopathies are.

A very interesting observation was recently reported by Fujita et al. (1980), who obtained a fluorescein angiogram of the ocular fundus of an infant with Norrie's disease. It revealed a tissue mass in the vitreous space which contained numerous dilated blood vessels from the disc area. The posterior pole of the fundus was not clearly visible. The peripheral choroid showed poor vascularization. Peripheral retinal vasculature was not angiographically demonstrable.

It can be stated in summary that there are clinical and histopathological indications that Norrie's disease is a proliferative retinopathy. Whether the primary disorder underlying the changes is a developmental disorder of the retinal vasculature, as in DEVR, is uncertain. In view of the abovementioned observation reported by Fujita et al. (1980), however, this is not improbable.

So far, no ocular anomalies have been observed in carriers of Norrie's disease. It cannot be excluded, however, that some of them may have minor fundus changes. Contact lens examination and fluorescein angiography of the peripheral fundus in carriers may contribute to our knowledge of the pathogenesis of this disease.

### 9.2.d Differential diagnosis

Norrie's disease should be differentiated from other neonatal affections which can lead to bilateral leucocoria, e.g. retinoblastoma, RLF and Coats' disease. The neonatal history and the ophthalmological family history are of course of importance in this respect.

Neonatal leucocoria is observed also in the Reese-Blodi-straatsma syndrome and trisomy 13 (to be discussed later). These syndromes, however, are characterized by far more severe malformations of other organs.

Norrie's disease is less readily distinguishable from manifestations known as "congenital encephalo-ophthalmic dysplasia" which, like Norrie's disease, may be accompanied by mental retardation and convulsions. The hereditary transmission of this syndrome is obscure, but certainly is not X-chromosomal, as Norrie's disease is.

Differential diagnosis from incontinentia pigmenti of course poses no problem, because the latter occurs only in females.

DEVR, finally, rarely manifests itself with bilateral leucocoria shortly after birth. Yet in rare more severe cases differentiation from Norrie's disease may be more difficult, particularly because in the latter condition cerebral anomalies are not always manifest in an early stage. Severe fundus changes were present shortly after birth in IV-1 F (Chapter 3). In this case the diagnosis of Norrie's disease was rejected on the basis of the absence of cerebral anomalies, the asymmetry of the ocular anomalies, and the presence of the fundus changes in the mother.

### 9.3 Reese-Blodi-Straatsma syndrome and trisomy 13

The syndrome described as "retinal dysplasia" by Reese and Blodi (1950) and Reese and Straatsma (1958) is characterized by severe bilateral ocular anomalies and general malformations. The latter usually lead to a fatal issue within a few months of birth. They mainly involve the central nervous system and cardiovascular system, but other malformations (cheiloschisis, palatoschisis, polydactylia) have been observed as well.

The following ocular symptoms have been observed in the syndrome: microphthalmia (usually mild), shallow anterior chamber, posterior synechiae, coloboma of the iris, cataract (usually not total), and a white vascularized tissue mass close behind the lens in the vitreous space. In some cases elongated ciliary processes are seen whose central parts are attached to the retrolental tissue mass.

In 1960 Patau and co-workers demonstrated the presence of an additional chromosome in patients with symptoms like those described by Reese, Blodi and Straatsma. The ocular changes subsequently described in this syndrome (which is associated with trisomy of chromosome 13) by Cogan and Kuwabara

(1964) and Miller et al. (1963) likewise corresponded with the symptoms described by Reese et al. It is therefore likely that the Reese-Blodi-Straatsma syndrome is based, at least in a number of cases, on trisomy 13.

### 9.3.a Histology

The histopathological features of the RBS syndrome are known very well because, as already pointed out, most patients die relatively soon after birth. Symptoms of dysembryogenesis of cornea, iris and iridocorneal angle have been frequently found in eyes examined. The neuroretina is partly detached from the pigmented layer. Not infrequently a retinal fold extends from the disc to a tissue mass in the anterior part of the vitreous space. Such tissue masses have often been regarded as persistent elements of the primary vitreous (Hopener and Yanoff, 1972). The detached parts of the neuroretina show proliferations of glial tissue and rosettes. The latter are traversed by tubular structures which often connect with the subretinal space. Photoreceptors and elements of the outer retinal layers are found arranged around the lumen of these structures. These dysplastic rosettes differ in variety of form, dimensions and structure from the neoplastic rosettes which characterize retinoblastoma. The latter are small, circular and of uniform structure and morphology. Unlike non-neoplastic rosettes, moreover, they lack Müller cells (Fulton et al. 1978).

### 9.3.b Pathogenesis

In view of the microscopic changes in retinal structure the above described syndrome was called "retinal dysplasia" by Reese and Blodi (1950). This term was later criticized because similar dysplastic changes can be histologically demonstrated in several other conditions and are therefore not specific for the RBS syndrome (Hunter and Zimmerman, 1965). Moreover, the term emphasizes only the retinal changes in a syndrome with many other severe malformations (Waardenburg, 1963).

It is of great importance that dysplastic rosettes are no longer regarded as a specific manifestation of primary neuro-ectodermal dysplasia of the eye. Similar neuroretinal structural changes and the presence of rosette-like structures have been observed in cases of congenital retinal fold (Mann, 1935), choroidal coloboma (Badtke, 1960; Lahav, 1973) and persistent hyperplastic primary vitreous (Lahav et al., 1973). Non-neoplastic rosettes have been observed in test animals after intra-uterine damage of the neuroretina caused by röntgen irradiation (Pagenstecher, 1916), perforating trauma of the eyeball (Silverstein, 1974) and after viral infection (Silverstein, 1971; Albert et al., 1977).

That rosette-like structures can develop late in the course of embryonic development and even after birth, is demonstrated by their presence in RLF

(Klein, 1949). Similar microscopic features can even develop in adults after neuroretinal detachment due to trauma or proliferative organizations resulting from diabetic retinopathy or occlusion of the central retinal vein, as demonstrated by Lahav et al. (1975). To put it succinctly: rosettes with a non-neoplastic pathogenesis are a rather non-specific manifestation of virtually any damage to the neuroretina, whether during or after completion of embryonic development.

Although some of the ocular changes observed in the RBS syndrome (e.g. dysembryogenesis of the anterior segment and colobomas of the iris) indicate an early disturbance of embryonic development, the retinal changes are partly compatible with a late developmental disorder, and more specifically with disturbed vascular development with secondary vascular proliferations in the vitreous space, as can be observed also in, say, anencephalia. Microscopic examination of the retinal vasculature in eyes with relatively little retinal deformity may yield additional information on the pathogenesis of the ocular anomalies in the RBS syndrome.

### 9.3.c  Differential diagnosis

Congenital non-attachment of the retina with similar rosette-like structures has been observed in Meckel's syndrome, which like the RBS syndrome is associated with multiple malformations of the central nervous system and numerous other organs (Lahev and Albert, 1973; Warburg, 1978), and in other rare chromosomal anomalies such as trisomy 18 (Fulton et al., 1978).

Differential diagnosis from DEVR of course poses no problem at all, because general symptoms are totally absent in DEVR.

### 9.4  Congenital encephalo-ophthalmic dysplasia

The term encephalo-ophthalmic dysplasia was introduced by Krause (1946), who described 18 patients with a variety of cerebral anomalies in combination with RLF-like ocular symptoms. Krause's exhaustive study was published at a time when the role of oxygen in the aetiology of RLF was yet to be established. The fact that several of Krause's patients had been prematurely born and had received neonatal oxygen administration, has subsequently raised doubt about the presence of the ocular symptoms at birth in a number of these cases.

Several subsequent studies, however, described infants not given neonatal oxygen administration in whom similar symptoms were found, which were confined to the eyes and the central nervous system. The similarity in clinical features between these cases and the lack of an alternative term justifies maintenance of the original term — congenital encephalo-ophthalmic dysplasia — for the time being.

### 9.4.a    Clinical symptoms

The anomalies described by Krause were hydrocephalus and microcephaly, associated with a varying degree of mental retardation. The ocular symptoms were bilateral. Retinal detachment (usually in the form of funnel detachment) was frequently observed. Although some eyes showed possibly primary abnormalities of the iridocorneal angle, no signs of early embryonic close defects of the optic cup were observed.

Cases of hydrocephalus in combination with bilateral RLF-like ocular symptoms without a history of neonatal oxygen administration were subsequently described by Snell (1965), Karlsberg et al. (1973), Svedberg (1975) and Warburg (1978).

There are sound reasons to postulate that the ocular anomalies in this syndrome are based on a primary disturbance in the development of the retinal vascular system. The clinical features in most cases clearly indicate such a pathogenesis. The ophthalmoscopic findings in Warburg's patient (1978) suggested an only very partial vascularization of the retina. Histological examination, as performed in the case reported by Karlsberg et al. (1973) revealed unmistakable proliferations of retinal vessels through the internal limiting membrane to the vitreous space. The retina peripheral to these neovascularizations was entirely avascular.

Snell (1965) described a patient with hydrocephalus in whom he found fibrovascular proliferations and dysplastic rosettes in the detached neuroretina. As already mentioned, such rosettes are frequently found also in late developmental disorders. In this case, too, the fibrovascular structures were almost certainly derived from retinal neovascularizations.

The cause of the cerebral anomalies in these patients is obscure. Karlsberg et al. (1973) found not only the histological signs of bilateral hydrocephalus but also bilateral subdural haematomas, a haematoma of the posterior fossa and a vestigial cerebellum. In the cases so far examined histologically, no evidence of cerebral vascular developmental disorders has been found.

The syndrome has been observed in either sex, and nearly always in sporadic cases. Autosomal recessive transmission is not improbable, for parental consanguinity was established in a few cases (Warburg, 1978).

Krause described RLF-like ocular symptoms in a few patients with microcephaly. It seems to me that the symptoms of the patient described in Chapter 7 — with microcephaly and bilateral falciform retinal folds — also belong to the syndrome of congenital encephalo-ophthalmic dysplasia. In both fundi of this girl it was evident that retinal vascular development had hardly occurred outside the posterior pole.

## 9.5 Proliferative retinopathy in anencephalia.

Cogan (1963) demonstrated anomalies of the retinal vasculature in anencephalia. Anencephalia is not a rare malformation, and not compatible with life; its histopathological features are therefore wellknown. The histopathological features are therefore wellknown. The histopatholical findings described by Cogan (1963) were massive proliferations of endothelial cells at the "advanced border of the retinal vasculature", and proliferations of neuroglial cells in the peripheral fundus.

Andersen et al. (1961) described light-microscopic findings obtained in 40 eyes of ancephalic patients. A characteristic feature in their specimens was hypoplasia of the ganglion cells and nerve fibre layer of the retina, and hypoplasia of the axons in the optic nerve. They considered these changes to result from the cerebral malformations. Unmistakable proliferative changes of the type seen in RLF were found in only one eye: that of a full-term anencephalic neonate.

Addison et al. (1972) found RLF-like vascular proliferative changes in 9 out of 73 histologically examined eyes of anencephalic persons. The changes ranged from marked proliferation of capillaries in the inner layers of the retina to distinct intraretinal neovascularizations extending to varying levels in the vitreous space. In all eyes the neovascularization had occurred at the demarcation between vascular and avascular retina, as in RLF.

### 9.5.a  Pathogenesis

The descriptions published by Cogan (1963), Andersen et al. (1961) and Addison et al. (1972) clearly show that the histological changes in some anencephalics closely resemble those of RLF. Since the fibrovascular proliferations cannot be a result of oxygen administration, however, the term RLF does not apply. Addison et al. (1972) rightly used the term proliferative retinopathy.

These publications show that the neovascularization observed in anencephalics is associated with incomplete vascularization of the (peripheral) neuroretina. The logical implication is that, as in DEVR, a primary developmental disorder of the retinal vasculature has been complicated by reactive neovascularization. The extensive proliferations which Addison et al. (1974) found in premature anencephalics aged 26 and 28 weeks, respectively, indicate that the disorder can occur fairly early in the course of development.

The cause of the disorder in retinal vascular development in anencephalics is obscure. The inner retinal layers are probably already hypoplastic even before development of the retinal vasculature, due to subnormal development of the ganglion cells and their axons. This hypoplasia of the nerve fibre layer may have led to disturbed vascular development in these cases.

### 9.6  Familial unilateral proliferative retinopathy

It was difficult to classify the condition observed in two members of the following family (Figure 145).

294

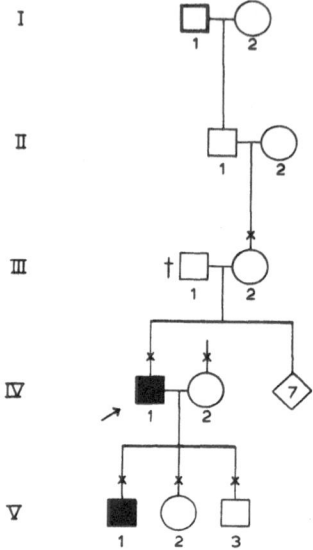

Figure 145. Pedigree of the family with unilateral proliferative retinopathy.

*Subject IV-1 (29-03-47)*

*History*
VOD had been poor since early infancy, but no treatment had been given in childhood. At age 21 the patient was referred to our department for correction of the elevated position of OD. The fundus changes were tentatively ascribed to previous chorioretinitis. In 1971, recession of the superior rectus muscle was performed to correct the eye position. General health had reportedly always been good. No record of premature birth or neonatal oxygen administration.

*Family history*
Diminished VOD in the eldest son; paternal great-grandfather was reported to have had diminished visual acuity in one eye.

*Ophthalmological examination*

| | |
|---|---|
| Visual acuity | VOD: 4/300; projection in the nasal visual field incorrectly indicated. |
| | VOS: S + 0.5 1.0. |
| Eye position | Virtually straight; latent nystagmus. |
| Anterior segments | ODS: Normal. |
| Vitreous | ODS: Normal retrolental vitreous structure. A few delicate white particles are visible. |
| Fundi | OD: From the disc, the temporal retinal vessels |

take a stretched course through the centre of the posterior pole to the inferior temporal quadrant. Some traction on these vessels has produced the features of dragged disc. The macula is no longer clearly distinguishable among the closely packed parallel retinal vessels in the posterior pole. Immediately temporal to the posterior pole an extensive sharply defined area with extensive pigmented layer atrophy and some pigmentations is visible (Figure 146). The retina in this area shows fibrovascular proliferations slightly raised in the preretinal vitreous space. The retinal vessels which extend beneath these proliferations show local deformation due to traction exerted by this tissue. The retinal periphery anterior to the temporal equatorial zone showed extensive white without pressure and seems avascular. The nasal periphery shows similar changes. There are no retinal defects or exudates.

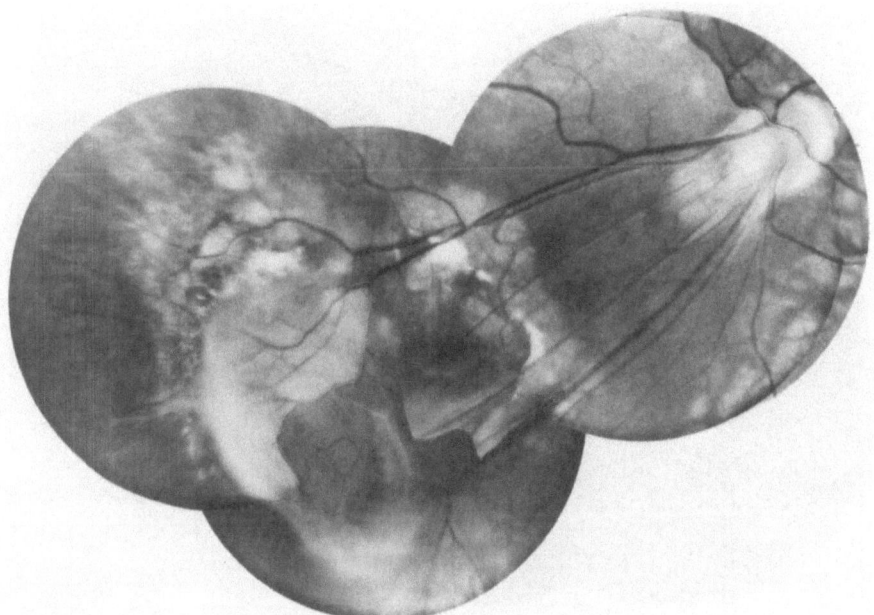

Figure 146 (IV-1). Fundus OD.

Fluorescein angiogram

OS: The posterior pole presents an entirely normal appearance. The peripheral fundus shows a normal configuration of retinal vessels and is otherwise also normal.

OD: The early phase of the posterior pole very clearly shows the abnormal configuration of the retinal vasculature. Inferior and temporal to the posterior pole there is a hypofluorescent area, obviously due to poor perfusion of the choriocapillaris, surrounded by a hyperfluorescent corona of atrophic pigment epithelium. Peripheral to this, the retinal vessels show marked deformation, and an area about the size of one disc diameter in which preretinal neovascularizations cause intensive fluorescein leakage (Figure 147). Slightly peripheral to this lies an interesting area near the equator, where the retinal vessels terminate in a few aberrant and leaking terminal ramifications. The retina peripheral to this area is totally avascular (Figure 147).

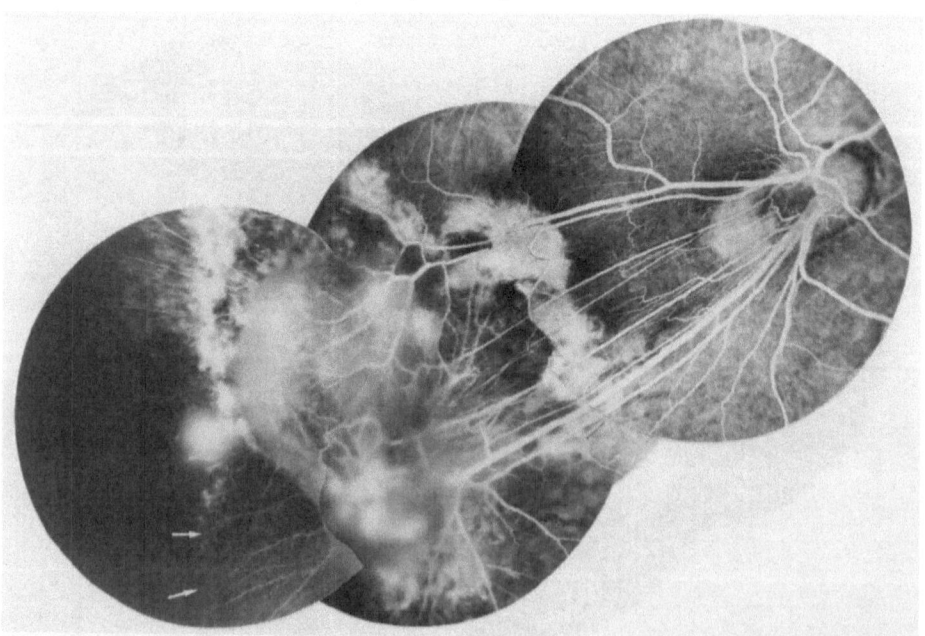

Figure 147 (IV-1). Fluorescein angiogram fundus OD. At a few sites, intensive leakage from small neovascularizations. The arrows indicate the demarcation between vascular and avascular retina.

OS: The late phase of the posterior pole shows some hyperfluorescence of the disc. The peripheral fundus near 3 o'clock shows no anomalies.

## Conclusion

OD shows unmistakable symptoms of incomplete vascularization of the temporal and the nasal retinal periphery with distinct neovascularizations. The fundus OS shows no abnormalities.

*Subject V-1 (24-01-71)*

## History

At age 5 the school medical officer diagnosed diminished VOD. The ophthalmologist consulted found fundus changes in OD at examination under anaesthesia. The patient was referred to our department for further diagnosis.

## Ophthalmological examination

| | |
|---|---|
| Visual acuity | VOD: S + 1.0/Cyl. − 2.5 axis 50° 0.2. |
| | VOS: S − 0.5 1.0. |
| Cycloplegic refraction | OD: S + 2.0/Cyl. − 2.5 axis 50°. |
| Eye position | Straight. Slight temporal displacement of the corneal reflex OD. |
| Anterior segments | OD: A few small posterior synechiae in the superior nasal quadrant. |
| | OS: Normal. |
| Vitreous | OD: The centre of the retrolental vitreous is of normal structure, without cells. |
| | OS: Normal structure, without cells. |
| Fundi | OD: In the posterior pole, a small atrophic area of the pigmented layer lies immediately temporal and superior to the disc. The configuration of the retinal vessels near the disc is abnormal: the macula and the blood vessels of the posterior pole show distortion in superior nasal direction (Figure 148). A strand of grey tissue extends from the disc in superior direction and ends in the are of the pars plana near 1 o'clock in a mass of white glial tissue. This mass is localized immediately posterior to the lens equator, but not attached to it. Only at the disc and in the extreme periphery is the strand attached to the retina; otherwise it extends preretinally in the vitreous space. No |

298

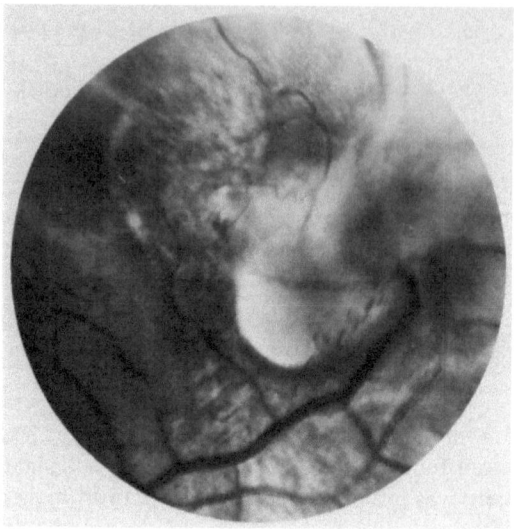

Figure 148 (V-1). OD. The blood vessels on the disc show superior nasal distortion.

vessels are visible in the strand. In the extreme periphery near 12 o'clock, a dark green raised structure is localized close to the glial tissue mass at the distal end of the tissue strand. The nature of the tissue of this swelling is not readily identifiable. The retinal periphery outside the glial structures shows no distinct vascular changes.

OS: The posterior pole and periphery of the fundus are entirely normal.

*Conclusion*

Mass of proliferative tissue in the extreme fundus periphery and vitreous strand to the disc in the right eye.

*Discussion*

The symptoms observed in the two above described members of one family suggest a peripheral proliferative retinopathy confined to one sector of the fundus. History and clinical features suggest that the condition is congenital in both cases. The fluorescein angiogram of OD in IV-1 reveals an avascular retinal periphery. The configuration of the most peripheral retinal vessels near the central demarcation of the avascular retina is suggestive, not so much of secondary occlusions in a normally developed vascular system as of a vascular developmental disorder.

The condition in this family is not readily classifiable. DEVR seems to be the primary consideration in differential diagnosis. The fundus changes in OD of IV-1 and the father-to-son transmission are quite consistent with DEVR.

Although the severity of changes can differ widely in the two eyes of a patient with DEVR, I have not observed a unilateral form of this disease. The localization of the proliferative changes in V-1 (superior nasal quadrant) is likewise not readily compatible with DEVR.

CHAPTER 10

# OBSERVATIONS ON WAGNER'S SYNDROME, SEX-LINKED JUVENILE RETINOSCHISIS AND JUVENILE RHEGMATOGENOUS RETINAL DETACHMENT

## 10.1 Wagner's syndrome

After presenting a brief survey of the clinical and pathological manifestations of Wagner's syndrome, this chapter discusses the vascular anomalies of the peripheral fundus in this syndrome. Symptoms suggestive of a developmental disorder of the peripheral choroid, retinal pigment epithelium and retinal vasculature in Wagner's syndrome have been discussed in a previous publication (Van Nouhuys, 1981b). The results of this study are again presented and discussed in this chapter.

### *10.1.a Clinical symptoms*

The most conspicuous symptoms of Wagner's syndrome are to be found in the vitreous and the peripheral fundus. A characteristic finding is the absence of any vitreous structure in most parts of the vitreous space, as a result of which this space is optically empty. A few filamentous vitreous structures, however, are visible at some sites and show considerable mobility.

Another characteristic feature, which is virtually pathognomonic of Wagner's syndrome, is the circular attachment of a delicate vitreous membrane to the retina slightly posterior to the equator of the fundus, which is often visible in all quadrants. Gross pigment deposits are localized superficially in the retina in the peripheral fundus (Figure 158). In some cases they are radially arranged along the retinal vessels, which often show white vascular sheaths (Wagner, 1938; Jansen, 1966; Frandsen, 1966; Alexander and Shea, 1965).

Small white atrophic areas, often surrounded by a pigment zone in the equatorial fundus region, are frequently observed (Jansen, 1966), as also are lattice degeneration and white without pressure. In the posterior fundus the large choroidal vessels and the sclera are often clearly visible.

Some authors (Jansen, 1966; Frandsen, 1966) have pointed out the abnormal retinal vascular pattern near the disc (inversed disc) (Figure 149). This phenomenon is sometimes accompanied by nasal ectopia of the macula. Refraction anomalies are frequently found, the most common being myopia or myopic astigmatism.

Retinal defects and rhegmatogenous retinal detachment have been described as a complication of Wagner's syndrome in many reports (Cibis, 1965; Jansen,

1965; Alexander and Shea, 1965; Delaney et al., 1963; Van Balen et al., 1970; Hirose et al., 1973; Knobloch, 1975). There are often small multiple defects, which lead to retinal detachment at an early age (Hirose et al., 1973).

Cataract is another frequent complication, which likewise can occur at an early age. The opacities begin in the posterior cortex, where they form an irregular stellate pattern. Subsequently, progressive sclerosis of the nucleus of the lens is often observed.

Open iridocorneal angle glauoma is not a rare complication after age 30. Jansen (1966) found increased intraocular pressure in about 33% of patients.

*Retinal functions*

Corrected visual acuity is good in most patients as long as complications such as lens opacities, retinal detachment or glaucoma have not yet developed.

The visual fields are often concentrically limited, or show annular scotomas (Jansen, 1966).

The ERG is usually abnormal. Böhringer et al. (1960) found a slightly reduced amplitude of the scotopic B-wave, while Jansen (1966) recorded a subnormal response of both the photopic and the scotopic ERG in most eyes. He found no distinct changes in dark adaptation in most of his patients.

Colour vision is normal in most patients in whom no significant media opacities have developed (Pinckers, 1970).

The EOG often shows a subnormal ratio (Pinckers, 1970).

*10.1.b Histopathology*

Only a few specimens from patients with Wagner's syndrome have been examined histologically. The specimens described by Alexander and Shea (1965) showed severe changes resulting from late complications such as retinal detachment, haemorrhages, and probably glaucoma. Böhringer et al. (1960) described specimens in a much better condition, obtained from two members of the family described by Wagner. The same specimens were examined in detail by Manschot (1971). Histologically, the circular white rim ophthalmoscopically observed around the mid-periphery of the fundus proved to be the site at which a preretinal membrane which centrally adhered to the retina, curved away from the retina to end freely in the periphery of the vitreous space. Manschot (1971) wrote: "It appears as if the preretinal membrane originates from a splitting within the nerve fibre layer or — at the periphery — from a detachment of almost the whole nerve fibre layer".

Most of the retina showed a normal structure. No structures were histologically visible in the centre of the vitreous space. The retina showed areas of cystic degeneration and atrophy. The retinal periphery contained pigmentations, especially along the retinal vessels. The atrophic retinal changes were very variable: beside histologically nearly intact retinal areas there were areas which showed pronounced atrophy. The few vessels visible in the retinal periphery showed a swollen vascular wall. The choroid was likewise atrophic. At no site were inflammatory changes found (Böhringer et al., 1960).

### 10.1.c General manifestations: clefting syndromes

Apart from the ocular symptoms, the family described by Wagner showed no general symptoms which might be related to the eye disease. In later descendants in the same family, Böhringer (1960) found no general manifestations either. The two families described by Jansen (1966) likewise showed no general symptoms.

In 1939 Friedman described a family with Wagner-like changes of the peripheral fundus, retinal detachment and cataract, in which several members also showed craniofacial peculiarities: prominent lower jaw, hypertelorism and dental anomalies.

In the past two decades, several publications have described families with Wagner-like fundus and vitreous changes and cataract, in which widely diverse general abnormalities were found. The pedigrees of most of these families are compatible with autosomal dominant transmission.

The most common accompanying general abnormalities include palatoschisis, mid-facial flattening, hyperextensible joints and mild spondyloepiphyseal dysplasia (Delaney et al., 1963). The general and ocular symptoms can be found combined in one family or in one patient. In such cases the condition is currently often described as Stickler syndrome (Stickler et al., 1965; Van Balen and Falger, 1970; Blair et al., 1979).

Several families or individuals show only a few of the abovementioned general symptoms. In view of this, some authors divide the patients into subgroups. The presence of general symptoms such as dwarfism or hearing loss (Maumenee, 1979) can make the classification of symptoms very complex. Görlin and Knobloch (1972) distinguished a great many hereditary syndromes which can be associated with retinal detachment. Several of these syndromes show autosomal dominant transmission, but in others autosomal recessive transmission seems likely.

It has so far remained uncertain whether the families in which only ocular symptoms are described, are genetically related to or identical with families in which general symptoms occur in addition to the vitreoretinal lesions.

Knobloch's conclusion (1975) that Wagner's syndrome is associated with "generalized epiphyseal dysplasia" does not seem to be justified in all families. The chance that general symptoms were present but not identified in the large families described by Wagner (1938), Böhringer et al. (1960) and Jansen (1966) seems very small.

I personally examined several members of the families described by Jansen (1966) as well as patients in three other families with Wagner's syndrome: none of them showed distinct symptoms of the Stickler syndrome.

At this time it seems justifiable, as Deutman (1977) pointed out, to regard Wagner's syndrome and the clefting syndromes as different entities, however similar the ocular symptoms may be. For the time being the designation Stickler syndrome should be reserved for families which, in addition to the vitreoretinal changes, show the non-ophthalmological abnormalities of the syndrome.

### 10.1.d Fluorescein-angiographic study of the circulation of the equatorial retina and choroid in Wagner's syndrome

*Subjects and methods*

From three pedigrees with Wagner's vitreoretinal degeneration we selected patients not older than 30. In order to ensure sufficient quality of equatorial fundus photography we accepted only subjects without lens opacities (a rather frequent complication even in young patients with Wagner's syndrome), who were capable of full mydriasis. We succeeded in obtaining adequate fluorescein angiograms of the peripheral fundus in six cases.

Colour photographs and fluorescein angiograms were made of the posterior pole and peripheral fundus in different quadrants. In all cases the early exposures of the angiograms were made of an equatorial region selected after examination by indirect ophthalmoscopy.

Our patients 1, 2 and 3 were three affected sisters from a large pedigree with Wagner's syndrome. Our patient 4 and her mother, patient 5, had only recently been seen for the first time, and their pedigree had not yet been studied. Patient 6 was a member of the large family described by Jansen (1966).

None of our patients showed orofacial or skeletal symptoms of the kind seen in the Stickler syndrome. Our six patients all showed an optically empty vitreous space, pervaded by a few vitreous membranes of the type characteristically found in Wagner's vitreoretinal degeneration.

The results of this study have been recently published (Van Nouhuys, 1981b).

*Case histories*

*Patient 1 (15-01-56)*
In both eyes of this 24-year-old woman the larger choroidal vessels were clearly discernible in the regions adjacent to the disc on the nasal side. The vessels at the head of the optic nerve showed an inverse pattern (Figure 149). Large greyish-white areas of chorioretinal atrophy were visible along a circumferential white line in the temporal half of both fundi. Several clumps of pigment and small circular strophic spots with pigmented edges were observed in these areas.

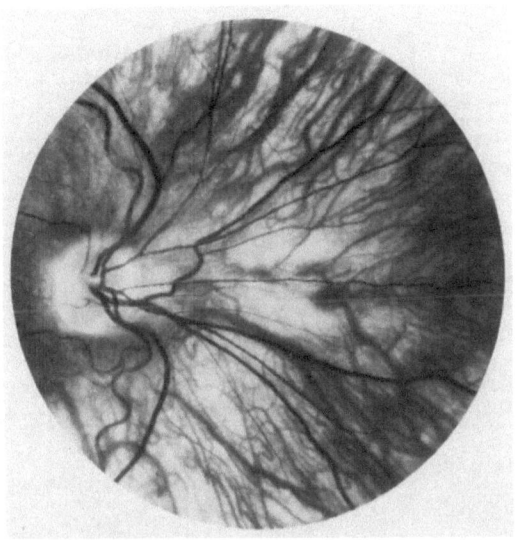

Figure 149. Patient 1. OD. Retinal vessels exiting from the disc in nasal direction.

The early phase of the fluorescein angiogram of the temporal equatorial zone of OD showed, at 10 o'clock, a normal flush of the choriocapillaries central to the equator, but no filling of the choriocapillaris in the atrophic areas; consequently the larger choroidal vessels were clearly visible (Figure 150). The retinal vessels central to the equator showed normal perfusion but their pattern was abnormal: the superior temporal vessels curved down and the inferior temporal vessels showed an upward deviation as they approached the posterior border of the atrophic areas. The terminal branches of these vessels ended abruptly near this border, the peripheral retina being completely avascular (Figure 151).

Fluorescein angiography of OS likewise revealed extensive areas of atrophy of the choriocapillaris and pigment epithelium in the temporal half, with non-perfusion of the retina (Figure 152). On the nasal side the retina showed a normal vasculature in equatorial regions, and no visible areas of atrophy of the choroid and pigment epithelium.

*Patient 2 (08-07-61)*

Both fundi of this 18-year-old sister of patient 1 showed several oblong, whitish, sharply defined lesions in the temporal periphery (Figure 153). The retina in these areas was very thin and atrophic, and showed a few small defects. Early-phase fluorescein angiography at 3 o'clock of OS revealed poor filling of the choriocapillaris anterior to the equator. There was no discernible perfusion of the retina in and anterior to the atrophic areas (Figure 154).

306

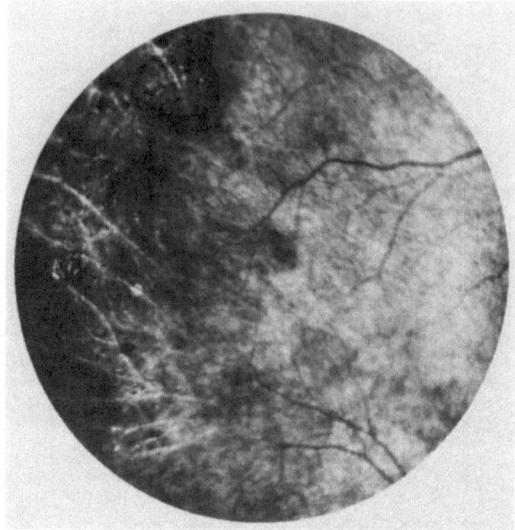

Figure 150. Patient 1. OD. Absence of the flush of the peripheral choriocapillaris in the early phase of the angiogram.

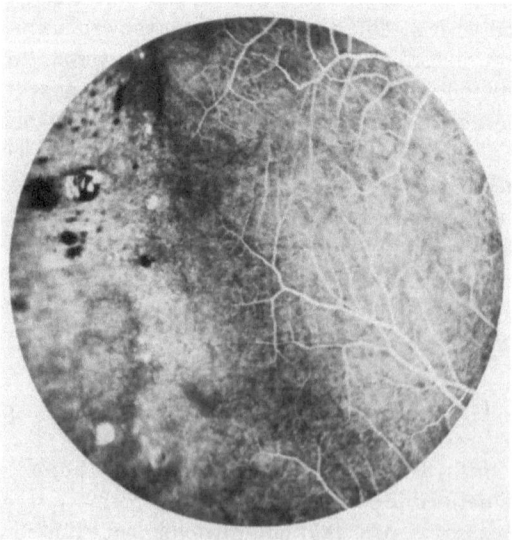

Figure 151. Patient 1. Same area as in Figure 150. Late phase of the angiogram showing atrophic changes of the retinal pigment epithelium and non-perfusion of the retina peripheral to the equator.

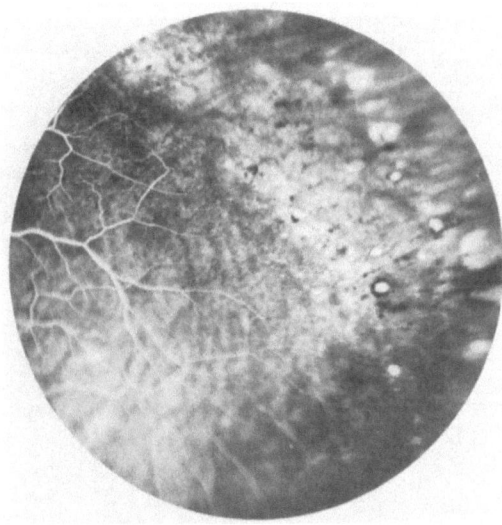

Figure 152. Patient 1. OS. Late phase of the angiogram showing non-perfusion of the temporal retinal periphery.

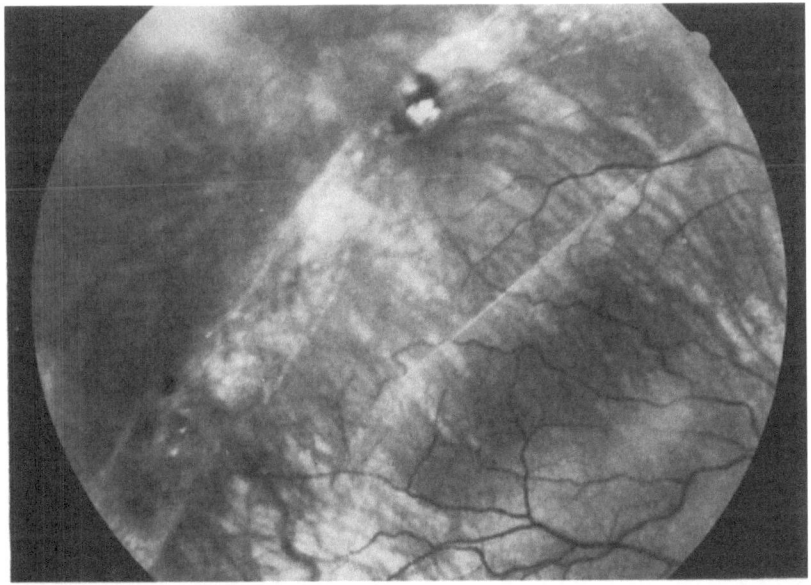

Figure 153. Patient 2. OD. Sharply defined white lesions near the temporal equator. Retinal vessels terminate central to these lesions.

308

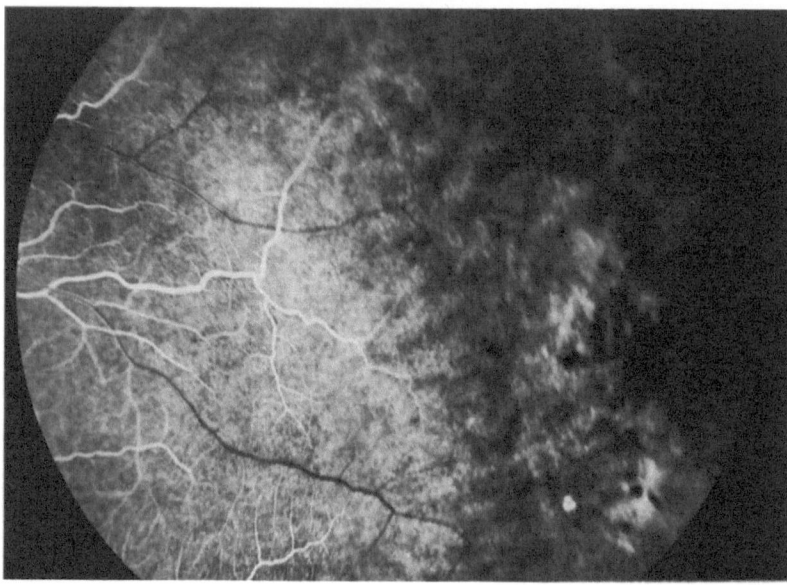

Figure 154. Patient 2. OS. Early venous phase of the angiogram of the temporal equatorial zone.

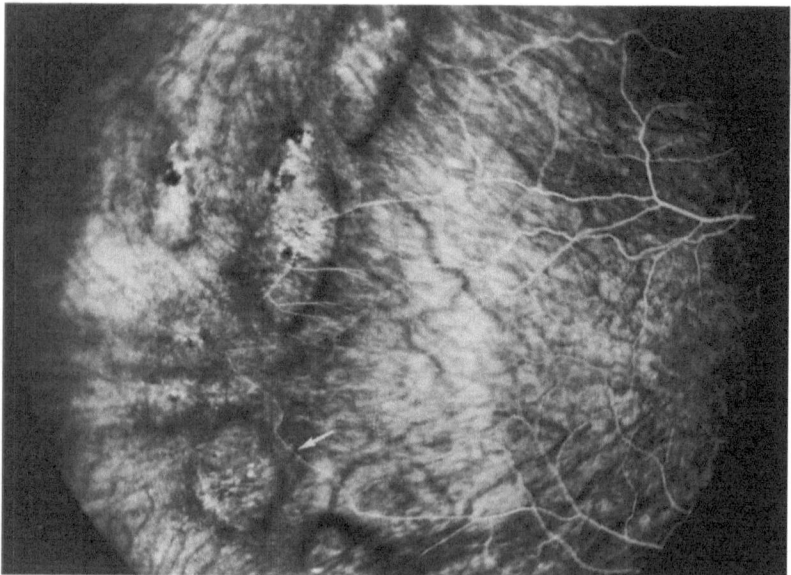

Figure 155. Patient 2. OD. Late phase of the angiogram showing aberrant course of retinal vessels central to the atrophic lesions (arrow).

Late-phase angiograms of the temporal equatorial fundus of OD showed a deviating course of the retinal vessels near the central margin of the atrophic areas. One vessel, however, extended through part of an atrophic area (Figure 155), produced a few ramifications in posterior direction and took an aberrant recurrent course. The retina anterior to the equator was not perfused.

*Patient 3 (06-03-64)*

This 16-year-old sister of patients 1 and 2 showed extensive whitish areas of chorioretinal atrophy, confined almost exclusively to the temporal half of the fundi anterior to the equator. Only a few delicate clumps of pigment were visible in these areas. We selected the mid-periphery of OD at 10 o'clock for fluorescein angiography.

Figure 156A shows the early exposures of this area: central to the equator the larger choroidal vessels and part of the choriocapillaris were already filled, but no fluorescein had entered the peripheral choroid. A normal choroidal flush was visible centrally 3 seconds later. There was filling of some large choroidal vessels in the equatorial zone as well as of a few smaller vessels with terminal ramifications to remnants of the almost totally absent choriocapillaris (Figure 156B). Figure 157 shows a late-phase exposure of the same region: anterior to the equator there was hyperfluorescence due to depigmentation of the pigment epithelium. Retinal vessels were arranged more or less parallel to the central margin of the atrophic periphery. Only two vascular branches extended through the otherwise avascular peripheral retina. Fluorescein angiography of similar regions in OS was not performed because the patient became nauseated after injection of fluorescein.

*Patient 4 (04-09-69)*

This 10-year-old girl was referred to our department with retinal detachment OD, caused by a round hole in a peripheral area of chorioretinal atrophy at 9 o'clock. Fluorescein angiography was performed a few days after a successful encircling operation. The inverse pattern of the vessels at the disc was very pronounced. In both eyes the macula showed ectopia to a position very close to the disc. Marked atrophy of the choriocapillaris and pigment epithelium was visible in the posterior fundus on the nasal side of the optic nerve head.

Peripheral areas of chorioretinal atrophy were seen in the equatorial zone of the temporal half of both fundi (Figure 158A). Some of these areas were also found in the superior nasal quadrants. We selected the equatorial region of OS at 2 o'clock for fluorescein angiography.

Early-phase exposures revealed a nearly absent choriocapillaris and very atrophic pigment epithelium (Figure 158B). The late phase showed hyperfluorescence in the atrophic area and deviant retinal vessels posterior to its central margin (Figure 158C). An interesting finding was that part of the whitish atrophic area showed hyperfluorescence in the late-phase exposures (compare Figure 158A with Figure 158C). No pigment clumps were found in this part, with an apparently normal pigment epithelium.

*Patient 5 (08-10-49)*

Both peripheral fundi of this 30-year-old mother of patient 4 showed more extensive temporal areas of chorioretinal atrophy with sharply defined margins. Figure 159 shows the early-phase fluorescein angiogram of OS at 2 o'clock: no flush of the choriocapillaris and depigmentation of the retinal pigment epithelium anterior to the equator. The more central vessels were deflected and arranged more or less parallel to the posterior margin of the aberrant zone.

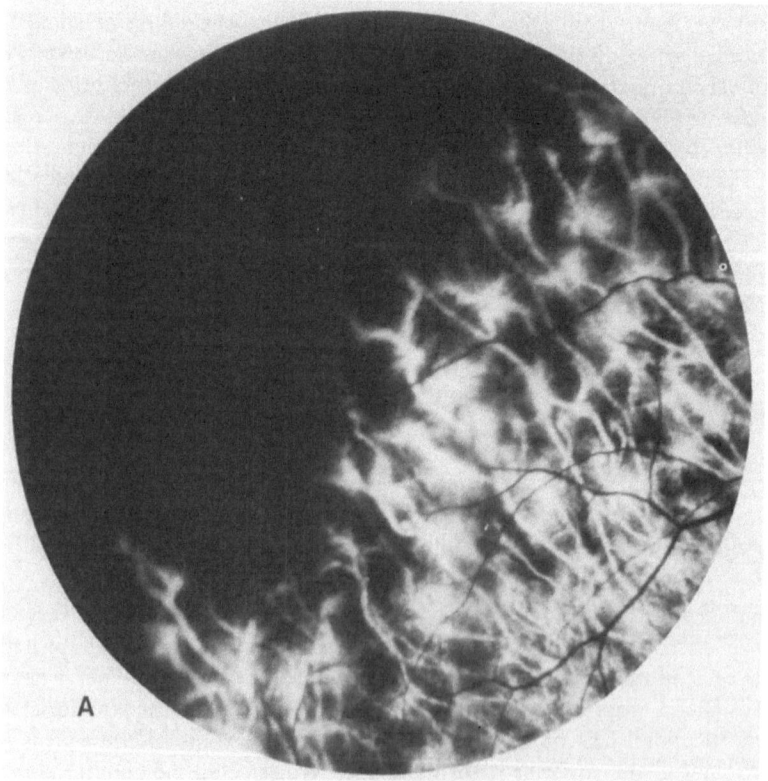

Figure 156. Patient 3. A) OD. Early phase of angiogram of superior temporal quadrant.

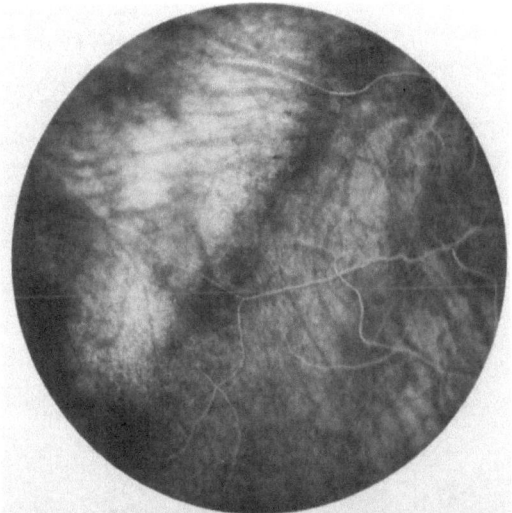

Figure 157. Patient 3. Late phase of the angiogram of the same area as in Figure 156.

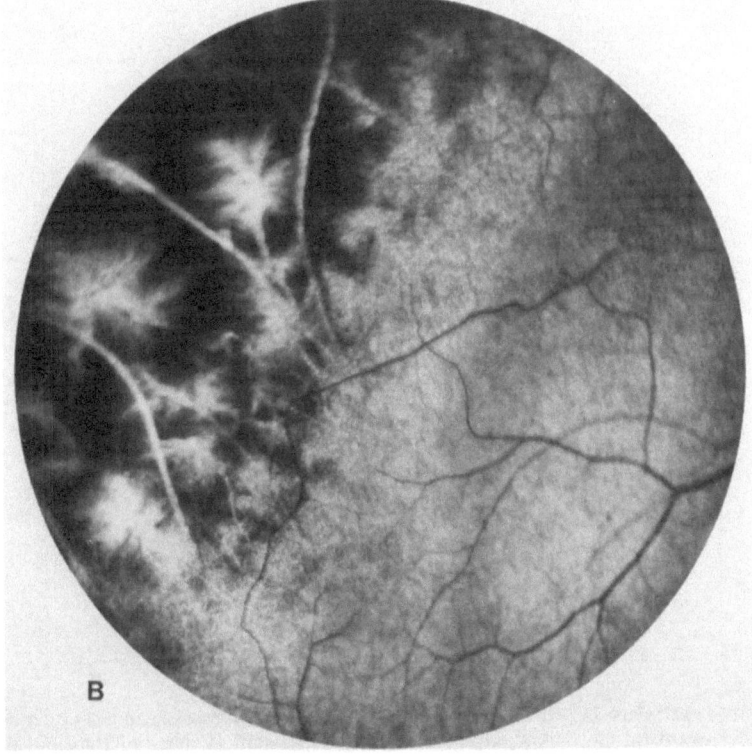

Figure 156. B) Same area as in 156A, but 3 seconds later: disturbed perfusion of the peripheral choriocapillaris.

312

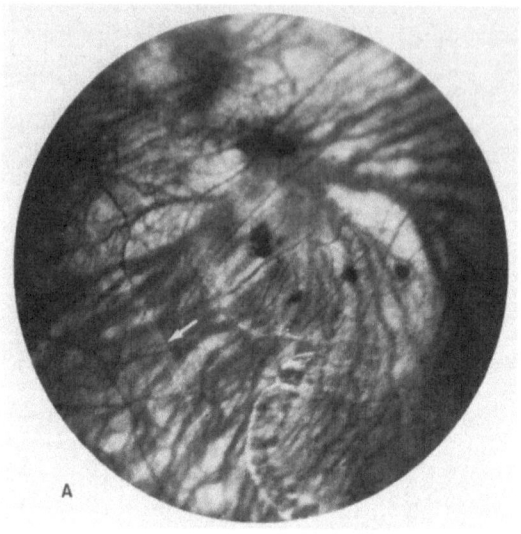

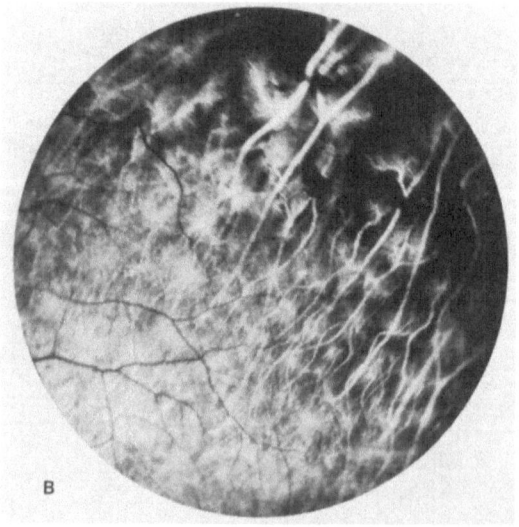

Figure 158. Patient 4. A) OS. Sharply defined white areas encompassing pigment deposits in the equatorial zone of the superior temporal quadrant. Central to these areas, a vitreous membrane attaches to the retina (arrow). B) The same area as in 158A. Early phase of the fluorescein angiogram. C) The same area as in 158A and 158B. Late phase of the angiogram.

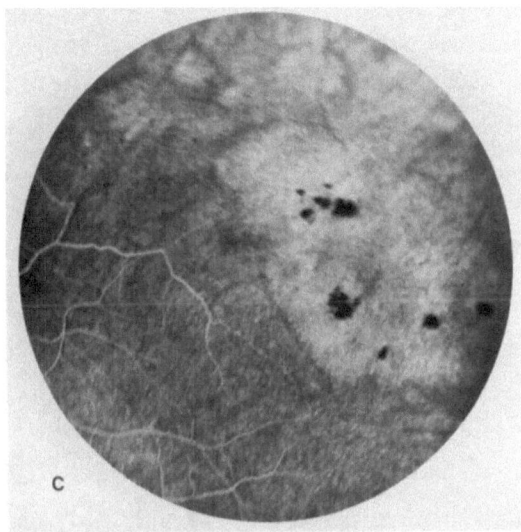

Figure 158. C) The same area as in 158A and 158B. Late phase of the angiogram.

However, a single arterial branch took a radial course through the area of chorioretinal atrophy. Anterior to this lesion the vessel curved back, bifurcated and ended in a few short terminal ramifications at the posterior margin (Figure 160). Argon laser photocoagulation of the upper temporal quadrant of OD was performed in view of retinal degeneration, although no breaks were found. As in OS, retinal vessels were found arranged parallel to the posterior margins of almost avascular areas of chorioretinal atrophy.

*Patient 6 (09-01-62)*

This 18-year-old male was an effected member of a large family with Wagner's vitreoretinal degeneration. The posterior poles of both eyes showed only a slightly abnormal vascular configuration at the disc, and scanty areas of choroidal atrophy were seen in the peripheral fundi; these were virtually confined to the temporal side. No retinal breaks were visible within these areas. Early-phase fluorescein angiograms of OS at 2 o'clock showed delayed, incomplete filling of the choriocapillaris. In this area the larger choroidal vessels were not visible (as they were in the other patients), probably because the pigment epithelium showed less marked depigmentation. Late-phase angiograms revealed very slight leakage from some retinal vessels – a phenomenon not observed in the other patients (Figure 161). The configuration of the vessels, with their deflection at the central margin of the atrophic areas, leaving them devoid of vasculature, was similar to the pattern observed in the other patients.

*Discussion*

The peripheral fundi in our six patients with Wagner's vitreoretinal degeneration showed areas with an aberrant choroidal and retinal structure. The characteristic features of these areas can be summarized as follows.

314

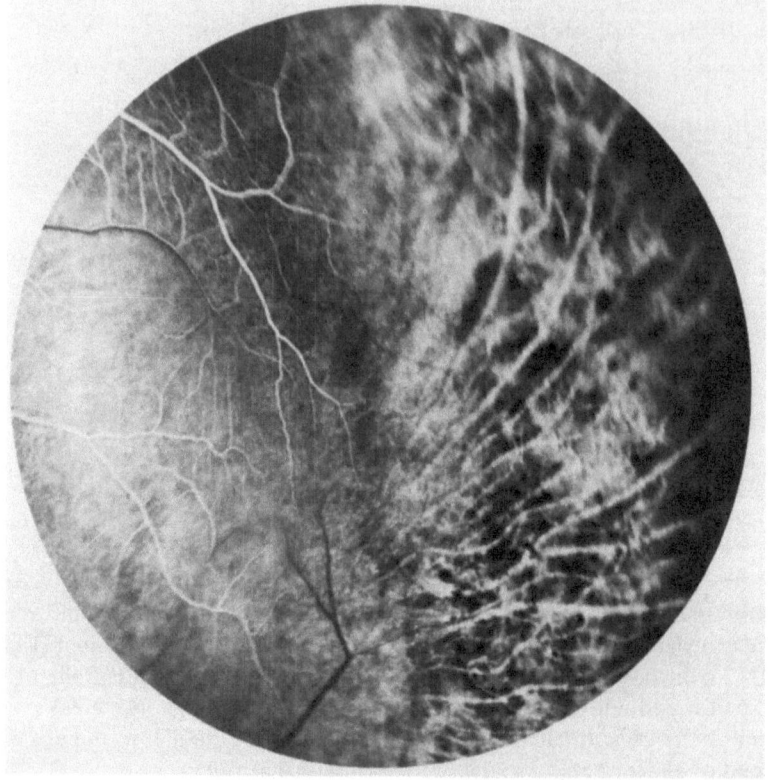

Figure 159. Patient 5. OS. Arteriovenous phase of the fluorescein angiogram showing marked anomalies of the choroid and retinal pigment epithelium anterior to the equator. Non-perfusion of the peripheral retina. Note the abnormal configuration of the retinal vessels.

They were localized mainly in the temporal equatorial zone of the fundus, mostly in the superior quadrant, and always anterior to circumferential white line. Along this line – which is a well-known feature in Wagner's syndrome – vitreous was attached to the retina.

The neuroretina presented a whitish appearance, often in well-defined areas. The preretinal vitreous was liquefied, and consequently it was impossible to distinguish vitreoretinal adhesions along the margins of these areas.

Gross pigment deposits were always present in at least some of the areas, but no pigmentations were found outside the areas in the cases described. In other patients with Wagner's syndrome, however, we have observed clumps of pigment in more posterior parts of the fundus, often in association with degenerated retinal vessels.

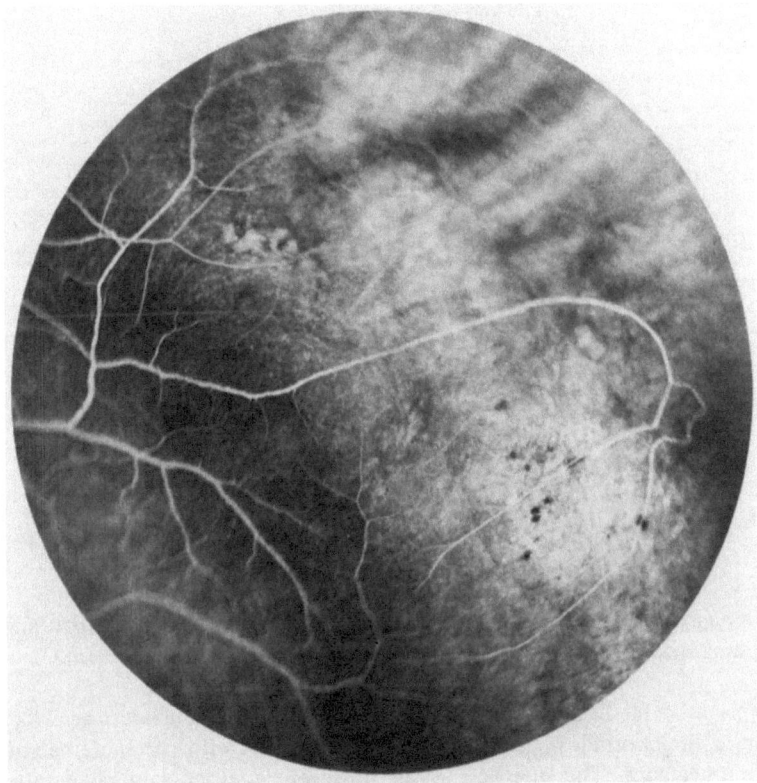

Figure 160. Patient 5. OS. Late phase showing curved and recurrent vascular branches in the equatorial retina.

The following findings were most prominent at fluorescein angiography:

Absence of retinal vessels and consequently non-perfusion of the retina in and anterior to the aberrant areas. In a few cases some of the areas showed the presence of a single retinal vessel. The course and ramifications of such a vessel were usually abnormal (Figures 155 and 160). No signs of vascular occlusion were found in the areas of non-perfusion.

Abnormal retinal vascular pattern central to the posterior margin of the peripheral atrophic areas. In most cases these vessels deviated from a more or less radial course to the periphery to a course which paralleled the posterior margin of the atrophic areas (Figures 151 and 159). Some of the smallest branches ended abruptly at the central margin of the aberrant areas.

Poor filling of the choriocapillaries was clearly observed on the early-phase angiograms of the equatorial fundus (Figures 156B, 158B and 159). The larger choroidal vessels were visible in these areas.

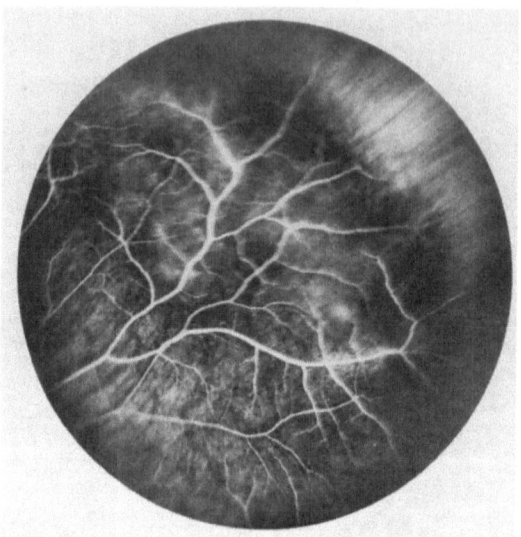

Figure 161. Patient 6. OS. Slight leakage from peripheral retinal vessels.

Depigmentation of the retinal pigment epithelium, the late-phase angiograms showing hyperfluorescence of the atrophic areas (Figure 158C).

I have so far described the abnormal peripheral fundus areas as atrophic because the choroid, pigment epithelium and neuroretina presented an atrophic appearance. The question arises, however, whether these changes were really caused by degeneration of a once normal choroid and retina or resulted from a developmental disorder. There are two important arguments in favour of the latter possibility.

The aberrant areas were equally evident in all our patients, even in the youngest. This suggests a developmental disorder.

The completely abnormal configuration of retinal vessels at the posterior margin of these areas could only be explained by disturbed development. The absence of occluded vessels in the non-perfused temporal periphery also demonstrated that retinal vasculature never developed in this part of the fundus.

I consider these findings to be evidence in support of the conclusion that the aberrant areas in the temporal equatorial zone of the fundus were caused by underdevelopment, and that these areas were therefore dysplastic rather than atrophic.

What remains to be established is the mechanism which effects the blockade of developing retinal vasculature at the equator in Wagner's syndrome. The early-phase fluorescein angiograms of some of our patients (3, 4 and 5) showed that the smaller choroidal vessels and choriocapillaris were poorly developed in the peripheral dysplastic areas.

Before it is vascularized, the retina depends for its nutritional supply on the choriocapillaris, once regression of the hyaloid system has occurred. In my opinion, one of the primary lesions in the fundus of our patients must be hypoplasia of the choriocapillaris in equatorial areas. This hypoplasia probably causes damage to the pigment epithelium and neuroretina (due to hypoxia) before retinal vessels develop in this part of the fundus during the final months of gestation. When the retinal vessels reach the posterior margins of the dysplastic areas, the structure of the damaged neuroretina is probably too inferior to permit them to develop in it. The aspect of the retinal vasculature central to the dysplastic areas suggests that there can be no question of a primary disorder of these vessels themselves, as in the case of, for example, DEVR.

The structure of these vessels was generally normal in our patients, and leakage was seen in only one case. The vitality of the vessels was demonstrated by the fact that most of them extended central to the blockade of the dysplastic areas or grew back in central direction. They had pushed away the more posterior vessels. This process had led to a more or less parallel arrangement with increased packing of retinal vessels at the posterior margin of the dysplastic areas (Figures 151 and 159).

It is important to distinguish the peripheral areas of chorioretinal dysplasia from lattice degeneration, which is a rather frequent finding in Wagner's syndrome. In view of the equatorial localization, the whitish retinal thinning with sharp demarcations and the pigment deposits, lattice degeneration may be mistaken for chorioretinal dysplasia. In lattice degeneration, however, an aborizing network of small white blood vessels is nearly always seen, whereas no remnants of degenerated vessels are found in areas of chorioretinal dysplasia (this is due to non-development of retinal vasculature in these areas, as previously pointed out).

The areas of chorioretinal dysplasia are usually larger than the elongated oval lesions of lattice degeneration. A third difference is the absence of an abnormal configuration of adjacent retinal vessels in lattice degeneration.

The occurrence of chorioretinal dysplasia as well as lattice degeneration demonstrates the ambiguous character of Wagner's syndrome: it is a developmental as well as a degenerative disorder.

The most conspicuous finding in Wagner's syndrome is extensive liquefaction of the vitreous. Wagner (1938) always regarded this abnormality as a developmental disorder because it was present even in the youngest patients. Although there is still some speculation about the origin of the secondary vitreous, most investigators hold that it is produced by retinal Müller cells. The dysplastic peripheral retinal areas may have contributed to the production of aberrant vitreous.

Retinal breaks are frequently observed in Wagner's syndrome. Of 70 eyes examined by Hirose et al. (1973), 59 (75%) showed a retinal break with or without retinal detachment, and surprisingly many were found in young patients. Retinal breaks were much more common in the temporal half of the fundus (67%) than in the nasal half (33%). Many patients showed multiple breaks at different distances from the ora serrata.

This predilection of breaks for the temporal periphery is probably a consequence of the temporal localization of the peripheral areas of chorioretinal dysplasia. In these areas the retina is very thin due to the combination of poor choroidal and absent retinal blood supply. This atrophy of all retinal layers can easily give rise to a break. In our patients 2 and 4 we observed small circular retinal holes in the peripheral dysplastic areas. The retinal detachment in our patient 4 was caused by such a break. The frequent occurrence of retinal breaks in young patients supports my theory that these breaks are caused by congenital failure of the circulation in the peripheral choroid and retina. In older patients, however, equatorial and lattice degeneration may contribute to the formation of retinal breaks.

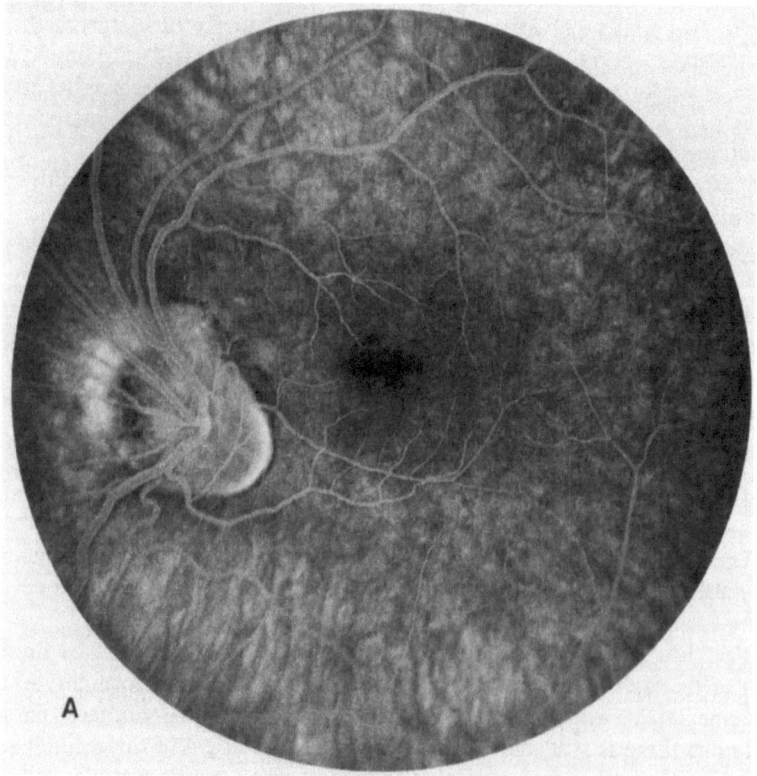

Figure 162. Patient 5. OS. Fluorescein angiogram. A) The configuration of retinal vessels in the posterior pole and the macular ectopia suggest nasal displacement of these structures during development.

### 10.1.e Pathogenesis of the aberrant configuration of retinal vessels in the posterior pole and ectopia of the macula

An aberrant configuration of retinal vessels in the posterior pole is a frequent finding in Wagner's syndrome. This anomaly is often especially pronounced near the disc: the large ramifications of the central retinal artery and vein exit over the lamina cribosa in nasal direction. Particularly the temporal branches deflect in temporal direction at some distance from the disc (Figure 149). The incidence of this aberrant configuration of retinal vessels near the disc varies widely in Wagner's syndrome, and ranges from hardly discernible to pronounced forms as shown in Figure 162A. The vessels exiting from the disc always extend in nasal direction. This is why some authors use the term "inversed disc" (Jansen, 1966). The disc itself, however, is normally implanted, and the abnormalities involve only the retinal vessels. The position of the macula can be normal, but extopia of the macula is often seen when the changes in the vascular pattern are very marked. In cases known to me, the macular ectopia was always also in nasal direction.

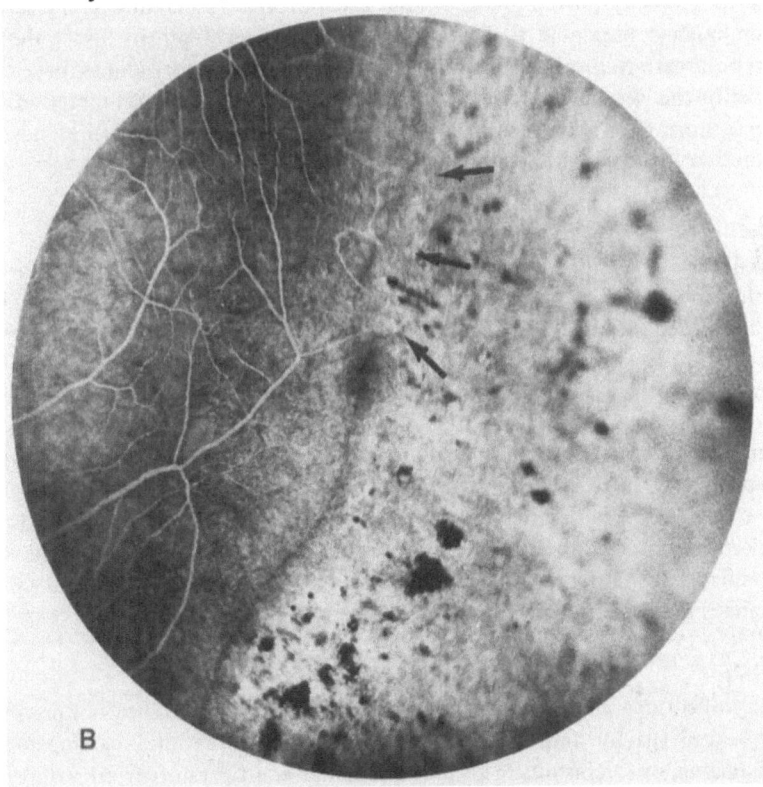

Figure 162. B) Closely packed parallel vessels in the temporal fundus. These vessels have been unable to develop in the dysplastic zone (right half of photograph), as clearly demonstrated by the course of one vessel along the central boundary of this zone (arrows).

The posterior pole of OS in our patient 4 showed the most extreme macular ectopia I have ever observed in Wagner's syndrome: in this case the foveola was seen close to the temporal margin of the disc.

The aberrant vascular configuration in the posterior pole and the macular ectopia in Wagner's syndrome indicate displacement of the blood vessels and probably also of other structures of the neuroretina in nasal direction.

In Wagner's syndrome the preretinal vitreous contains no structures which might have caused significant tractional deformation of the retina (the only discernible structure in the vitreous is the delicate vitreous membrane central to the equator, which causes no retinal deformation even near its attachment to the retina).

There are therefore sound reasons to assume that the anomalies in the posterior pole are not acquired but result from a developmental disorder.

In my opinion the deformation of the retinal vasculature in the posterior pole in Wagner's syndrome has developed in response to the inability of the more peripheral ramifications to grow in the dysplastic zones (Figure 162B). We have already mentioned the abnormal arrangement of retinal vessels central to these dysplastic areas, where parts of the vasculature seem to have been pushed back due to lack of room during development. Since the dysplastic areas are localized mainly in the temporal equatorial zone, developing parts of the vasculature have been pushed back mostly in nasal direction. This displacement has not confined itself to the peripheral vessels but has continued into the posterior pole of the fundus (Figure 163).

## 10.2 Sex-linked retinoschisis

Sex-linked juvenile retinoschisis is a hereditary condition of the neuroretina which involves both the posterior pole and the periphery of the fundus. Jager (1953), Balian and Falls (1960), Ricci (1961), Ewing and Ives (1969) and Deutman (1971). Many other authors have described smaller families or individual patients.

I do not intend to present a detailed discussion of all aspects of this disease, but rather refer to relevant publications by Franchescetti et al. (1963) and Deutman (1971).

However, a few less widely known symptoms sometimes observed in sex-linked juvenile retinoschisis merit special attention. They are: ectopia of the macula, deformation of the retinal vessels in the posterior pole, and vascular changes in the peripheral retina.

### 10.2.a Clinical symptoms

Sex-linked juvenile retinoschisis as a rule manifests itself in boys of pre-school or school age by diminished visual acuity ODS, sometimes accompanied by nystagmus or strabismus. The reduced visual acuity results from retinoschisis in the macula. The changes in the posterior pole are often subtle, and fundus

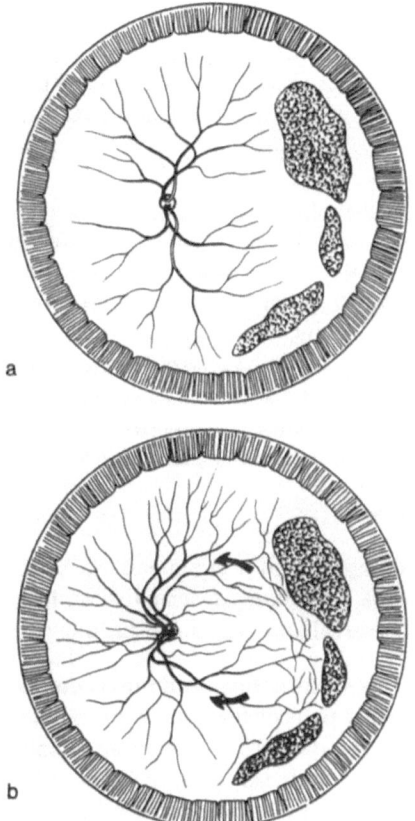

Figure 163. Schematic representation of the pathogenesis of the nasal displacement of retinal vessels in Wagner's syndrome (fundus OS). A) Situation by about the 6th–7th month of foetal development. A few dysplastic areas in the temporal fundus. Development of retinal vessels has so far been normal. B) During the final months of intra-uterine development the temporal vascular branches have reached the central boundary of the dysplastic zones. Further growth pushes more central parts of the vascular network in nasal direction (arrows).

examination with slit-lamp and contact lens is indispensable in identifying the lesions. A characteristic feature is the presence of a delicate, wheel-like structure at the centre of the posterior pole, within which small cysts are often visible in the superficial retinal layers. Around this structure the internal limiting membrane shows delicate radial folds extending in all directions in the posterior pole.

The changes in the posterior pole usually disappear gradually with increasing age, while less specific atrophic changes of the macula persist (Deutman, 1971).

Nearly always there are glittering white areas throughout the fundus. They are reminiscent of Berlin's oedema (Bengtson and Linder, 1967). True retinoschisis as a rule occurs bilaterally in the periphery of the inferior temporal quadrant. Although changes in the posterior pole were found in virtually all cases of sex-linked juvenile retinoschisis, peripheral retinoschisis was observed in only about 50% of cases (Ewing and Yves, 1969). Gross pigment deposits may be found scattered in the fundus (Sabates, 1966), and fluorescein angiography often clearly reveals changes of the pigment epithelium (Constantaras et al., 1972).

Movable veils are often (but by no means always) found in the vitreous. They are usually attached to the retina and sometimes encompass parts of the retinal vasculature. In such cases these structures are quite unmistakably loosened parts of the inner retinal layers which, due to ruptures in these layers, often show hardly any connection with the retina. The detached avascular veils sometimes found in the vitreous probably also originate from the inner retinal layers. Detachment of the posterior vitreous membrane is a very common finding in sex-linked juvenile retinoschisis. Anterior vitreous detachment can also occur (Bailian and Falls, 1960; Lisch, 1968).

### 10.2.b Vascular changes

Although vascular changes are not prominent in sex-linked juvenile retinoschisis, the condition is sometimes associated with interesting phenomena in the retina. The retinal vasculature may show the following changes.

Deformation of the vascular bed. Abnormal configuration of the blood vessels in the loosened parts of the neuroretina is of course to be expected, because these retinal structures are themselves subject to morphological changes. Rupture of vessels can sometimes cause haemorrhages between the separated retinal layers (Conway and Welch, 1977).

A more interesting feature is the vascular deformation which occurs in attached parts of the retina. Figure 164 is a fluorescein angiogram of an area in the inferior temporal quadrant of the left fundus, central to the equator. It shows temporally extending stretched vessels which merge into the central part of the cleavage. The posterior poles ODS in this case show a vascular configuration highly reminiscent of that of DEVR, with pronounced inferior temporal ectopia of the macula (Figure 165A and B). It seems likely that the deformation in the posterior poles results mainly from traction exerted by the peripheral retinoschisis. The literature has so far paid scant attention to such phenomena in sex-linked juvenile retinoschisis, probably because pronounced changes of the kind described here are rare. Nevertheless, examination of fundus photographs in these cases shows that slight macular ectopia is not rare. In some exceptional cases of sex-linked juvenile retinoschisis there may even be a small radial fold in the posterior pole (Figure 166).

Degeneration of the vascular wall. White vascular sheaths are not uncommon in sex-linked juvenile retinoschisis. Identical changes are sometimes observed in Wagner's syndrome, but not in DEVR.

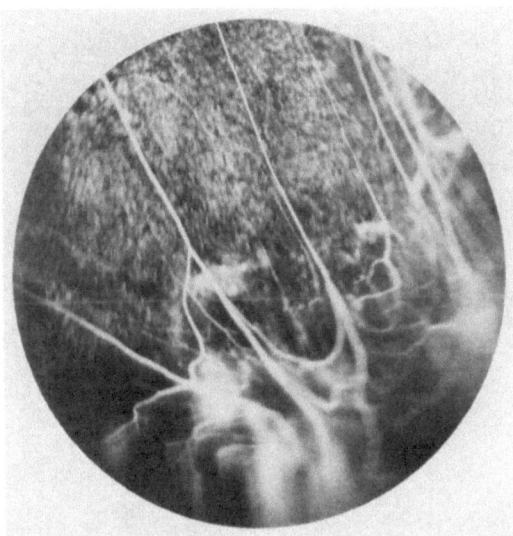

Figure 164. OS. Stretched vessels in the retina central to the retinoschisis (top). The blood vessels bottom right are localized within the region of retinal cleavage.

Incomplete vascularization of the peripheral retina is an interesting pheno-menon, observed only in a minority of patients with sex-linked juvenile retinoschisis. The avascular temporal retinal periphery is bounded on the central side by a zone of aberrant, underdeveloped capillaries (Figure 167). These vessels are often sclerotic and present themselves as the whitish, den-drite-like structures described by Balian and Falls (1961) and Cibis (1965). Ewing and Ives (1969) considered these structures to originate from vessels. Identical whitish degeneration of the most peripheral capillaries can also be seen in DEVR (Chapter 3, Figure 20). Fluorescein angiography of such areas in sex-linked juvenile retinoschisis can sometimes reveal exactly the same features as in DEVR (see Bec et al., 1980).

The above described findings imply that some cases of sex-linked juvenile retinoschisis involve premature arrest of the development of the peripheral retinal vasculature which closely resembles that observed in DEVR.

A possible explanation of the peripheral retinal vascular developmental dis-order in some patients with sex-linked juvenile retinoschisis is that the retino-schisis in these cases occurs before completion of retinal vascularization during the intra-uterine period. It is quite conceivable that the cleavage in the nerve fibre layer of the retina, which in the peripheral retina contains the majority of the blood vessels, precludes further development of the latter. It is beyond doubt that the vascular network can become severely damaged in sex-linked juvenile retinoschisis, and that the connections between the superficial blood vessels and those localized at a slightly deeper level in the nerve fibre layer,

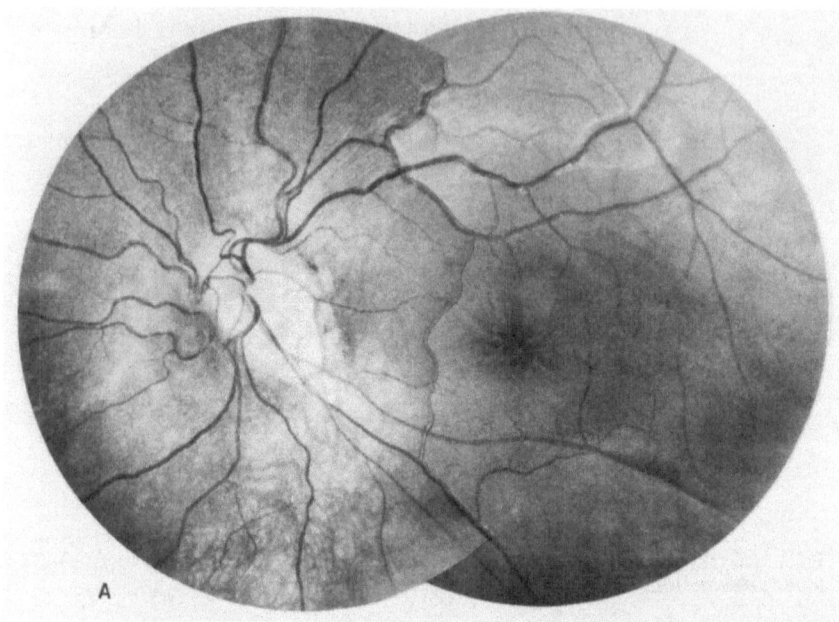

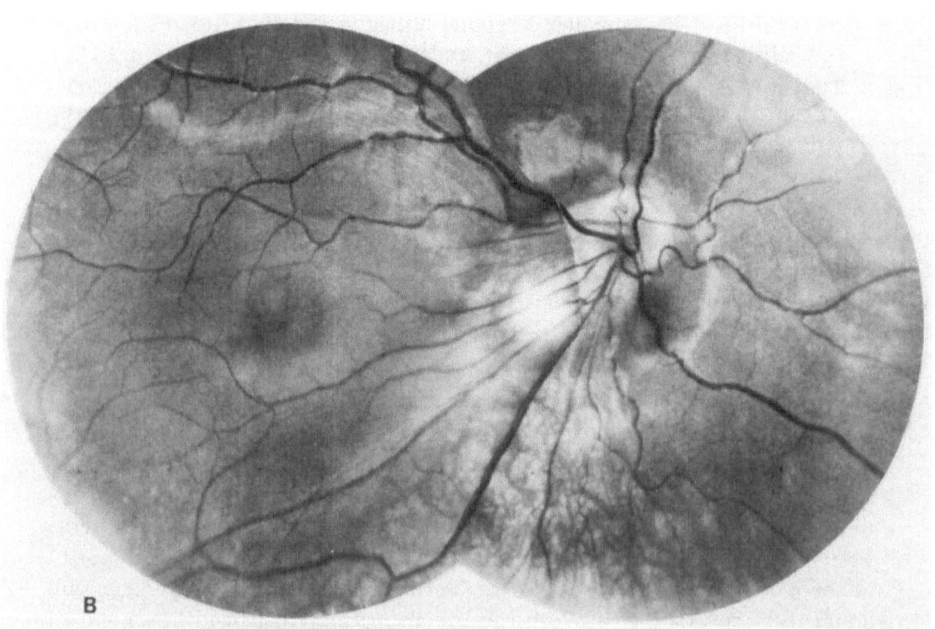

Figure 165. Macular ectopia in OS (A) and OD (B) of a patient with sex-linked juvenile retinoschisis.

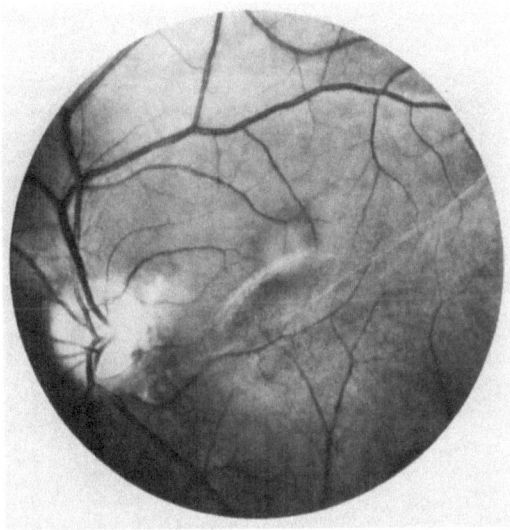

Figure 166. OS. Small retinal fold in the macular region in sex-linked juvenile retino-schisis. Slight superior ectopia of the macula. Similar changes were present in OD.

can be disrupted. Symptoms of such disruption are visible in Figure 167, where some blood vessels seem to terminate abruptly. Should such incidents occur in the course of the intra-uterine period, they should certainly interfere with the development of the peripheral retinal blood vessels.

### 10.2.c Histology and pathogenesis

Yanoff et al. (1969) were the first to describe the histopathological changes in sex-linked juvenile retinoschisis. They established that the cleavage of the neuroretina occurs in the nerve fibre layer. The site of the cleavage distinctly differs from that in senile retinoschisis, in which the changes are mostly confined to the outer plexiform layer. Microscopic changes of the retinal vessels were not observed.

The pathogenesis of the cleavage of the inner retinal layers has so far remained obscure. The primary defect may be localized in the Müller cells, as Yanoff et al. (1968) suggested; but it cannot be excluded that the nerve fibres play a role in the pathogenesis of the changes (Manschot, 1972).

The ERG always shows abnormalities in sex-linked juvenile retinoschisis (Ricci, 1960; Forsius et al., 1963). The B-wave is clearly reduced in many cases. Since the B-wave probably originates largely from the Müller cells (Miller and Dowling, 1970), the ERG abnormalities might be compatible with a primary defect of these cells.

The role played by the retinal vessels and peripheral retinal circulation in the pathogenesis of the retinoschisis is not clear. Some authors (Ewing and

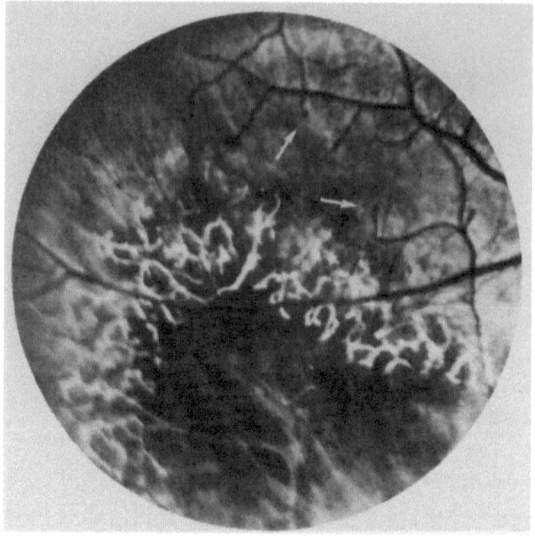

Figure 167. Vascular anomalies in the equatorial retina in sex-linked juvenile retinoschisis.

Ives, 1969) consider it possible that vascular changes might be of primary importance for the retinal cleavage. In my opinion it is more likely that the retinal vascular changes are a result of the retinoschisis rather than its cause.

## 10.3  Juvenile rhegmatogenous retinal detachment

Several authors have reported on fluorescein-angiographic examination of the peripheral fundus in patients with non-traumatic rhegmatogenous retinal detachment and/or their relatives. Amalric (1969) presented peripheral angiographic changes found in a 15-year-old sister of a 17-year-old female with rhegmatogenous retinal detachment as a result of multiple retinal defects. The aberrant configuration of the peripheral retinal vessels with abnormally numerous terminal ramifications ending in a zone which comprised leaking neovascularizations and the familial occurrence of the peripheral retinal anomalies, strike me as highly suggestive of DEVR.

Rosen (1968) demonstrated angiographic perfusion disorders in three patients with rhegmatogenous retinal detachment. Their retinal detachment resulted from a horseshoe rupture, multiple small retinal defects, and disinsertion of the retina, respectively. The angiographic changes in these eyes varied widely, and in no case was the fluorescein angiogram suggestive of an abnormal development of the retinal vasculature.

Tatsuyama and Shimizu (1972) performed fluorescein angiography in 26 patients with rhegmatogenous retinal detachment of different age and with different clinical symptoms. The authors generally found disturbed perfusion in equatorial degenerative areas which comprised retinal defects. They regarded these circulatory disorders as due to obliteration of peripheral retinal vessels. No angiographic findings suggestive of DEVR were obtained in this series of patients.

Wessing (1974) made some interesting observations in patients with retinal detachment. He described "fan-shaped formations abruptly ceasing posterior to the degenerative area". The peripheral ramifications of retinal vessels were abnormally stretched and very closely packed, giving the impression of an increased number of blood vessels. The angiograms (Wessing, 1974) strike me as suggestive of DEVR, or at least of disturbed vascular development. By virtue of the absence of fluorescein leakage from these vessels, the angiographic features were identical with those found in our H family (Chapter 3).

Wessing's observation (1974) that the formations of peripheral retinal vessels were mainly found in young patients, is quite compatible with the theory of a developmental disorder.

Minoda and Kanagami (1976) performed fluorescein angiography in 100 patients with rhegmatogenous retinal detachment, and in many eyes found total avascularity of the peripheral retina. The retinal vasculature ended in numerous terminal ramifications and arteriovenous anastomoses from which fluorescein leaked. The demarcation between vascular and avascular retina was well-defined; it was straight in some cases, but meandered in others. A similar pattern was often observed in the contralateral eye with an attached retina.

Several angiographic illustrations in the article published by Minoda and Kanagami (1976) are identical with the angiogram of vascular anomalies in our patients with DEVR. In my opinion the findings suggest disturbed vascular development rather than changes secondary to retinal detachment. Identical changes can result from RLF. The article presents no information of the patients' neonatal histories, nor on ocular symptoms (if any) in members of their families.

Numaga and Miyakubu (1981) found fluorescein-angiographic evidence of peripheral retinal vascular anomalies in 20% of 51 eyes of 45 patients with retinal detachment who were younger than 20. The lesions very closely resembled those of RLF, but none of the patients had been born prematurely. The authors rightly concluded that the symptoms indicated a vascular developmental disorder as a factor in the pathogenesis of the retinal detachment. In my opinion the angiographic findings in their patients are identical to those obtained in DEVR. In their summary at least, the authors make no mention of a family study.

### 10.3.a Personal observations

Our experience with peripheral fluorescein angiography in younger patients (not over 25) with non-traumatic rhegmatogenous retinal detachment is limited to about 10 cases. In one of these patients the fluorescein-angiographic findings were an important aid in diagnosing DEVR (IV-6 H). The remaining 9 patients included 8 in whom the peripheral retina showed no angiographic changes clearly suggestive of retinal vascular developmental disorder. In one 18-year-old patient with recent rhegmatogenous retinal detachment, perfusion of the peripheral retina was abnormal in both eyes. The findings obtained in this patient and his nearest relatives are reported below.

*Patient II-1 (14-01-62)*

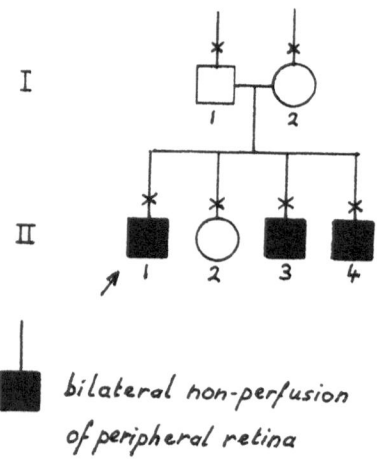

bilateral non-perfusion
of peripheral retina

Figure 168. Pedigree of the family of patient II-1 (14-01-62)

*History*
Visual complaints OS since two weeks. No trauma. No eye diseases known in the family. No record of premature birth or neonatal oxygen administration.

*Ophthalmological examination*

| | |
|---|---|
| Visual acuity | VOD: Cyl. − 2.0 axis 3° 1.0. |
| | VOS: 0.1, uncorrected. |
| Vitreous | OD: Mild syneresis. |
| | OS: Mild syneresis; pigment particles. |
| Fundi | OD: Whitish degenerative area in the superior temporal quadrant with a few small retinal defects. |
| | OS: Rhegmatogenous retinal detachment in both temporal quadrants. A whitish retinal area in the superior temporal quadrant contains a few small circular defects. |

Fluorescein angiogram      OD: No retinal perfusion peripheral to the equator in the temporal equatorial zone. The configuration of the vessels central to the equator is not clearly abnormal.

OS: Fluorescein leakage in the area posterior to the temporal equator in the detached retina. No perfusion of the peripheral retina (Figure 169).

*Family study*

All family members were ophthalmologically examined, including biomicroscopy of the peripheral fundus in full mydriasis. The patient's father (I-1) showed marked syneresis of the vitreous ODS, but no other abnormalities. The patient's mother (I-2) and sister (II-2) showed no abnormalities. The retinal periphery in both brothers showed no distinct retinal vasculature anterior to the equator in the temporal half, but a vascular configuration of the type seen in DEVR was not found. One of the brothers (II-4) showed a few small white spots in the inferior temporal quadrant of the retinal periphery OD.

*Examination of II-3 (19-12-65)*

Fluorescein angiogram      OD: The retinal vasculature in the inferior temporal quadrant seems to terminate anterior to the equator. The peripheral boundary is partly formed by curved venous branches which

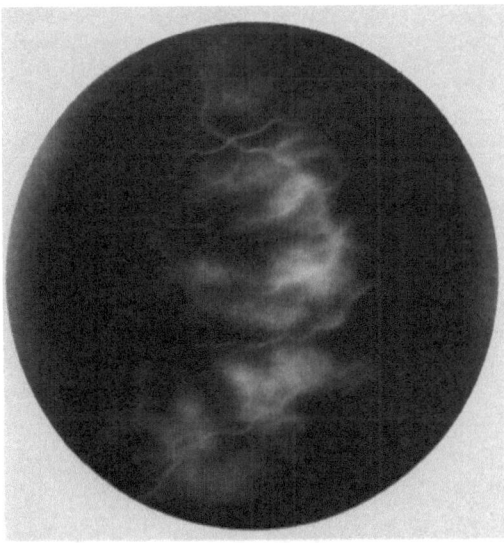

Figure 169. **II-1. OS.** Late phase of angiogram showing leakage from equatorial vessels in the detached retina. The peripheral retina seems to show non-perfusion.

present the appearance of arcade vessels. No fluorescein leakage from these vessels (Figure 170).

OS: The inferior temporal quadrant shows virtually the same abnormal features as in OD.

*Examination of II-4 (10-05-67)*

Fluorescein angiogram

OD: The temporal retinal vasculature ends anterior to the equator. The most peripheral parts of the vascular network are of very low density. Arcade vessels form the peripheral demarcation (Figure 171).

OS: The peripheral retinal vessels again seem to end anterior to the equator. A few scars of the pigment epithelium are seen in the non-perfused zone.

*Discussion*

The fluorescein angiograms of the three brothers all suggest a somewhat anomalous vascular development of the peripheral retina. Near the equator the retinal vascular network is of strikingly low density, and the vasculature ends slightly peripheral to the equator. A striking finding is that the most peripheral parts of the vasculature shows a normal configuration even with the presence

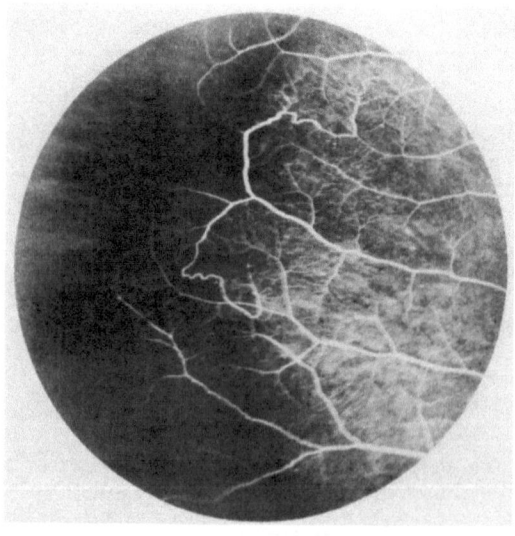

Figure 170. II-3. OD. Fluorescein angiogram of the temporal periphery.

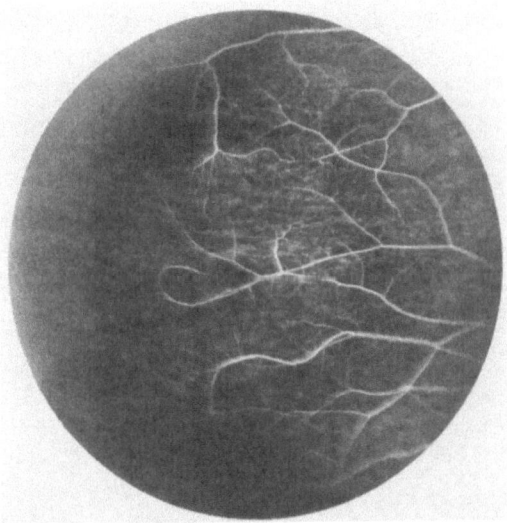

Figure 171. II-4. OD. Fluorescein angiogram of the temporal periphery.

of arcade vessels, which, however, are not localized in the region of the ora serrata but only slightly peripheral to the equator.

The extent to which these anomalies have been the cause of the retinal defects and retinal detachment in II-1 cannot be established with certainty. It is certain, however, that the retinal defects in this patient were found in the non-perfused part of the retina, and that consequently the non-perfusion of this part of the retina has probably played a role in their pathogenesis.

The presence of these anomalies in the three brothers of course suggests that the condition is hereditary. The type of transmission is a matter of speculation in this small family. DEVR merits primary consideration in differential diagnosis from this condition, in which the configuration of the peripheral retinal vasculature differs from that in DEVR in that underdeveloped capillaries are not visible anywhere, there is no fluorescein leakage, and the vascular pattern central to the equator is normal.

CHAPTER 11

# CONGENITAL BILATERAL ARTERIAL ANASTOMOSIS BETWEEN THE CHOROID AND THE PERIPHERAL RETINA

Vascular anastomoses between the choroid and the retina can be either acquired or congenital. Acquired anastomoses have been described in conditions associated with lesions of Bruch's membrane, e.g. chorioretinitis due to toxoplasmosis (Saari et al., 1975), photocoagulation (Galinos et al., 1976), senile disciform degeneration of the macula (Green and Gass, 1971) and trauma (Goldberg, 1976a).

Congenital anastomoses between the choroidal and the retinal circulation occur as asymptomatic vascular variants, e.g. cilioretinal arteries and opticociliary arteries and veins near the disc.

In a case recently reported by Slusher and Tyler (1980) there was a cilioretinal artery which did not communicate with the retinal circulation via a capillary bed, as usual, but showed a direct anastomosis with a retinal arterial branch.

Daicker (1968) likewise reported on asymptomatic congenital retinochoroidal anastomoses in the peripheral fundus.

Van Nouhuys and Deutman (1980) described a female patient with congenital bilateral anastomoses between the peripheral choroid and retina which in one eye had led to significant visual loss. This patient's case history is presented here.

*Case history*

A 26-year-old woman was referred to us two weeks after she had noticed blurred vision OS. Her general medical history was unremarkable.

*Ophthalmological examination*

| | |
|---|---|
| Visual acuity | VOD: 1.25, emmetropia. |
| | VOS: 0.12, emmetropia. |
| Anterior segments | ODS: Normal cornea, anterior chamber and iris. Clear lenses. With a fully dilated pupil the inferior margins of both lenses are visible from 4 to 8 o'clock, where they are somewhat irregular. No gap is visible in the zonules. |
| Vitreous | ODS: A few punctate opacities. |

Fundi

OD: Normal posterior pole. A local not prominent retinal detachment in the inferior periphery of the fundus extends in central direction slightly posterior to the equator. The retinal vessels in the detached area are deformed and irregular. Exudates are seen beneath the central part of the retinal detachment (Figure 172). No retinal breaks are visible.

OS: The posterior pole shows preretinal gliotic membranes giving rise to an evident pucker of the macula. A few small retinal exudates are visible beneath this area (Figure 173). The inferior periphery shows exudative retinal detachment very similar to that in OD. The retinal vessels in the detached area are tortuous. A few small retinal haemorrhages are seen next to these vessels (Figure 174).

Fluorescein angiogram

OD: The early phase of the inferior equatorial area shows no filling of the choriocapillaris beneath the detached retina. One choroid artery in this area appears to be filled by fluorescein in centripetal direction (Figure 175A). Near the equator this artery produces several branches connected with dilatated, abnormal retinal

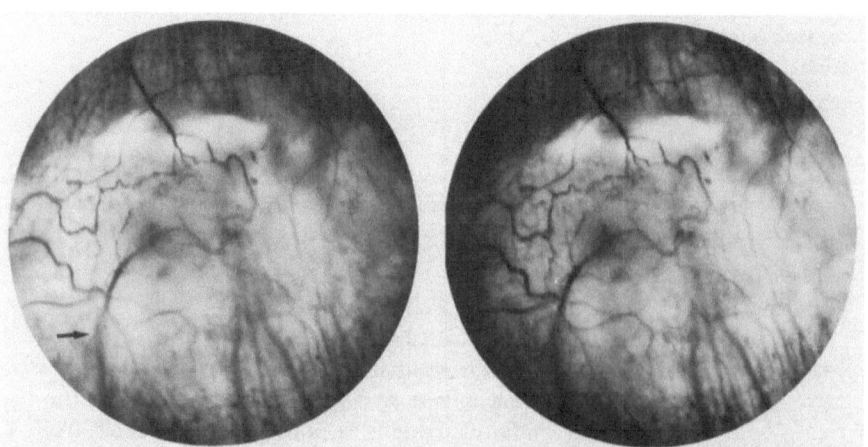

Figure 172. OD. Stereo-photograph showing local exudative retinal detachment in the equatorial zone near 6 o'clock, and tortuous blood vessels. Note the choroidal blood vessel (arrow).

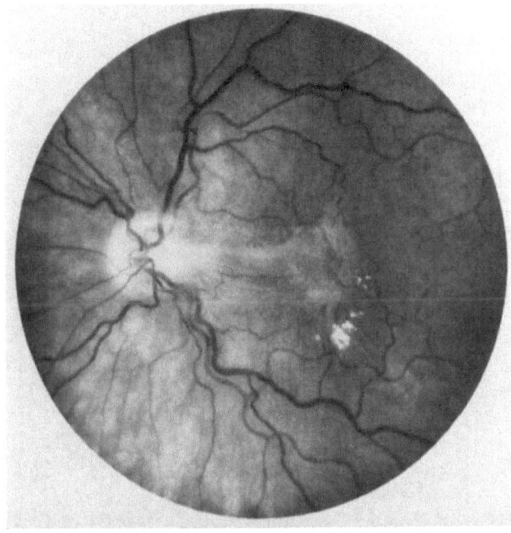

Figure 173. OS. Posterior pole with macular pucker.

vessels (Figure 175B). Profuse leakage from these vessels rapidly stains the retina and subretinal fluid (Figure 175C).

OS: A separate fluorescein angiogram was made for early-phase exposures of the area of exudative detachment. A large choroid artery fills

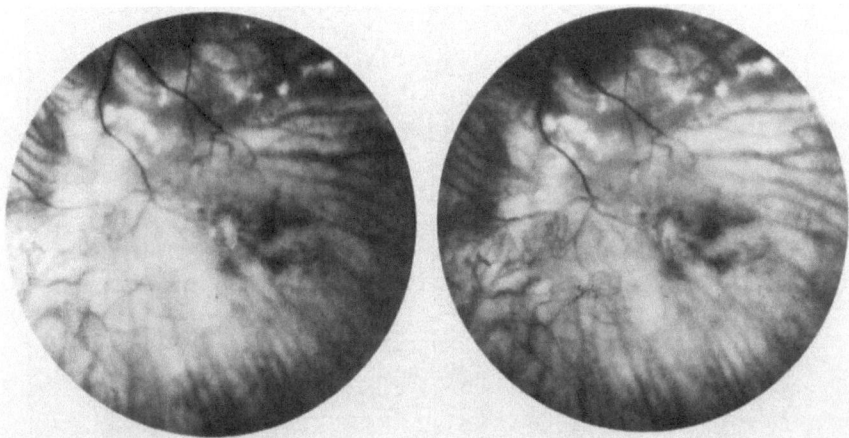

Figure 174. OS. Stereo-photograph showing local exudative retinal detachment near the equator (6 o'clock position).

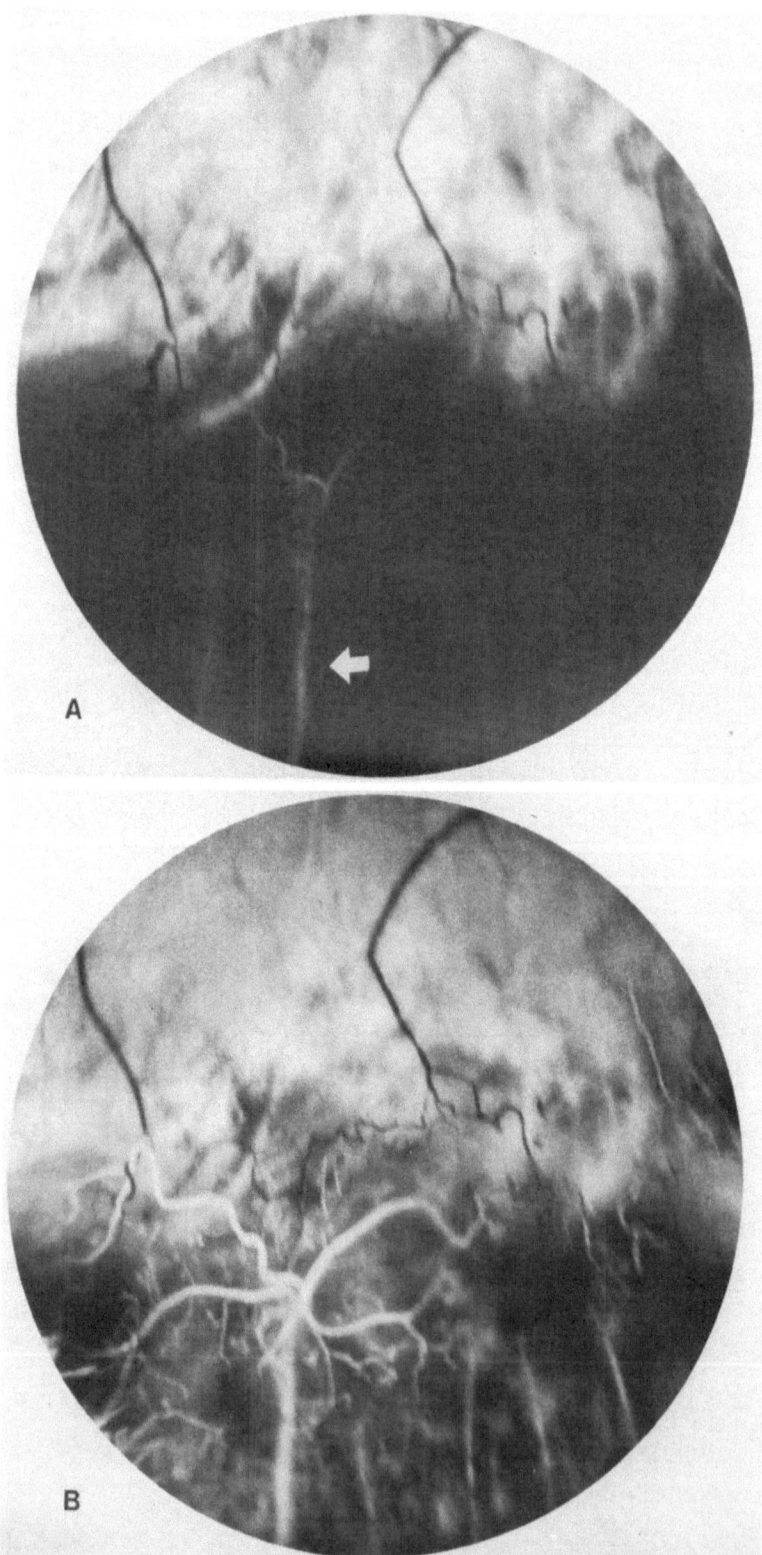

with fluorescein in centripetal direction (Figure 176A). Several branches of this artery are connected with aberrant retinal vessels in the equatorial retina (Figure 176B).

ERG and EOG       ODS: Normal.

### General physical and laboratory findings

General physical examination revealed no abnormalities. Laboratory findings (ESR, complete blood count, serum electrolytes, glucose, urea, nitrogen and alkaline phosphatase, Rose test, latex test, agglutination tests for toxoplasmosis, VDRL, serum protein electrophoresis and tests for abnormal haemoglobins) were normal. So were X-rays of the chest and paranasal sinuses.

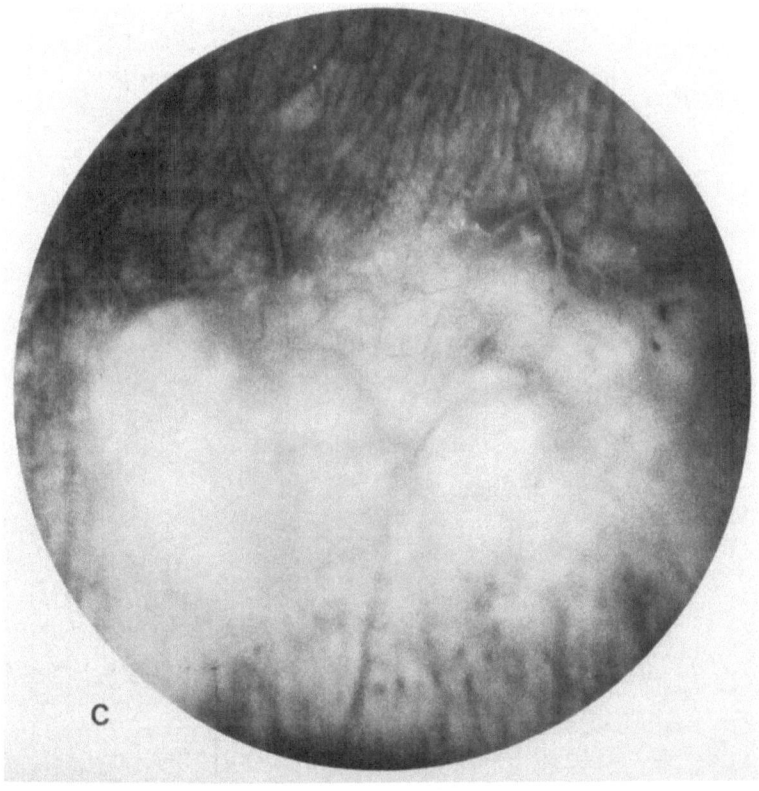

Figure 175. OD. Fluorescein angiogram of the region shown in Figure 172. A) Centripetal filling of choroid artery (arrow) in the early phase. B) Slightly later exposure showing filling of several ramifications of the choroid artery. These ramifications communicate with retinal vessels. C) Diffuse fluorescein leakage into the subretinal fluid.

338

*Family study*
Four sisters and one brother underwent complete ophthalmological examination, which revealed no abnormality at all. The patient's mother showed diabetic retinopathy.

*Follow-up and treatment*
The patient's visual acuity and fundus lesions remained unchanged during about a year after her first visit to our department. Subsequently, however, we observed a slight increase in subretinal exudates and the area of serous retinal detachment in the direction of the posterior fundus.

An attempt was made to close the anastomosing choroid artery by cryo-coagulation in order to arrest the process of continuous intraretinal and subretinal leakage: 15 months after the initial examination cryocoagulations were applied to the sclera OD overlying the peripheral segment of the main

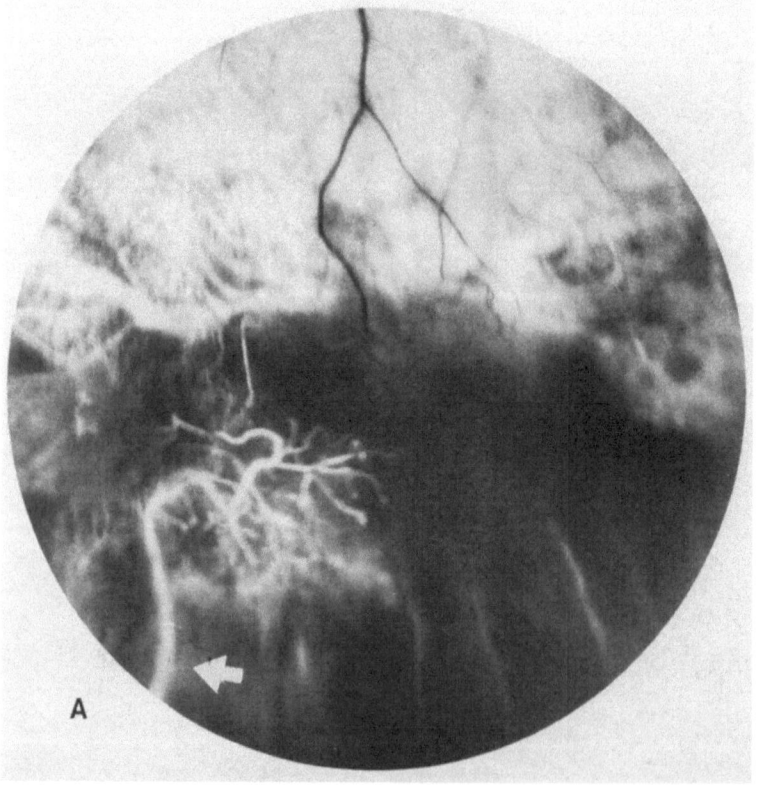

Figure 176. OS. Fluorescein angiogram of the region shown in Figure 174. A) Early phase showing filling of a large choroid artery in centripetal direction (arrow); this artery produces several branches to the retina.

anastomosing choroid artery. No complications occurred during and after this treatment, but fluorescein angiography 6 and 10 months later clearly revealed a patent anastomosis and undiminished leakage. No further attempts to close the anastomosis have since been made.

*Discussion*

The choroid arteries which form the anastomoses in our patient's eyes, are quite evidently "recurrent ciliary arteries". The fluorescein angiogram clearly showed that the blood flow came from the anterior choroid in central direction. Angiographic demonstration of these peripheral arteries is generally impossible, but in our case we succeeded by virtue of the non-perfusion of the peripheral choriocapillaris.

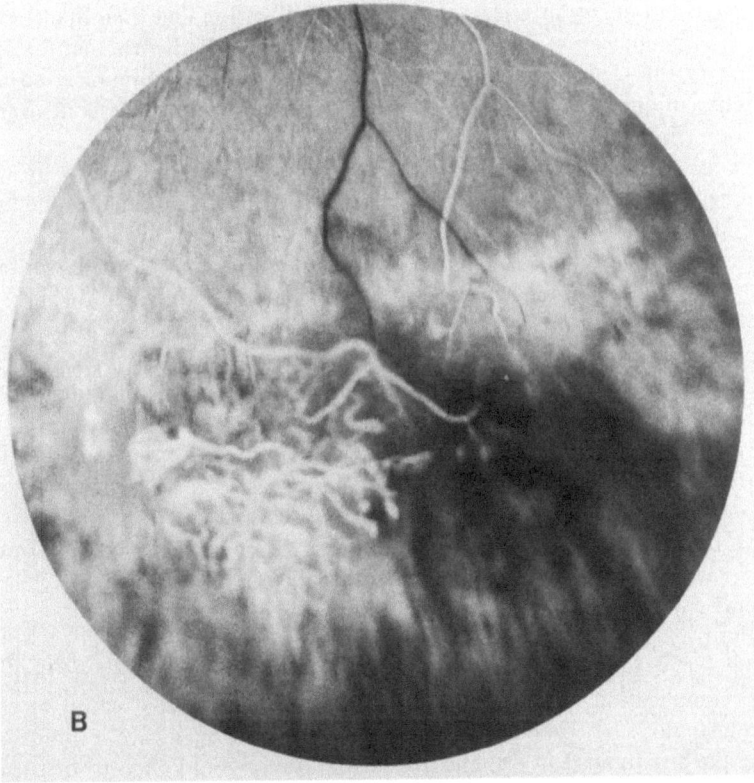

Figure 176. B) Slightly later exposure showing network of intraretinal vessels which communicate with retinal arteries and veins. The afferent choroid artery is no longer visible.

The hypoplasia of the choriocapillaris and the localization of this abnormality near 6 o'clock indicate that the primary anomaly probably is a partial coloboma of the anterior choroid and the retinal pigment epithelium.

Partial colobomas of the choroid always show a defect of the choriocapillaris, Bruch's membrane and the retinal pigment epithelium, but as a rule the layer of larger choroidal vessels is primordially present, as it was in our patient. Apart from the fact that the inferior margins of the lenses were visible when the pupils were fully dilated (possibly as a result of minimal flattening), no colobomatous lesions of the ciliary body, iris and zonules were seen.

The defect in Bruch's membrane and the retinal pigment epithelium must have created a continuity between choroid and retina which enabled the anatomosing recurrent ciliary artery to grow through.

This blood vessel is the last in the embryonic development of the choroid. Its primoridum, which arises from the primary arterial circle of the iris, is formed from the 6th month of intra-uterine development on (Heimann, 1972). The recurrent ciliary arteries grow in central direction and their branches establish communication with the peripheral choriocapillaris. Whether the main branch of the recurrent ciliary artery establishes direct communication with branches of the posterior ciliary arteries near the equator, is a controversial question (Francois et al., 1955; Wybar, 1954).

We assume that, in the final months of intra-uterine development, growing branches of a recurrent ciliary artery in our case could not establish the usual communications with the peripheral choriocapillaris near 6 o'clock because the latter's primordium had failed to form at the site of the coloboma. Through the local defect in Bruch's membrane and the retinal pigment epithelium, the branches of the recurrent ciliary artery could grow into the neuroretina, in which they formed anastomoses with small retinal vascular branches. The latter were in communication with retinal veins into which they drained the blood, as the fluorescein angiogram revealed.

Evidently the considerable luminal width of the recurrent ciliary artery ensured a large supply of blood to the anastomosing retinal vascular ramifications. The leakage from the latter undoubtedly resulted from decompensation caused by this large blood supply and the consequent high pressure in these vascular branches. The leakage in turn gave rise to subretinal exudates, oedema and serous retinal detachment.

The pucker in the posterior pole of OS must be a phenomenon secondary to the longstanding peripheral retinal detachment. There is a risk that the same complication will develop in OD, especially because attempts to close the anastomosis by cryocoagulation have failed. More aggressive techniques to close the anastomosis — e.g. electrocoagulation — would seem to merit consideration if the exudative retinal detachment should expand, although the procedure entails a certain risk.

Differential diagnosis in the probably very rare instances of this anomaly should take into account other conditions which can be associated with peripheral exudates, e.g. Coats' disease and retinal angiomatosis. The localization near the 6 o'clock position clearly distinguishes the condition from DEVR and RLF, which also produce quite different clinical symptoms. The peripheral retinal oedema and the position of the lesions in the inferior part of the fundus might cause confusion with posterior cyclitis. The vascular lesions and the absence of preretinal snowballs and cyclitic membranes, however, are not suggestive of this inflammatory condition.

CHAPTER 12

# COATS' DISEASE AND RETINAL ANGIOMATOSIS

## 12.1 Coats' disease

Coats' disease is probably based on a developmental disorder of, especially, the peripheral retinal vasculature. This is why this disease should be discussed here. There is another argument for presentation of this disease: in some cases the fundus features of Coats' disease may resemble those of DEVR. It is therefore important also to consider the differential diagnosis.

### 12.1.a Clinical symptoms

Coats' disease is characterized by intraretinal or subretinal exudates and malformations of the retinal vessels, while intraretinal haemorrhages are not a rare feature (Figure 177). The condition is usually discovered in children of pre-school or school age, and mostly in boys. The disease is as a rule unilateral, although bilateral cases are by no means an exception.

The vascular lesions of the disease are multiple lesions of arterioles as well as venules and capillaries. They are usually found in the smaller vessels outside the posterior pole. The irregular, sausage-like dilatations of arterioles and venules are ophthalmoscopically evident. Aneurysms of the same vessels often show a glittering white surface due to secondary degeneration of the vascular wall. The capillary lesions are especially readily detectable in fluorescein angiography: the capillary network shows a general coarsening of its structure, and the individual capillaries have an abnormally large luminal width (Figure 178). Saccular microaneurysms of these capillaries are frequently seen in the angiograms. Fluorescein leakage from affected parts of the vascular bed is a general phenomenon, but often very limited. In some cases the fluorescein angiogram reveals total non-perfusion of the peripheral retina (Figure 179). More often, avascular zones are seen which are surrounded by perfused retinal areas.

Exudates in the deeper layers of the retina are usually found near the vascular lesions. In a later stage, extensive subretinal exudates may be seen which lift the retina off its pigment epithelium.

Although retinal detachment in Coats' disease is nearly always exudative, rhegmatogenous retinal detachment has been described as a complication of this condition (Kelley and Danzinger, 1979). The deformed vessels and bright red

344

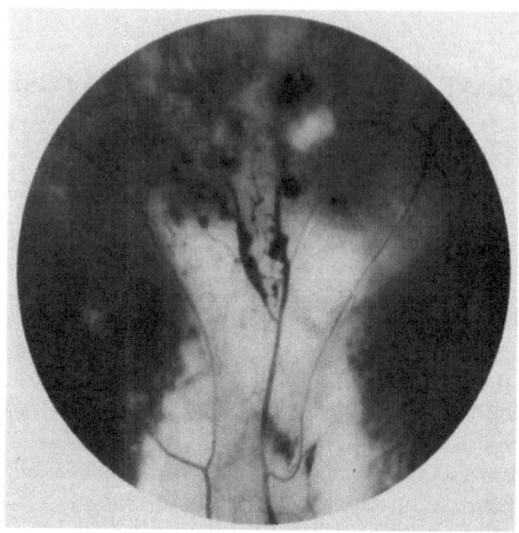

Figure 177. Telangiectases and subretinal exudates.

haemorrhages often contrast clearly against the white or yellow background of the massive exudates. In some cases the exudates assume a darker, greyish colour due to a mixture of blood. It is an established fact that, in Coats' disease, exudates can be found in parts of the fundus in which no distinct vascular lesions are discernible; and in some cases there is no vascular deformation observable at all. Coats himself described the various findings in great detail (1908, 1911 and 1912). On the basis of these findings he divided his patients into two groups.

Type 1: Massive subretinal exudates without distinct vascular lesions.
Type 2: Massive subretinal exudates with vascular lesions.

He distinguished originally a third type, but this is not longer regarded as Coats' disease but as probably identical to retinal angiomatosis.

We know that some adults can develop vascular deformations and exudates which closely resemble those of Coats' disease. Moreover, telangiectases of retinal vessels have also been described in combination with other eye diseases such as retinitis pigmentosa (Morgan and Crawford, 1968; Schmidt and Faulborn, 1972) or with systemic syndromes such as the epidermal naevus syndrome (Burch et al., 1980).

Although some authors describe these retinal vascular changes as Coats' disease, this is not justifiable, and can give rise to confusion. The term Coats' disease should be confined to cases of telangiectasia observed in children (Manschot and De Bruijn, 1967). This opinion seems to be entirely acceptable,

although it is not always possible to differentiate between a congenital telangiectasia and an acquired vascular anomaly.

Several authors describe telangiectasia discovered at an adult age as "idiopathic retinal telangiectasia". For the category accompanied by other general
or ocular symptoms, the term "symptomatic" or "secondary retinal telangiectasia" would seem to me to be suitable.

### 12.1.b Histology

Coats himself described many histopathological changes in detail: conspicuous
dilatation of the smaller vessels and hyaline degeneration of vascular walls,
intraretinal and subretinal haemorrhages and exudates, foam cells, cholesterol
crystals and subretinal fibrosis. According to Woods and Duke (1963) the sub-

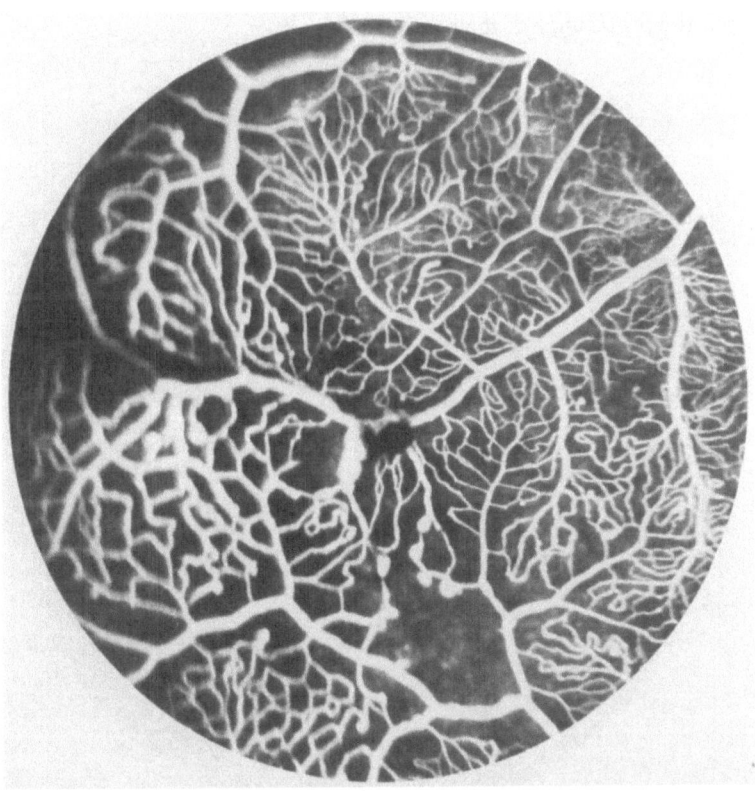

Figure 178. OD. Fluorescein angiogram of the retina temporal to the posterior pole.
The coarsening of the structure of the vasculature increases to the periphery. Small avascular areas.

retinal exudates contain free cholesterol, cholesterol esters and fatty acids, and thus differ from the exudates found in diabetic retinopathy, which mainly consist of neutral fats (Figure 180).

The wall of the dilatated retinal vessels often consists only of endothelial cells, with a thin PAS-positive basement membrane surrounding them (Manschot and De Bruijn, 1967). The somewhat larger vessels often show hyaline swelling of the vascular wall, in which PAS-positive matter, erythrocytes and pigment can be found (Tripathi and Ashton, 1972).

There is oedema of the retinal stroma around the affected vessels, and infiltrates of mononuclear cells and eosinophile granulocytes are often observed (Figure 181). The deeper retinal layers often contain PAS-positive exudates.

The origin of the lipoid macrophages (ghost cells) has long remained obscure. In microscopic specimens of eyes with Coats' disease, Manschot and De Bruijn (1967) and Takei (1976) found proliferation of pigment cells and observed transitions from pigment epithelium cells to foam cells which demonstrated the probability of their relatedness.

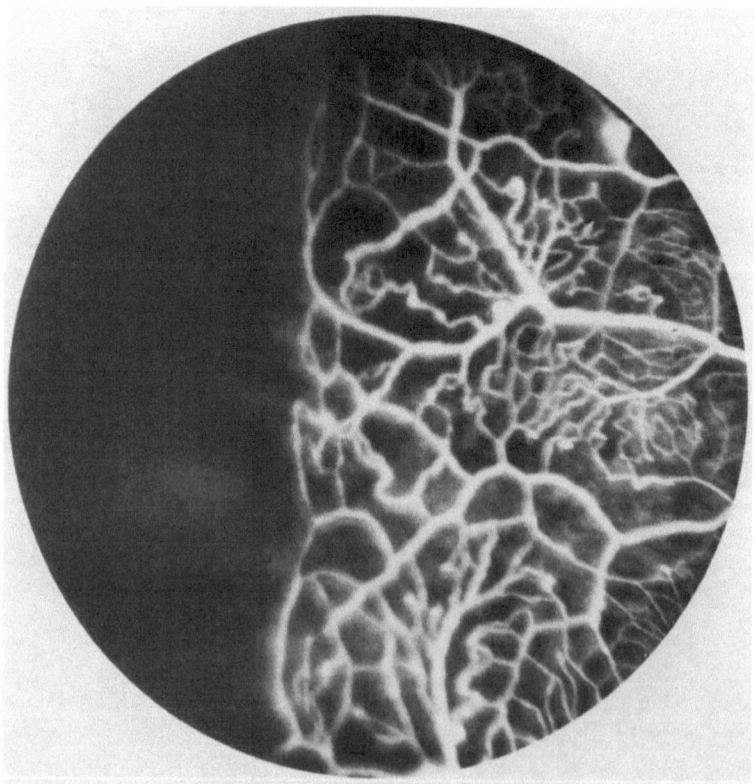

Figure 179. OD. More peripheral exposure showing non-perfusion of the equatorial zone in the same eye.

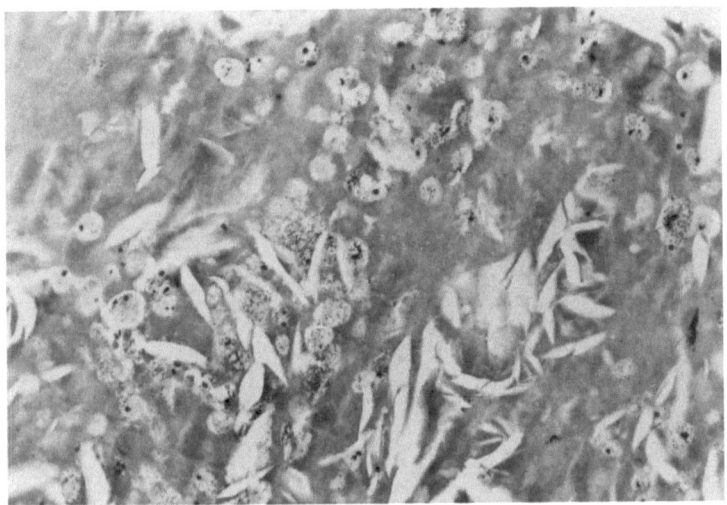

Figure 180. Cholesterol crystals and ghost cells in subretinal exudate (× 200).

It is interesting to note that Coats already suggested the possibility of this relatedness of these cells in 1912. The origin of fibrocytes in the subretinal plaques is not quite certain, but these cells are probably also derived from the pigment epithelium (Manschot and De Bruijn, 1967).

### 12.1.c Pathogenesis

Nearly all authors who have reported on Coats' disease in the past few decades agree that the retinal vascular anomalies must be the cause of the exudate formation. This concept implies that a purely exudative affection without vascular lesions does not exist. Both the microscopic features of the vessels and the leakage observed at fluorescein angiography indicate a disturbed function of the blood-retina barrier, as a result of which plasma constituents and sometimes blood cells can enter the retinal stroma.

Many investigators have concerned themselves with the fact that intraretinal exudates can develop at a considerable distance from the areas with vascular anomalies. In some cases there are capillary anomalies in the region of such exudates, but these can only be detected by fluorescein angiography. The exudates develop at a significant distance from the leaking retinal vessels in most cases. This phenomenon can also be observed in other conditions associated with loss of function of the blood-retina barrier.

A site of predilection is the perimacular layer of Henle, where a radial pattern of exudates can develop. The retina near the vascular malformations is usually oedematous.

It is a wellknown phenomenon, in other conditions as well, that the exu-

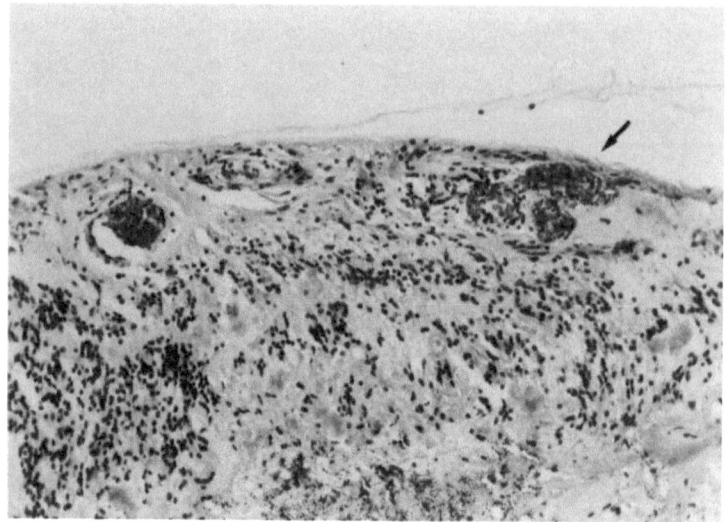

Figure 181. Cross-section through the neuroretina in Coats' disease. The retina is swollen due to glia proliferations and oedema. Several thin-walled blood vessels of fair luminal width are seen in the inner layers (arrow) (X 140).

dates do not readily form in an oedematous part of the retina but develop preferably at the boundary of such areas, thus giving rise to a so-called circinate local exudative process. Exudates of this type are also observed at some distance from the vascular lesions in the initial stage of Coats' disease.

Virtually nothing is known about the pathogenesis of the vascular lesions of Coats' disease. Most authors postulate a congenital telangiectasia, but whether the primary vascular lesions of Coats' disease are always present at birth has not been established.

A very important question to tbe raised is: did the anomalous vascular areas arise from an initially more or less normal network of retinal vessels, or were the vessels primarily deformed? The development of Coats-like anomalies at a later age suggests the former possibility, but does not mean that this is also involved in juvenile patients with Coats' disease.

The non-perfusion of retinal areas may result exclusively from disturbed development, but equally well from occlusion and retraction of vessels. Microscopic studies have revealed vessels with an unmistakably swollen wall, with a constricted lumen (Tripathi and Ashton, 1971), or with a normal lumen (Manschot and De Brujin, 1967); but occluded vessels are not a histopathological feature of Coats' disease.

An important phenomenon given but scant attention in the literature is the rare occurrence of neovascularizations of the kind seen in numerous conditions associated with non-perfusion of the retina. True neovascularization, arising from parts of the retinal vasculature and extending into the vitreous space, is a rare finding in Coats' disease, although areas of retinal non-perfusion are often observed.

Wise (1961) regarded the ingrowth of fibrovascular tissue from the deeper retinal layers into the subretinal space as a reaction to the hypoxia of these layers, resulting from the formation of exudates between the neuroretina and the nutrient choriocapillaris and pigment epithelium. Wise was also among the few authors who described the presence of neovascularizations of retinal vessels with growth into the preretinal vitreous space. Generally, however, neither clinical nor pathological examination reveals such neovascularization in Coats' disease.

The aetiology of Coats' disease has so far remained obscure. Nearly all cases of the disease so far described were sporadic cases, but some authors have described familial cases. The family described by Schmidt and Faulborn (1972) showed telangiectasia combined with tapetoretinal degeneration and, as already pointed out, cannot be regarded as showing Coats' disease. The familial cases reported by Pajtas (1950) and Campbell (1976) strike me as not quite suggestive of Coats' disease. Particularly the clinical features described by the former author might well be compatible with DEVR.

In my opinion, no convincing evidence has so far been offered that genetic factors play a role in the aetiology of Coats' disease. I made an interesting clinical observation which excludes such factors in one of a pair of monozygotic twins, whose case history follows.

*Case history*

Marcel P. (19-05-69) was referred to our department at age 7 with a one-week history of diminished VOS. Marcel was one of a pair of twins (described as monozygotic by the mother), who spent the first two weeks of life in the incubator. The birth weight of both neonates was some 2000 g. Marcel's postnatal condition was good; his brother's was slightly less but still fair. The amount of oxygen administered was unknown. Both children were in good general health. No family history of ocular symptoms.

*Ophthalmological examination (Marcel)*

| | |
|---|---|
| Visual acuity | VOD: 1.25, uncorrected. |
| | VOS: 2/60, uncorrected. |
| Anterior segments | ODS: Normal. |
| Fundi | OD: Only small scattered exudates in the temporal mid-periphery of the fundus, and some irregular dilatations of retinal vessels (Figure 182). Entirely normal posterior pole. |
| | OS: Extensive subretinal exudates in all quadrants of the fundus with irregular malformations of the retinal vessels and telangiectases. The |

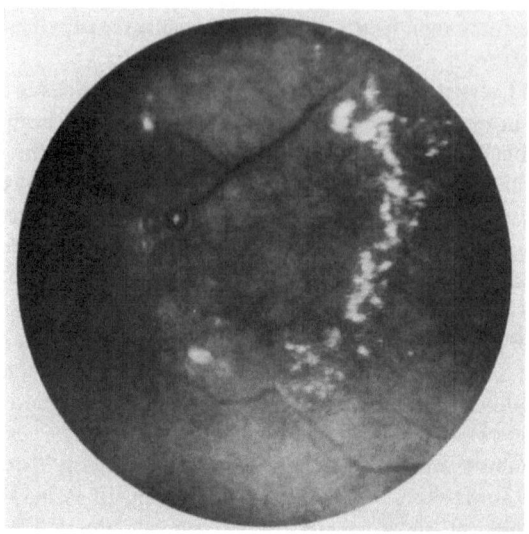

Figure 182. OD. Telangiectases and intraretinal exudates temporal to the posterior pole.

Fluorescein angiogram

inferior temporal sector of the retina was evidently detached by the extensive subretinal exudates (Figure 183).

OD: The region temporal to the posterior pole is shown in Figure 178. The structure of the retinal capillary bed is evidently coarsened. There are occasional areas of retinal non-perfusion. The smaller vascular branches, both arterial and venous, show irregular variations in luminal width. The late phase shows relatively little fluorescein leakage. The somewhat more peripheral exposures clearly show non-perfusion of the retina in the temporal equatorial zone.

*Conclusion*
Bilateral Coats' disease.

*Treatment*
Patient was treated by intensive photocoagulation (under anaesthesia) of all effected areas in the temporal part of the fundus OD. OS was not treated.

Ophthalmological examination of the parents revealed no abnormalities. The twin-brother Ronnie was of course also examined carefully, but fundus examination in mydriasis failed to reveal a single abnormality.

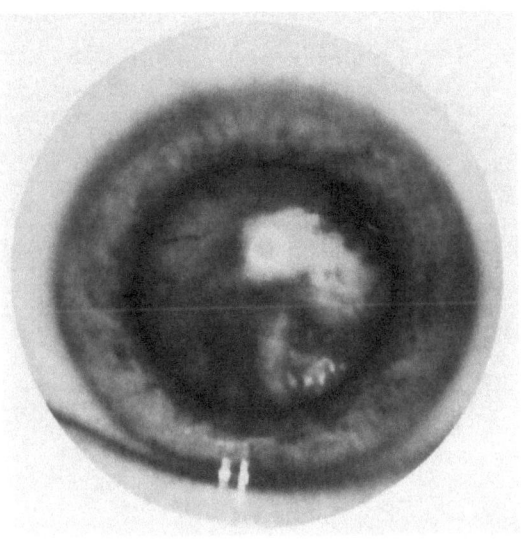

Figure 183. OS. Retinal detachment caused by massive subretinal exudates.

Although the two brothers closely resembled each other, extensive blood typing was done. The identical blood typology found in the two children was as follows:

ABO; C c D  E e;  M N;  S s Pl;  K k;  Kp$^a$  Kp$^b$;  Fy$^a$  Fy$^b$;  Jk$^a$  Jk$^b$;

A+  +−+  −+  − +  −+ +  − +  −  +  −  +  +

Lu$^a$  Lu$^b$;  Le$^a$  Le$^b$.

−  +  −  +

Fluorescein angiography three months after coagulation revealed destruction of significant parts of the aberrant retinal vascular network. In some areas there were still some patent capillaries and small afferent and efferent vessels, but perfusion in these vessels was diminished due to marked constriction of the lumen (Figure 184). In the course of the follow-up over 4 years, VOD remained unchanged and no complications developed. The follow-up on Ronnie over the same period failed to reveal any fundus changes.

The above case history of a boy with bilateral Coats' disease in whose monozygotic twin-brother no fundus changes were found, confirms the non-hereditary character of the disease. Our findings also exclude a mutation in the parental germ cells or in the zygote as a possible cause.

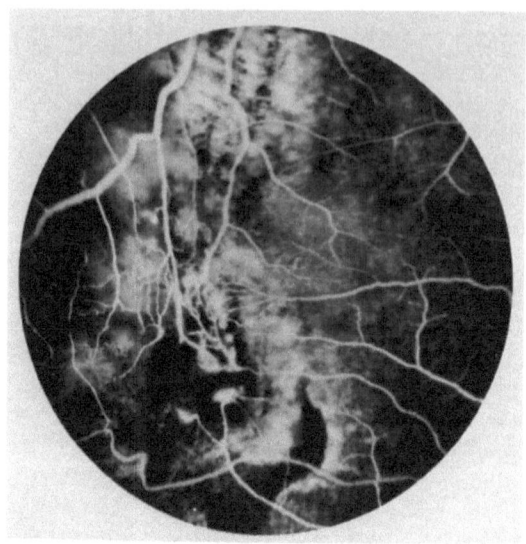

Figure 184. OD. Fluorescein angiogram after coagulation.

## 12.1.d Differential diagnosis

Much has been written about the relationship between Coats' disease and Leber's multiple miliary aneurysms (Leber, 1916). I have been unable to confirm the opinion of Chisholm et al. (1974) that the aneurysms in the latter disease are localized in the arterioles, unlike those in the former disease. I believe that the dilatations and aneurysms in Coats' disease are found in the arterioles as well as in the capillaries and venules, as demonstrated in Figure 178.

Many authors regard the two diseases as different stages of the same condition (Manschot and De Bruijn, 1967), and this strikes me as an acceptable postulate. It simply solves differential diagnostic problems as well. Far advanced stages of Coats' disease, in which massive subretinal exudates are in evidence, should be distinguished from all conditions which can cause leucocoria at an early age, at which time the possibility of retinoblastoma should always be considered. In addition to fundoscopic examination (under anaesthesia, if necessary), ultrasonography and, especially in older children, fluorescein angiography are important aids in diagnosis.

A discussion of the differential diagnosis of leucocoria is not within the scope of this study; in this respect I refer to the textbooks.

Differential diagnosis from DEVR is clinically important. Cases of DEVR which involve exudates might certainly be confused with Coats' disease. It should be borne in mind that the vascular anomalies in the two conditions differ significantly, and that the preretinal vitreous changes are far more prominent in DEVR, or at least in the severe cases. Ophthalmoscopically discernible telangiectases are not present in DEVR.

Family studies are indicated in dubious cases. Familial cases of Coats' disease, as reported in the abovementioned publications, are probably based on DEVR.

### 12.1.e Treatment

Coagulation is indicated in most cases of Coats' disease. Only if the posterior pole of the retina has already become detached due to extensive subretinal exudates can cryocoagulation or photocoagulation be regarded as futile. Small areas of slight vascular anomalies without surrounding exudates in the peripheral fundus can be left untreated as long as the condition remains stationary (but of course require frequent follow-ups).

Unfortunately, most children are not treated until visual acuity in the affected eye has diminished due to oedema and exudates in the macula. In such cases rapid extensive coagulation therapy (which nearly always must be given under anaesthesia) is indicated. In view of the presence of exudates between neuroretina and pigment epithelium, and oedema of the neuroretina, coagulations of long duration and high intensity are required. In young children under anaesthesia, it is important to make a careful examination of the fundus periphery of the contralateral eye, to ascertain that even very slight lesions are not overlooked.

The results of cryocoagulation or photocoagulation are fair if treatment is started early. Spitznas et al. (1975) reported improved visual acuity in 25% of the treated eyes in a large series of cases, and also noted that 54% showed no further diminution of visual acuity. In the categories with slight or moderate anomalies, the results were even significant more favourable.

### 12.2  Retinal angiomatosis

Retinal angiomatosis (Von Hippel-Lindau's disease) is an autosomal dominant condition of the retinal blood vessels often accompanied by central nervous symptoms and sometimes by symptoms from other organs, more specifically the kidneys and adrenal glands. Although the disease symptoms as a rule do not occur until after childhood, most authors regard the condition as a developmental disorder.

### 12.2.a Clinical symptoms

The fundus changes have been described in detail by Von Hippel (1895, 1904). Retinal angiomatosis becomes manifest in usually gradual visual loss resulting from oedema and exudates in the retina of the posterior pole. Ophthalmoscopy reveals a pinkish-red or sometimes whitish angioma, often outside the posterior pole but sometimes found quite near the disc or the macula. A characteristic feature of such an angioma is the communication with a dilatated and tortuous afferent and efferent blood vessel (Figure 185). These vessels are sometimes very inconspicuous, especially when the angioma is localized near the disc. Several angiomas may be found in one fundus, and not infrequently both eyes are affected.

Intraretinal haemorrhages and retinal oedema are frequently found near an angioma. They often obstruct the view on the vascular lesion (Figure 186). Vitreous haemorrhages are less common. Leakage often leads to exudate formation in the retina at some distance from the angioma. As in many processes associated with intensive leakage from parts of the retinal vasculature, exudates may accumulate in the centre of the posterior pole. If left untreated, the angiomas often increase in size, with progression of exudative changes. Finally, retinal detachment usually occurs as a result of the accumulation of subretinal exudates or due to traction exerted by glia proliferations in the vitreous space. Fluorescein angiography reveals fluorescein leakage from the angiomas, which is usually rapid and intensive. The afferent and efferent vessels, however, as a rule do not leak. The retinal capillaries near the angioma often (but not always) show dilatations and microaneurysms from which fluorescein may leak. Retinal areas of non-perfusion as a rule are not observed.

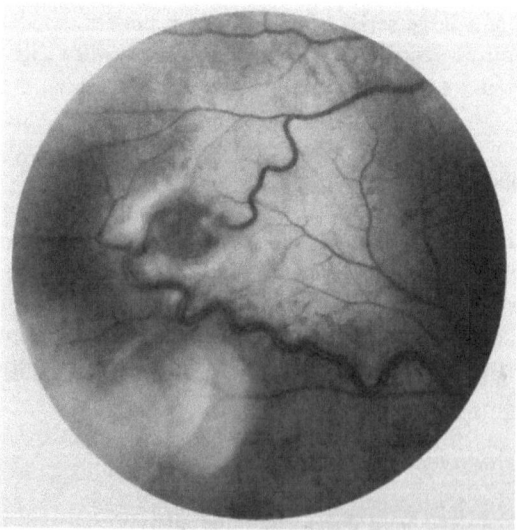

Figure 185. Retinal angiomatosis. Peripherally localized angioma without exudates or haemorrhages.

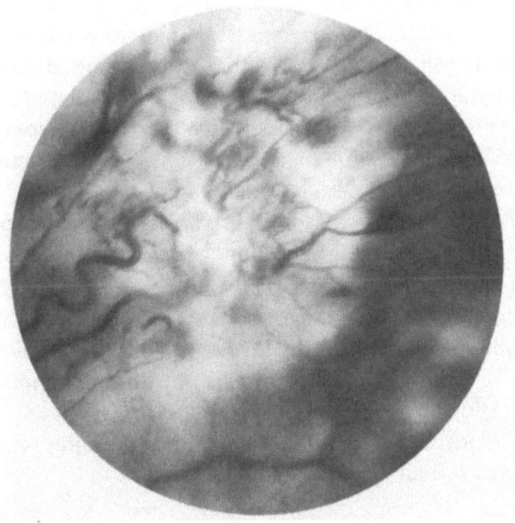

Figure 186. Angioma obscured by oedema, exudates and minor haemorrhages.

### General symptoms

Czermak (1905) already described a patient with retinal angiomatosis who developed clinical symptoms of an intracranial tumour. The postmortem disclosed a cerebellar cyst in this case. According to Lindau (1927), about 25% of patients with retinal angiomatosis develop central nervous system symptoms. They result from haemangiomas which are usually localized in the cerebellum. Such lesions cause symptoms like headache, dizziness, vomiting and other symptoms of cerebellar dysfunction. Haemorrhages from cerebellar haemangiomas are vitally dangerous complications, which unfortunately are not rare in Von Hippel-Lindau's disease. Tumours and cysts in numerous organs have been described in this disease. Particularly hypernephromas (Kaplan et al., 1961) and pheochromocytomas (Wise and Gibson, 1971) can be present, and general physical examination of patients with retinal angiomatosis should therefore specifically focus on possible symptoms of such tumours.

### 12.2.b Histology and pathogenesis

Microscopically, the retinal tumours are hamartomas which consist of hyperplastic, newly formed vascular canals separated by endothelioid cells (Jesberg et al., 1968). Particularly around the somewhat large angiomas, there is proliferation of glia cells in the neuroretina which may extend into the vitreous space. Haemorrhages and exudates with infiltration of macrophages in the retinal stroma are often observed.

Goldberg and Duke (1968) studied the histopathological features of the disease in a trypsin digest specimen of the retinal vessels, in which they found foci of endothelial cell hyperplasia in the walls of the afferent and efferent retinal vessels of the angioma. On the basis of this finding they considered it possible that the dilatation of these vessels was not secondary to haemo-dynamic changes caused by the angioma but indicated a hamartoma of arter-ioles, capillaries and venules.

It has not been established with certainty whether microscopic evidence of the retinal vascular anomalies of Von Hippel-Lindau's disease is already present at birth. Small nests of angioblastic cells are possibly already formed in the fetal retinal vasculature. These may subsequently proliferate and give rise to clinical symptoms. An argument in favour of this theory is the finding of angiomas of Von Hippel-Lindau's disease in infants (Appelmans, 1947). Jesberg et al. (1968) and Nicholson et al. (1976), however, hold that the lesions may have developed postnatally from ophthalmoscopically and angio-graphically normal retinal vascular areas.

### 12.2.c  Differential diagnosis

The fundus changes observed in retinal angiomatosis should be distinguished from the phenomena observed in Coats' disease. Differentation may be diffi-cult when the extensive intraretinal and subretinal exudates and haemorrhages obscure the primary vascular lesions. In both conditions, exudates can form in the centre of the posterior pole at a considerable distance from the ophthalm-oscopically visible vascular malformations, and both diseases can be bilateral as well as unilateral.

In most cases the angiomas are clearly distinguishable in dimensions and their typical dilatated, tortuous afferent and efferent vessels from the much smaller, more diffuse lesions in Coats' disease. The family history and exam-ination of family members are of clinical importance in retinal angiomatosis, and may have diagnostic significance as well in dubious cases.

Like retinal angiomatosis, however, DEVR is subject to autosomal domi-nant transmission with highly variable expression. Yet the vascular lesions in retinal angiomatosis are so different from tnose in DEVR that differential diagnosis between these two conditions seldom poses a problem. Extensive exudates can be present in both conditions, but retinal haemorrhages (quite common in retinal angiomatosis) are rarely observed in DEVR.

Dilatated and tortuous blood vessels may be observed on the surface of some retinoblastomas, often in association with haemorrhages. Such tumours may produce symptoms which closely resemble those of retinal angiomatosis.

### 12.2.d Treatment

Coagulation of the angiomas is the treatment of choice of the ocular mani-festations of Von Hippel-Lindau's disease. Early treatment is important be-cause most of these angiomas grow quickly and can cause a rapid increase in exudates and haemorrhages.

Smaller angiomas can as a rule be successfully treated by Xenon arc coagu-lation (Wessing, 1967) or with the Argon laser (Goldberg and Koenig, 1974) (Figure 187).

Results obtained in the treatment of larger angiomas are less favourable (Goldberg and Koenig, 1974), but of course much depends on the severity and localization of the secondary changes in retina and vitreous. Apart from the importance of early treatment, careful periodical posttherapeutic exam-ination of both fundi is important because fresh lesions can quickly develop, and recurrence of exudative changes caused by coagulated angiomas is like-wise possible.

The many aspects of the treatment of tumours of the central nervous sys-tem and of other organs which can occur in Von Hippel-Lindau's disease are not within the scope of this study.

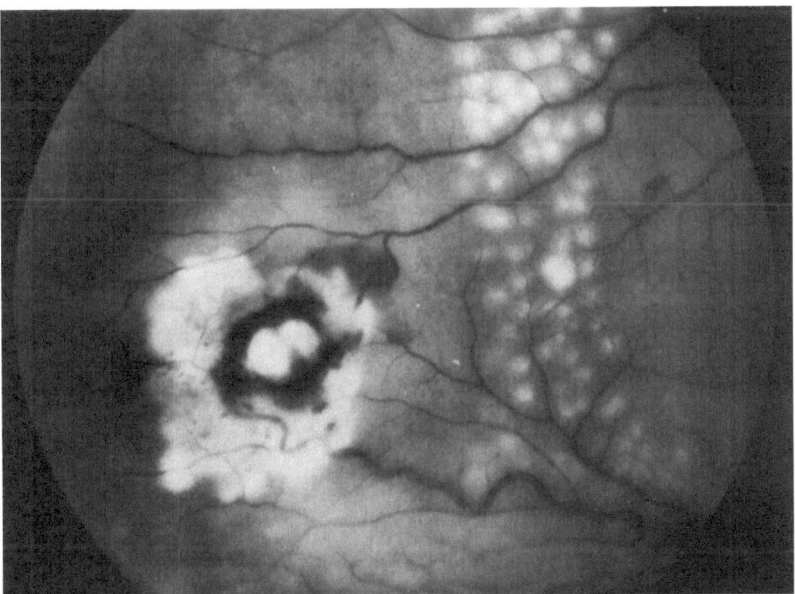

Figure 187. The same angioma as in Figure 185, shortly after laser coagulation.

## 12.3  Sturge-Weber's syndrome

Disorders of peripheral retinal perfusion have been incidentally observed also in Sturge-Weber's syndrome (Archer and Nevin, 1977). It remains uncertain whether this results from a developmental disorder of the retinal vasculature or from compression of the peripheral retinal vessels by an angioma of the choroid. This syndrome will not be discussed.

PART III

ADDITIONAL DIFFERENTIAL DIAGNOSES FROM DOMINANT
EXUDATIVE VITREORETINOPATHY

CHAPTER 13

# CONGENITAL CONDITIONS NOT ASSOCIATED WITH RETINAL VASCULAR DEVELOPMENTAL DISORDERS

## 13.1 Persistent hyperplastic primary vitreous

Although the clinical features of persistent hyperplastic primary vitreous (PHPV) are often typical and therefore readily identifiable, there are other manifestations not easily recognizable as based on PHPV. Manifestations of the latter category mainly develop in the posterior part of the vitreous space, and sometimes pose considerable problems of differential diagnosis, for example from DEVR. This is why this chaper focuses ample attention on the difficult, controversial subject of persistence of hyaloid elements in the posterior and preretinal parts of the vitreous space.

### 13.1.a  Clinical symptoms

*Anterior PHPV*

The clinical and histological features of this type of PHPV have long been known (Grolman, 1889; Parsons and Fleming, 1903; Collins, 1908).

The condition is characterized by nearly always unilateral leucocoria, usually noticed within a few weeks of birth. The affected eye is as a rule slightly smaller than normal, and sometimes has a shallow anterior chamber. In the characteristic case, radially arranged blood vessels extend across the iris; they emerge from beneath the iris in the pupillary aperture, and are remnants of the capsulopupillary part of the tunica vasculosa lentis (Figure 188). In many cases, however, no such vessels are found.

The lens is initially clear but sometimes slightly smaller than normal (Findlay, 1925). In a subsequent stage it becomes cataractous and may even be totally replaced by fibrotic tissue (Czermark, 1907). Immediately posterior to the lens, a white or pink tissue mass is visible which can vary in dimensions from a small plaque slightly nasal to the centre of the lens, to a structure which covers the entire posterior lens capsule (Reese, 1955). In this tissue one usually sees blood vessels which take a somewhat radial course (Von Winning, 1952). The retrolental tissue is thickest at the centre, and gradually becomes thinner towards the periphery (Reese, 1955). In adequate mydriasis (which cannot always be achieved), elongated ciliary processes are visible which are connected with the retrolental membrane. In eyes in which the retrolental

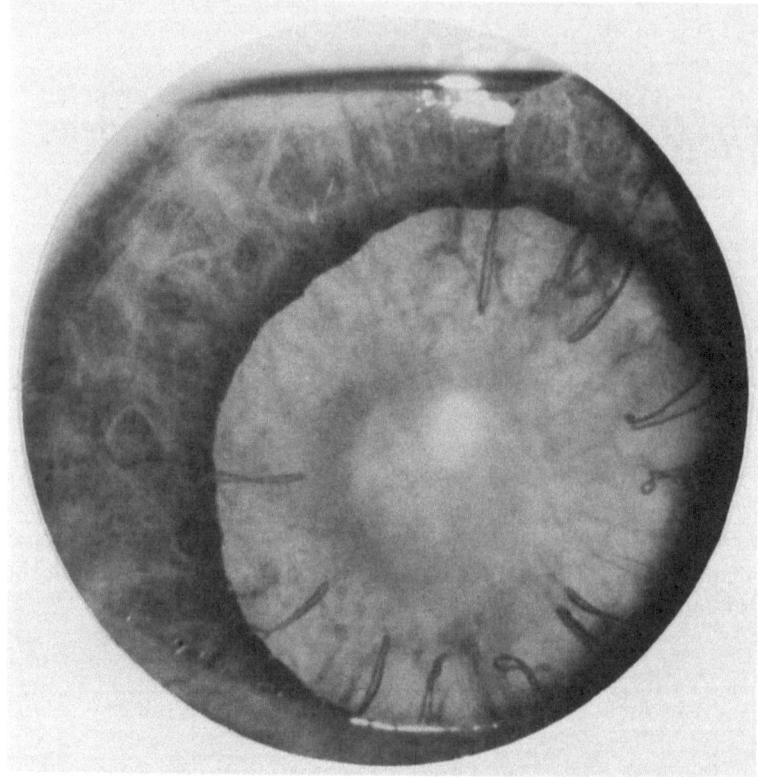

Figure 188. PHPV with persistent capsulopupillary vessels.

opacity is confined to the centre of the posterior capsule, a persistent hyaloid artery is sometimes clinically observed (Figure 189). In the case of lens luxation, too, the course of such a vessel from the disc is sometimes discernible (Straub, 1951).

The depth of the anterior chamber can be reduced due to oedema of the lens, contraction of retrolental tissue and haemorrhages in the vitreous space. Consequently, secondary glaucoma is a frequent complication even in the first years of life.

*Posterior PHPV*

Widely diverse anomalies associated with preretinal opaque structures and retinal folds have been ascribed to persistence and hyperplasia of the primary vitreous and the hyaloid system. As a rule, however, it is difficult to verify the diagnosis of such anomalies. Diagnosis is based mainly on the ophthalmoscopic findings, but the pluriformity of the fundus changes often renders the diagnosis of "posterior PHPV" rather speculative.

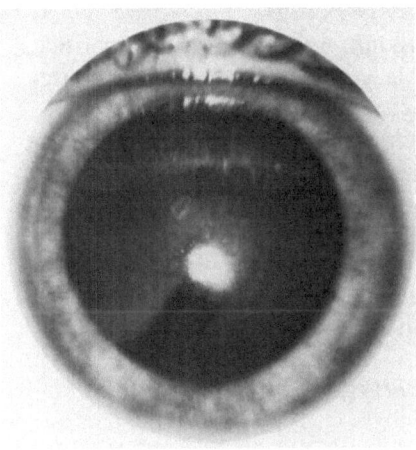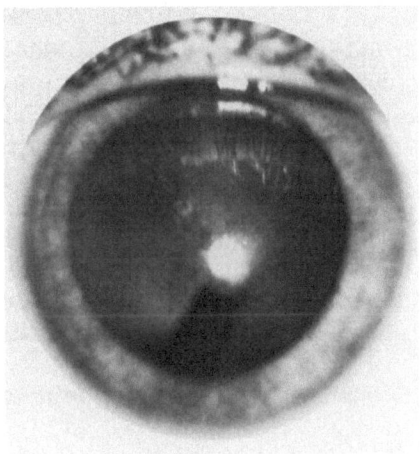

Figure 189. Stereo-photograph. Attachment of persistent hyaloid artery to the posterior lens capsule.

The congenital presence of white structures adherent to the disc in the pre-papillary vitreous space is probably a result of persistence and proliferation of embryonic vitreous elements in a number of cases. Such epipapillary membranes or tissue masses consist of glia cells, which probably originate from neuro-epithelial cells that envelop the proximal segment of the embryonic hyaloid artery (so-called Bergmeister's papilla). The presence of remnants of the hyaloid artery in combination with such glial structures confirms the hypothesis that the changes result from a disturbance in the regression of the posterior primary vitreous.

According to Scarlett (1922), De Beck (1890) already described 12 different types of clinical manifestations which in his view resulted from persistence of hyaloid elements. In five of these types there were strands, membranes and tissue masses which adhered to the disc.

Unilateral glial epipapillary structures ascribed to vestiges of the hyaloid vascular system were reported by Ten Doesschate (1916) and Danis (1921). In some cases the retinal vessels showed an abnormal course near the disc (Ten Doesschate, 1916), or vascular anomalies were observed on the disc (Scarlett, 1922).

The more recent literature shows that some confusion has arisen between posterior PHPV and congenital retinal fold (Van Nouhuys, 1981a). This subject is discussed in detail at the end of this section (13.1.d).

### 13.1.b Histology

Microscopic examination in cases of anterior PHPV has shown that the retro-lental structures consist of connective tissue in which many blood vessels are found (Rosen and Yamashita, 1964; Raskind, 1966). On the anterior side, this tissue is connected with the posterior lens capsule, through which it often passes into the stroma of the lens (Velhagen, 1912; Reese, 1955).

The extent to which microscopic examination can confirm the presence of persistent primary vitreous elements in the preretinal portion of the posterior segment is of great importance to our knowledge of PHPV. Eyes in which the changes are limited to local structures near the disc have, of course, rarely been enucleated; our histological data on such eyes are therefore limited. Seefelder (1909) found duplicature of the neuroretina near the disc in such an eye. The structure of the neuroretina in this area was abnormal.

*Retinal and preretinal changes in anterior PHPV*

At histological examination of ten eyes with severe retrolental PHPV, Manschot (1958) found preretinal structures extending from the retina to the posterior vitreous. In some eyes he observed deposits of amorphous matter in this part of the vitreous, which were connected with the innermost layer of the neuro-retina. Intraretinal and preretinal glia cell proliferations were also found. According to Manschot (1958), the various structures originated from the primary vitreous, which apparently was able to manifest itself also in the posterior parts of the vitreous space.

At light-microscopic examination of an eye with PHPV, Wolter and Flaherty (1959) found similar filaments and glia proliferations on the inner surface of the retina. Unlike Manschot (1958), these authors were unable to demonstrate any connection between the preretinal filaments and the Müller cells of the retina. But the structures did prove to be connected with retinal blood vessels.

Virtually identical filaments have since been described in PHPV by Spaulding and Naumann (1967), who identified a number of these structures as blood vessels which communicated with superficial retinal vessels. Vascular communications between retinal blood vessels and vascularized organizations in the vitreous space have also been demonstrated in PHPV by Gärtner (1964) and Stefani and Laszczyk (1976).

In my opinion the hypothesis that the abovementioned structures on the inner surface of the retina in eyes with anterior PHPV originate from the primary vitreous has become untenable with the discovery of vascular connections between this tissue and retinal vessels. Although it is possible that, as Gärtner (1964) and others believe, hyaloid vessels are localized close against the retinal surface in the foetal eye, and adhere to it in some cases, there are no indications that foetal connections between hyaloid vessels and retinal blood vessels can occur, as Pau (1957) suggested. The blood vessels in the epiretinal tissue on the inner surface of the retina in eyes with anterior PHPV, therefore, are in my opinion certainly not derived from the hyaloid system. A different explanation seems more logical.

The histological descriptions and illustrations in the abovementioned publications suggest that the epiretinal glia proliferations and blood vessels have been reactively produced by the retina. This hypothesis explains the connections between the vascular structures in the vitreous and the superficial retinal blood vessels.

The question why these reactive changes occurred in the retina seems easily answered: nearly all specimens in which the epiretinal structures were observed, showed unmistakable deformation of the retina due to traction exerted by the retrolental plaque of (anterior) persistent vitreous. Under these conditions the development of reactive intraretinal and epiretinal glia proliferations is to be expected.

In support of this hypothesis it can also be pointed out that persistence and hyperplasia of the primary vitreous in the posterior vitreous space cannot explain the extensive intraretinal glia proliferations repeatedly observed in anterior PHPV. These changes can only be understood as consequences of secondary changes in the retina.

It can be stated in conclusion that the changes of the retina and preretinal vitreous in the posterior segment of eyes with anterior PHPV cannot be readily explained by persistence of vitreous elements in these areas. The identification of preretinal structures not connected with the disc in the posterior part of the vitreous space as hyperplastic elements of the primary vitreous, is therefore insufficiently supported by histological findings at this time.

### 13.1.c  Differential diagnosis

Both PHPV and DEVR can cause leucocoria in young children. Only rarely, however, is leucocoria present at birth in DEVR, as it is in PHPV. In the case of unilateral leucocoria, examination of the fundus periphery of the contralateral eye is essential because DEVR, unlike PHPV, is nearly always a bilateral condition.

At this time it is impossible to establish the incidence of bilateral PHPV on the basis of data from the literature. Descriptions of unmistakable cases of bilateral anterior PHPV have been exceedingly rare. Reese (1955) briefly mentioned that the condition is unilateral in 90% of the cases, but it is not clear whether this percentage is based on personal observations or on a study of the literature.

Some patients described as suffering from PHPV (or, in older literature, as suffering from persistence of the tunica vasculosa lentis) showed symptoms highly suggestive of a peripheral proliferative retinopathy such as DEVR.

The patient described in detail by Magnus (1927) showed total funnel-shaped retinal detachment OD and a tissue mass in the inferior temporal fundus quadrant OS. With regard to this fundus (in which a falciform retinal fold was probably localized), Magnus (1927) noted that blood vessels were nowhere to be found in the attached part of the retina, and that several pigmented and depigmented cicatrices were present. In my opinion descriptions of this kind are far more consistent with DEVR than with PHPV.

Bilateral PHPV-like changes in various parts of the vitreous space and the fundus, as recently described by Loewer-Sieger et al. (1980), can be produced equally well by RLF and DEVR.

That not only the clinical but also the histological differential diagnosis between PHPV and advanced stages of neonatal proliferative retinopathies can be difficult, is demonstrated by the fact that the pathogenesis of RLF has for many years been erroneously sought in persistence and hyperplasia of the foetal tunica vasculosa lentis (Terry, 1942; Klien, 1949).

The results of a histological study of eyes with anterior PHPV by Stefani and Laszczyk (1976) are of particular interest in this context. In seven of eight eyes with PHPV, these authors found vascular retinal changes. In five eyes the retina was found to be incompletely vascularized, the retinal periphery (especially on the temporal side) being totally avascular. Neovascularizations were visible on the inner surface of this part of the retina. Although these neovascularizations showed connections with hyaloid vessels, vascular communications between retinal vasculature and vascular proliferations in the vitreous were discernible at least in some of the specimens.

On the basis of the detailed descriptions of Stefani and Laszczyk (1976), who clearly demonstrated the incomplete development of the retinal vasculature in their material, and in view of our current knowledge of the pathogenesis of DEVR, the microscopic features of several of the eyes described by these authors certainly seem compatible with the latter diagnosis. For further verification of this diagnosis, supplemental clinical studies of the patients and their family members would certainly be valuable.

PHPV is a non-familial condition, and the correctness of a diagnosis of PHPV is to be seriously doubted when several cases occur within one family.

Wang and Phillips (1973) described identical twins with unilateral leucocoria, which they ascribed to PHPV. No fundus changes were found in the contralateral eye in these children.

Gonvers et al. (1973) found bilateral fundus changes in six of seven children in one family, and ascribed them to PHPV. The symptoms were disparate: chorioretinal scars and exudates, radial retinal folds, retinal neovascularizations and exudates, cataract and vitreous organizations. The detailed descriptions and fundus photographs in my opinion leave no doubt that the changes in this family were based, not on PHPV but on DEVR.

The gravest problems of differential diagnosis, however, have evolved from the fact that posterior PHPV and congenital retinal fold have erroneously been regarded as identical concepts.

### 13.1.d  Posterior PHPV and congenital retinal fold

So far as I know, MIchaelson (1965) was the first to use the term "posterior persistent hyperplastic primary vitreous". His description of the syndrome was as follows. "This (posterior persistent hyperplastic primary vitreous), which probably represents a lesser degree of retinal fold, consists of persisting attachment of primary vitreous fibres to the retina at one or more places, with resulting progressive changes in the retina such as retinal holes and elevation. Weve (1935) and others indicated that it could be hereditary, transmitted as a recessive trait, possibly sex-linked, as the majority appear in males. This condition is described here as posterior persistent hyperplastic primary vitreous because developmentally it is a posterior manifestation of persistent hyperplastic primary vitreous as described by Reese, and clinically both manifestations may appear in the same eye or in the same patient, as will be shown.''

The above description strikes me as essential because it clearly shows that, according to Michaelson, the syndrome of congenital retinal fold described by Weve is based on persistence of the primary vitreous. This hypothesis is a variant of the theory of Salffner (1902) and Mann (1935) that congenital retinal fold is caused by an abnormal adhesion of the inner layer of the embryonic optic cup to elements of the hyaloid system.

After Michaelson (1965), Pruett and Schepens (1970) and Pruett (1975) used the term posterior PHPV as synonym of congenital retinal fold (ablatio falciformis congenita).

The principal argument against the postulate that the two conditions are identical is the finding of a falciform retinal fold in various conditions, and more especially in DEVR (Van Nouhuys, 1981). The pathogenesis of the retinal fold in the latter condition has been discussed in Chapter 7, and is not based on persistence of primary vitreous.

It is therefore an error to regard posterior PHPV and congenital retinal fold as identical conditions.

It cannot be excluded that, in some cases, the clinical features of a congenital retinal fold can develop in response to persistence and hyperplasia of the primary vitreous. However, the presence of hyaloid vessels or persistent primary vitreous in direct relation to the retinal fold is essential for this diagnosis. Moreover, it should be plausible that the tissue does not originate from fibrovascular proliferations of the retina, as it is in retinal folds observed in RLF, DEVR, etc. In my opinion few cases of congenital retinal fold can meet this criterion.

Pruett (1975) described 30 cases of posterior PHPV. No fold was found in 10 of the 22 eyes examined. More or less prominent retinal folds were reported in the remaining eyes. Changes of the kind Weve and Mann described as congenital retinal fold or ablatio falciformis congenita, are not recognizable in Pruett's publication, and none of the fundus photographs showed an elevated duplicature of the retina.

The cases of posterior PHPV described by other authors likewise rarely show the features of a congenital retinal fold. Joseph et al. (1972) described two patients with unilateral changes which they interpreted as posterior PHPV. No falciform retinal fold was found in these two cases. Of the 14 cases of posterior PHPV described by Rubinstein (1980), only one presented the fundus features of a falciform retinal fold. However, the aetiology of the changes found in this patient is quite obscure, for the fold had not formed until age 7.

These observations corroborate my impression that posterior PHPV is only rarely seen to produce the clinical features of congenital retinal fold.

## 13.2  Congenital toxoplasmosis

As already demonstrated in Chapters 3 and 4, some cases of DEVR show extensive atrophic and pigmented scars which can closely resemble the consequences of congenital toxoplasmosis. As in the latter, such scars can be localized in or near the posterior pole of the fundus in DEVR. However, in our families I have never found a large atrophic macular lesion of the kind frequently observed in congenital toxoplasmosis.

Whenever toxoplasmosis is suspected it is of course necessary to look for symptoms of this condition, e.g. cerebral calcifications, which in 5% of cases can be seen on X-rays of the skull (Schlaegel, 1976). Serological tests should be performed as well.

That differential diagnosis between DEVR and congenital toxoplasmosis can pose problems was demonstrated in our study in patient V-12 D (Chapter 3). The fundus changes in this patient, who was examined by several ophthalmologists and at two university institutes, have for years been regarded as a consequence of congenital toxoplasmosis.

Dekking (1949) described the presence of a congenital retinal fold or even of total retinal detachment in incidental cases of congenital toxoplasmosis.

## 13.3  Retinoblastoma

Cases of severe DEVR associated at an early age with large subretinal exudates and retinal detachment, can clinically resemble cases of retinoblastoma. One of our patients (IV-1 F) had been submitted to enucleation of one eye shortly after birth because this malignant tumour could not be excluded with certainty.

There is an extensive literature on the differential diagnosis of retinoblastoma, to which I may refer (Howard and Ellsworth, 1965; Ellsworth, 1976). This permits me to confine myself to a few important diagnostic differences between DEVR and retinoblastoma.

An essential diagnostic aid in cases in which one eyes shows extensive vitreous changes and retinal detachment is careful examination of the peripheral fundus of the contralateral eye. If this examination (which in young patients is always carried out under anaesthesia) reveals no changes, then DEVR is extremely unlikely. If changes are indeed found in the contralateral eye, then it is usually not difficult to differentiate between DEVR and retinoblastoma on the basis of the clinical findings.

Of course one should look for specific characteristics of retinoblastoma, e.g. tumour seedings in the vitreous, and calcifications which are often demonstrable on X-rays of the orbit. Other important aids in differential diagnosis are the ophthalmological history, a family study, and ultrasonographic examination. Quantitative analysis of the aqueous in an attempt to identify enzymes such as LDH is probably of importance in the diagnosis of retinoblastoma (Felberg et al., 1977), although increased LDH values have incidentally been found also in other conditions (Jacobiec et al., 1978).

CHAPTER 14

## ACQUIRED CONDITIONS

### 14.1 Eales' disease

It is not easy to define exactly which condition can be qualified as Eales' disease. It is evident that different authors have differently defined the condition in the literature. This is due to the fact that the aetiology of the condition is entirely obscure, and that the diagnosis is established mainly on the basis of the clinical symptoms. Some authors (Elliott, 1976; Donders, 1958) use the term Eales' disease to describe vasculitis of the retina of a type usually found in young adult males, which is associated with vascular occlusions, neovascularizations and vitreous haemorrhages and of which the cause is unknown.

Spitznass et al. (1975), however, maintained that the term Eales' disease should be reserved for a syndrome of peripheral vascular occlusions and neovascularizations which shows few (if any) pronounced symptoms of vasculitis. They held that the syndrome accompanied by marked signs of inflammation of especially the larger venous branches around the posterior pole (of unexplained origin) should be referred to as "idiopathic periphlebitis" rather than as Eales' disease (Figure 190). They find supportive arguments in Eales' description of changes, which does not mention inflammatory symptoms.

The difference in localization and in inflammatory symptoms often found between the two conditions would certainly seem to warrant this distinction. A problem, however, is that there are frequent cases in which the fundus shows both characteristics of phlebitis and of a peripheral occlusive vasculopathy.

In the following subsections I intend to use the definition of Eales' disease proposed by Spitznass et al. (1975).

### 14.1.a Clinical symptoms

Eales' disease is characterized by occlusions of retinal vessels outside the posterior pole, vascular sheaths around venules and sometimes also around arterioles, neovascularizations and retinal and vitreous haemorrhages. The latter are usually the cause of the first subjective manifestations.

The condition is often bilateral, shows a marked male predominance, and usually becomes manifest in young adults.

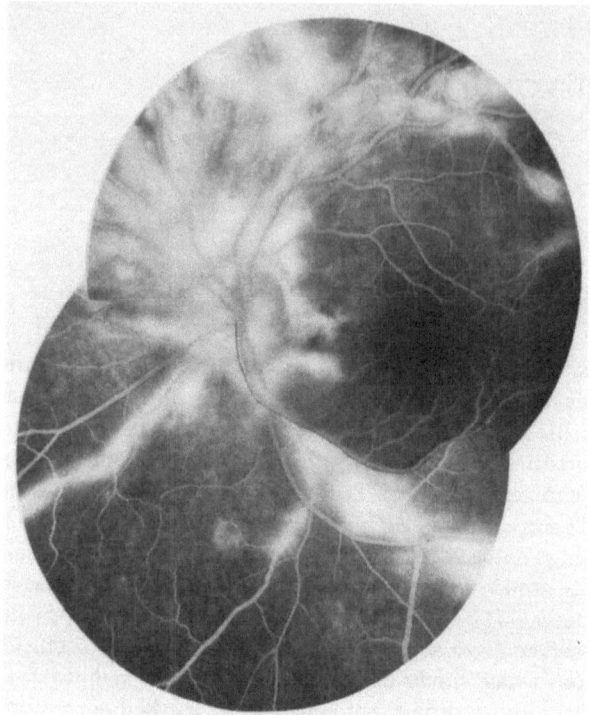

Figure 190. Fluorescein angiogram in "idiopathic periphlebitis". Intensive fluorescein leakage from larger vessels in the late phase.

The course shows considerable interindividual variation. In some cases vitreous haemorrhages can be absorbed spontaneously, without recurrent bleeding. In such cases the vascular proliferations often recede spontaneously, and visual function is permanently restored.

In many untreated cases, however, the vitreous haemorrhages relapse and considerable cicatrization in the vitreous space can lead to total retinal detachment. Rhegmatogenous retinal detachment has been observed as a complication in some cases of Eales' disease (Hulsbus et al., 1972).

### 14.1.b Differential diagnosis from DEVR

Most publications on DEVR mention Eales' disease as differential diagnosis. It seems to me that those who are familiar or at least acquainted with the clinical features of the two conditions should seldom encounter problems in this differential diagnosis.

Intraretinal and vitreous haemorrhages are frequently observed at an (early) adult age in Eales' disease, but are rare in DEVR; and white vascular sheaths along the veins are also exceedingly rare in the latter condition. The development of vascular occlusions and the progression of neovascularizations from the retina at an adult age likewise distinguish Eales' disease from a developmental disorder such as DEVR.

The difference in pathogenesis between the two conditions is quite apparent at fluorescein angiography. In both conditions the fluorescein angiogram reveals non-perfusion of the peripheral retina. In Eales' disease, however, the irregular demarcation of the perfused retina with the abrupt occlusions of large vessels clearly indicates that occlusive changes in an initially normal primitive vascular system are involved (Figure 191). This pattern clearly differs from the continuous marginal zone of incomplete vessels found in DEVR.

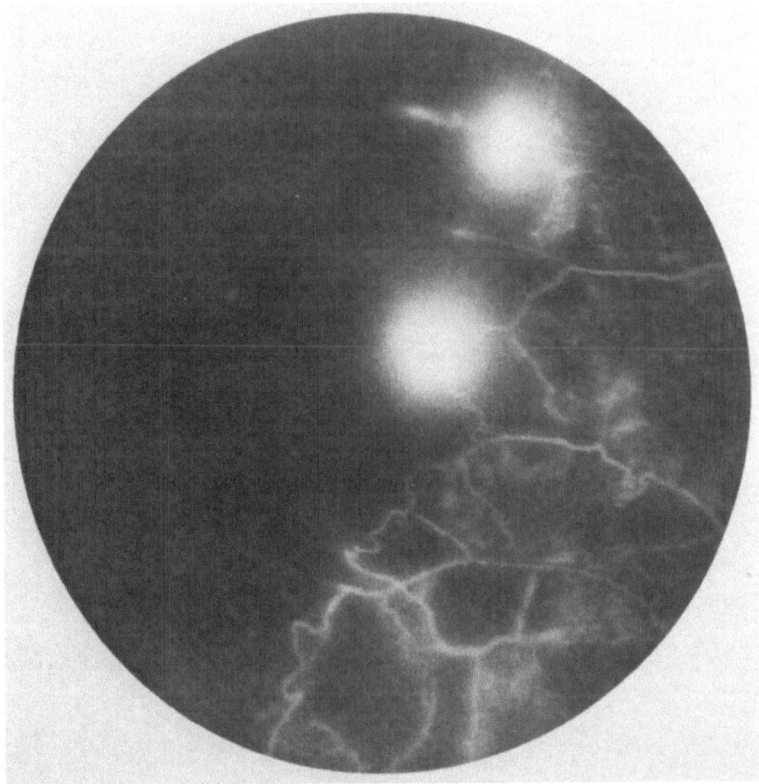

Figure 191. OD. Eales' disease. Non-perfusion of the peripheral retina due to vascular occlusions. Leakage from small neovascularizations.

## 14.2  Sickle cell retinopathy

Non-perfusion of the peripheral retina, with or without complicating neovascularization, is a frequent symptom of sickle cell retinopathy. This retinopathy is usually observed in persons with a combination of haemoglobins S
and C or a combination of haemoglobin S with the haemoglobin of thalass-
aemia (Goldberg, 1976).

### *14.2.a  Differential diagnosis from DEVR*

Differential diagnosis between sickle cell retinopathy and DEVR can seldom
pose problems. In some cases the symptoms of sickle cell retinopathy can
develop at an early age, like those of DEVR, and even lead to fibrovascular
organizations and retinal detachment. In actual practice the differential diagnosis is considered only when the changes are found in a black person, and of

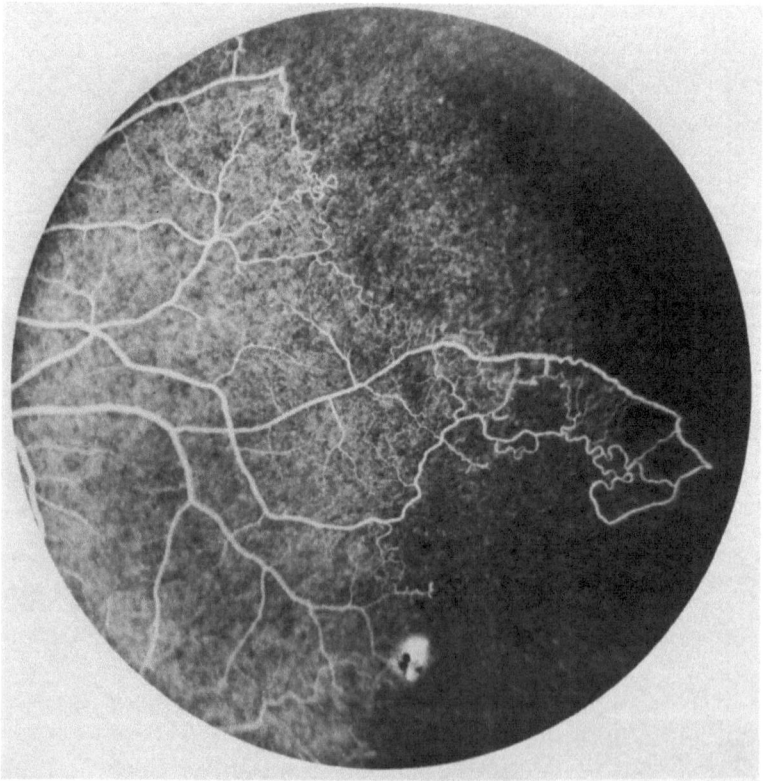

Figure 192. Sickle cell retinopathy OS. Fluorescein angiogram reveals non-perfusion of
the temporal retina.

course identification of the haemoglobin is essential in establishing the correct diagnosis.

Fluorescein angiography reveals non-perfusion of the peripheral retina in both conditions. The primary lesion in sickle cell retinopathy is arteriolar occlusion. As a result, capillaries which arise from the arterioles at a site central to the occlusion and form an arteriovenous anastomosis (Figure 192). This angiographic pattern is quite different from that of DEVR.

Unlike DEVR, sickle cell retinopathy is characterized by a normal configuration of the vasculature of the posterior pole of the retina, although some tortuosity of medium-size vessels is not rare. Neovascularizations and vitreous haemorrhages from these vessels are far more prominent in sickle cell retinopathy than in DEVR (Figure 193).

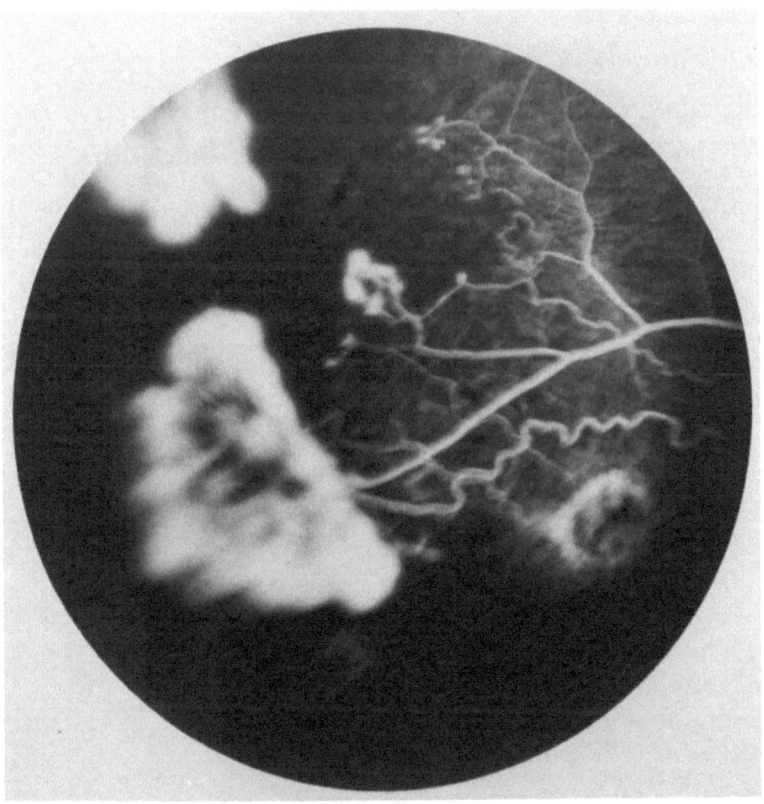

Figure 193. OD. Sickle cell retinopathy complicated by neovascularizations.

### 14.3 Pars planitis

#### 14.3.a Clinical symptoms

Pars planitis (Welch et al., 1960), otherwise known as peripheral uveitis (Brockhurst et al., 1960), posterior cyclitis (Hogan and Kimura, 1961) or idiopathic peripheral uveoretinitis (Tasman and Shields, 1980), is a chronic inflammation manifested by the presence of white "snowbanks" on the inner surface of the extreme periphery of the retina and the pars plana, and of cells in the vitreous. The changes are usually most pronounced in the periphery of the inferior fundus quadrants. The condition is often bilateral (Welch et al., 1960).

Pathological anatomical examination of eyes with pars planitis has revealed fibroglial tissue on the inner surface of the peripheral retina and the pars plana, and lymphocyte infiltration of the wall of retinal vessels (Pederson et al., 1978).

#### 14.3.b Differential diagnosis from DEVR

The clinical features of pars planitis undoubtedly show similarity to those of DEVR: both conditions usually manifest themselves with bilateral peripheral fundus changes in otherwise healthy young persons.

Preretinal opacities in the peripheral vitreous space and delicate white particles in the anterior vitreous space are features frequently found in both conditions.

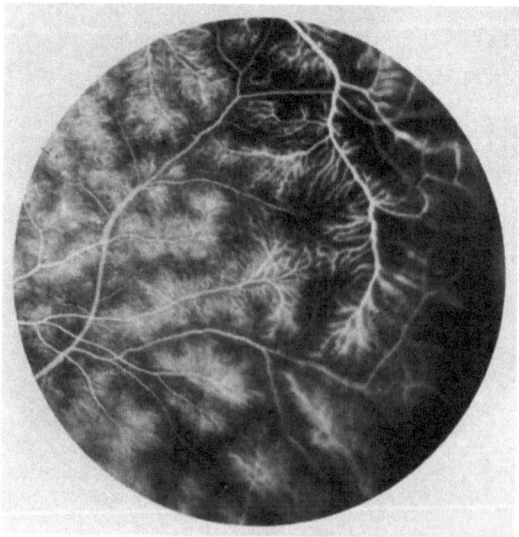

Figure 194. Pars planitis OS. Diffuse leakage of fluorescein from capillaries and veins.

The delicate vitreous opacities in pars planitis are generally far more pronounced than those in DEVR. The preretinal veils in the temporal periphery and the white exudates of DEVR differ from the less well-defined "snowbanks" on the inner surface of the peripheral retina in pars planitis, which usually show maximum density near the 6 o'clock position.

The fluorescein angiogram shows staining of the walls of retinal capillaries and veins, and leakage from these vessels throughout the fundus, in pars planitis (Figure 194). Non-perfusion of the peripheral retina can sometimes be demonstrated (Figure 175). However, the fluorescein angiogram differs markedly from that in DEVR.

The peripheral perfusion disorders in pars planitis probably result from the inflammatory changes and the oedema of the peripheral neuroretina and the vessels contained in it.

Neovascularization on the disc is a rare complication in pars planitis, which has been observed also without significant disturbances of peripheral retinal perfusion (Shorb et al., 1976).

A recent report on familial occurrence of pars planitis is of importance in the differential diagnosis discussed above (Augsburger et al., 1981).

## 14.4 Toxocariasis

The symptoms of ocular toxocariasis can vary widely, and it is often difficult or even impossible to establish the diagnosis on the basis of clinical findings. When the lesions are localized in the fundus periphery, the ophthalmoscopic findings may closely resemble those in DEVR.

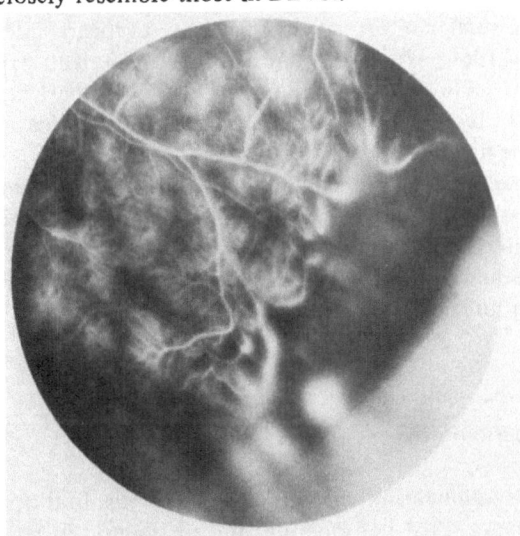

Figure 195. Same eye as Figure 194. Fluorescein angiogram of the temporal equatorial zone showing leakage from retinal vessels. Non-perfusion of the peripheral retina.

### 14.4.a Clinical symptoms

Intraocular symptoms of toxocariasis result from invasion of the second-stage larvae from the blood vessels into the eye. The condition is usually found in healthy children.

Toxocara infections of the eye can manifest themselves in a variety of ways. The following clinical symptoms have been ascribed to toxocariasis.

White granuloma in the posterior pole of the fundus.

Chronic endophthalmitis (or posterior uveitis) with prolific vitreous opacities.

Local white granulomatous or gliotic mass in the extreme fundus periphery. From this mass, vitreous strands or even falciform retinal folds can extend to the posterior pole of the fundus. Inflammatory changes are often discrete.

Apart from the abovementioned manifestations, toxocara has been regarded in incidental cases as a cause of optic neuritis (Bird et al., 1970) and iridocyclitis (Appelmans et al., 1965).

### 14.4.b Differential diagnosis

The presence of one or several gliotic masses in the extreme fundus periphery, usually accompanied by mild inflammatory changes in the vitreous, has been described by several authors and ascribed to toxocara infection (Perkins, 1966; Willetts, 1966; Wilkinson and Welch, 1971). This type of toxocara manifestation is reportedly not rare: in a series of 40 patients with probable toxocariasis, 17 presented with such peripheral lesions (Wilkinson and Welch, 1971). Only one had bilateral changes.

The abovementioned authors pointed out that the peripheral tissue masses, particularly in the presence of a radial retinal fold, might seem identical to the manifestations of cicatricial RLF and could also resemble the features of a congenital retinal fold. The following case history demonstrates that diagnosis can pose problems in such cases.

#### Case history

A healthy 6-year-old boy was referred to us because visual loss OS had been found at school.

The aqueous humour and vitreous contained cells. In the posterior pole of the fundus, some retinal deformation due to traction in temporal direction was visible (Figure 196). A white tissue mass was localized in the extreme inferior temporal periphery of the fundus. No vessels were visible in this tissue.

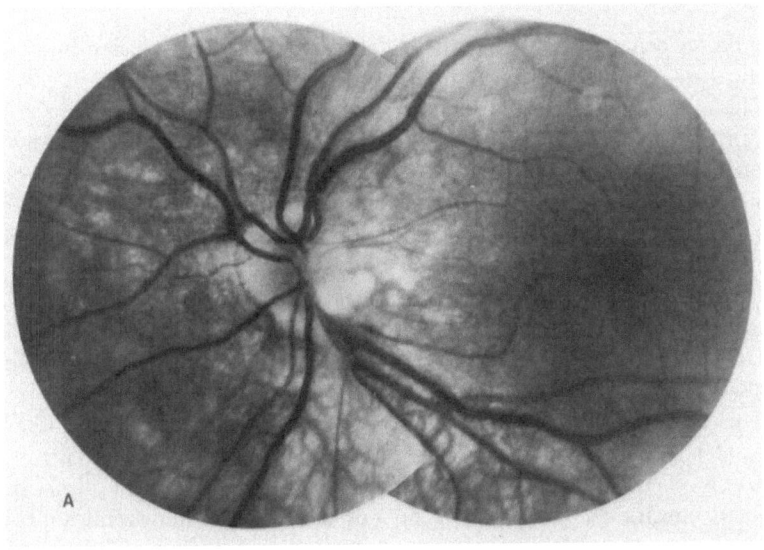

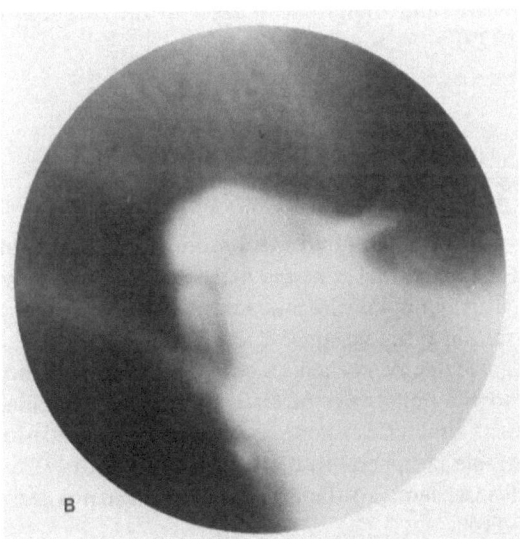

Figure 196. A) Mild deformation of the retina in the posterior pole. B) White tissue mass in the temporal periphery of the fundus.

The retina central to this mass was deformed and slightly raised in a radial duplicature. OD was entirely normal.

The clinical features in OS unmistakably resembled those found in several of our patients with DEVR. However, DEVR was virtually excluded by the absence of lesions in OD, and the absence of fundus changes in the other family members. RLF was eliminated on the basis of the neonatal history. The clinical features strongly suggested ocular toxocariasis, but complement fixation reaction and ELISA (vide infra) were both negative.

Particularly in (rarely described) bilateral cases of peripheral toxocara lesions (Wilkinson and Welch, 1971; Schlaegel and Knox, 1976), the possibility of DEVR should be taken into account and a family study should be made if necessary.

The case described by O'Connor (1972), with unilateral lesions, likewise illustrates the clinical similarity between DEVR and ocular toxocariasis.

Until recently, laboratory studies contributed little to the diagnosis of ocular toxocariasis. The parasites do not occur in the human intestine, and examination of stools is therefore useless. Blood eosionophilia is usually absent. Older serological assays and the skin test described by Duguid (1961) were not sufficiently specific to be of much value. Some authors maintain that the ELISA (enzyme-linked immunosorbed assay) introduced a few years ago, is more specific and therefore an asset in the diagnosis of toxocariasis (Pollard et al., 1979).

## 14.5 Myopia

### 15.5.a Perfusion disorders of the peripheral retina in myopia

At contact lens examination of eyes with moderate or high myopia, the retinal blood vessels in the equatorial zone are often almost or entirely invisible. This phenomenon is usually not confined to areas with distinct degenerative lesions but often involves the entire peripheral retina.

Fluorescein angiography in such cases reveals that the lumen of the retinal vessels central to the equator is often constricted. The filling phase of the peripheral retinal vessels is delayed, and retinal perfusion is often no longer clearly demonstrable peripheral to the equator (Figure 197). Such changes indicate the relative ischaemia of the peripheral retina in myopic eyes (Miyakubo and Numaga, 1980).

The disturbed perfusion of the peripheral retina in myopia differs from that in DEVR in that there is no zone of aberrant ramifications central to the area of non-perfusion, and no fluorescein leakage in the late phase. Consequently the lesions are not suggestive of a vascular developmental disorder but probably result from secondary changes and occlusions of peripheral retinal blood vessels.

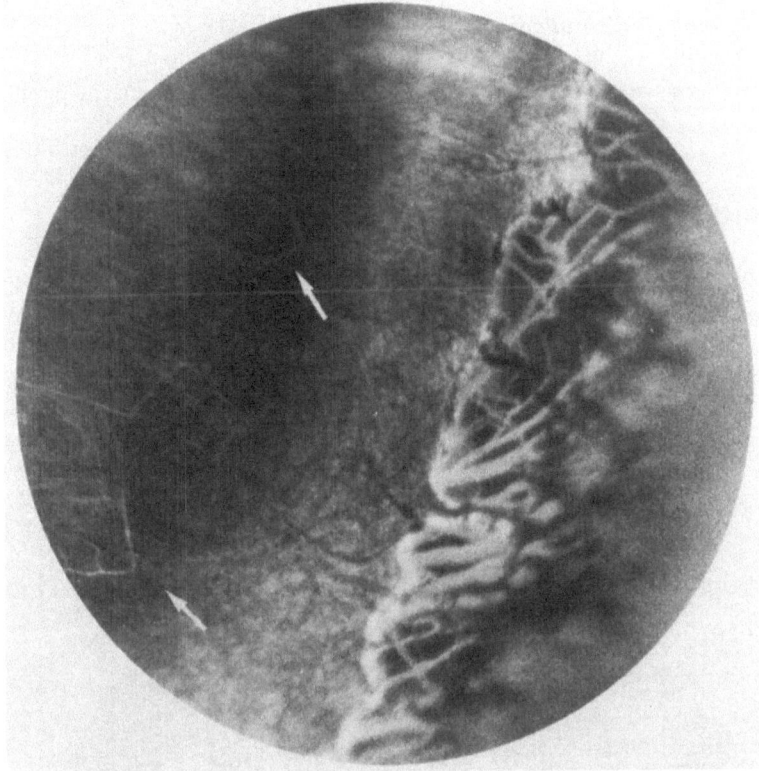

Figure 197. OS. Fluorescein angiogram of the temporal fundus periphery in high myopia. Cobblestones peripheral to the equator (on the right). Poorly perfused retinal vessels visible on the left (arrows). Non-perfusion of the equatorial retina (centre).

### 14.5.b Ectopia of the macula in high myopia

An abnormally stretched course of the retinal vessels in the posterior pole of the fundus is not infrequently observed in eyes with high myopia. In some cases, in which some temporal ectopia of the macula is present as well, there may be a close resemblance to posterior pole changes in DEVR.

*Case history HvK (06-02-26)*

*History*
A 54-year-old man was known to have high myopia before having undergone lens extraction OS at age 52. OD had become blind in childhood as a result of total retinal detachment. In view of slight intravitreous haemorrhage in OS, probably as a result of posterior vitreous detachment, a few vascular areas in the peripheral retina were coagulated. Birth had been premature but no supplemental oxygen had been given.

*Ophthalmological examination*

Visual acuity    VOS: S + 8.0/Cyl. − 3.5 axis 2° 0.5.

Anterior segments  OD: White, opaque tissue mass in the pupillary aperture.

OS: Aphakic pupillary aperture with sector iridectomy.

Vitreous     OD: Not assessable.

OS: Liquefaction with very little structure.

Fundus      OS: Abnormally stretched course of the temporal retinal vessels from the disc. Nearly all vascular branches exit from the temporal margin of the disc. Nasal ramifications of the central retinal artery and vein curve back in nasal direction. Distinct ectopia of the macula in temporal and also in slightly inferior direction (Figure 198).

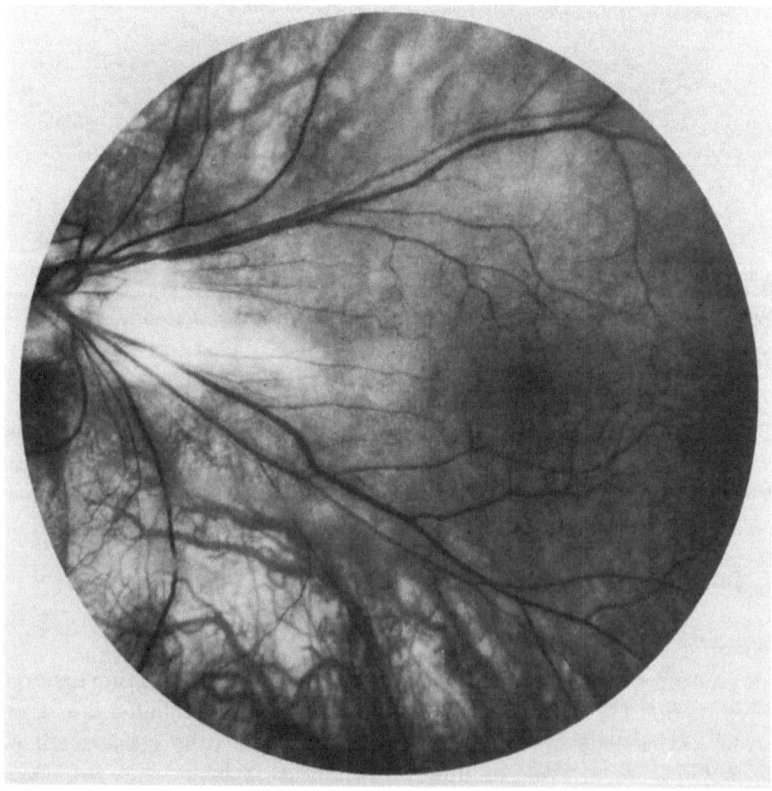

Figure 198. Abnormal vascular configuration in the posterior pole of the retina and macular ectopia in an eye with high myopia.

Outside the centre of the posterior pole the large choroidal vessels and sclera are clearly visible due to underdevelopment of choriocapillaris pigmented layer. Several pigmented scars of the laser coagulations are visible in the periphery. A delicate vitreous membrane attaches to the retina along the equator and is visible in both temporal quadrants. Nowhere in the retinal periphery are vascular changes seen that might indicate DEVR.

*Family study*
The brothers and sisters (three) of this patient all underwent examination of the fundus periphery in mydriasis. Apart from moderate myopia in one brother, no ocular anomalies were found. The patient's parents were no longer alive.

*Discussion*
The diagnosis of DEVR, suggested by the changes in the posterior pole of the fundus OS at the first examination, was not confirmed by the findings in the peripheral fundus, nor by the family study. A liquefied vitreous structure, myopia and a similar delicate vitreous membrane attaching along the equator are also observed in Wagner's syndrome, but the family study failed to reveal any evidence in this direction.

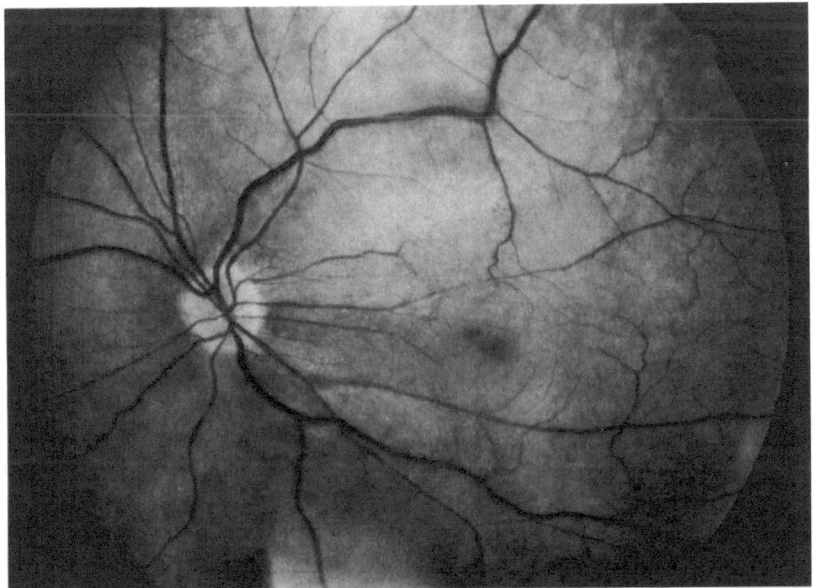

Figure 199. Deformation of the posterior pole of the retina.

## 14.6 Ectopia of the macula due to a pucker of the peripheral retina

*Case history BK-B (01-04-14)*

A 66-year-old woman was referred to our department by another hospital with the question whether the fundus changes in her left eye could be a manifestation of DEVR.

Metamorphopsia OS had existed for a few months. Ophthalmological examination had revealed a retinal defect and a preretinal membrane in the temporal fundus. There was no record of premature birth or neonatal oxygen administration. No family history of ocular anomalies.

*Ophthalmological examination*

| | |
|---|---|
| Visual acuity | VOD: S+ 0.75 1.25 |
| | VOS: S + 0.75/Cyl. − 0.5 axis 90° 0.4. |
| Intraocular pressure | ODS: 17 mm Hg. |
| Eye position | Straight. |
| Anterior segments | ODS: Normal. |
| Vitreous | OD: Normal. |
| | OS: Delicate white particles. |
| Fundi | OD: Normal posterior pole. Normal appearance of peripheral fundus, specifically no retinal vascular changes. |
| | OS: A few branches of the temporal retinal vessels take an abnormally stretched course from the disc in temporal direction. The macula is displaced in the same direction and in fact markedly deformed (Figure 199). The temporal equatorial zone of the retina shows preretinal membranes and retinoschisis at several sites. A large retinal defect is seen close to a pucker near 4 o'clock. |
| Fluorescein angiogram | OD: No anomalies of the posterior pole and the temporal equatorial zone in the late phase. |
| | OS: The early phase of the temporal equatorial zone shows severe deformation of the retinal vessels: near 4 o'clock a large arterial branch is distorted in inferior direction towards the centre of the retinal pucker. Consequently the ramifications of this vessel on the superior side are markedly stretched (Figure 200). Slightly higher, near 3 o'clock, a narrow zone with fairly intensively leaking retinal capillaries is visible. The late phase reveals significant leakage from these |

capillaries in an area bounded by epiretinal membranes. The posterior pole shows slight diffuse leakage from retinal capillaries.

*Discussion*

The configuration of the retinal vessels in the posterior pole and the macular ectopia are suggestive of DEVR. The absence of vascular changes in the peripheral retina OD, and the nature of the vascular changes in the peripheral retina OS, however, are not consistent with this diagnosis. Non-perfusion of the peripheral retina is not demonstrable in the fluorescein angiogram. Nor is the history suggestive of DEVR (in which the onset of symptoms is rarely in middle age).

The deformation of the retinal vessels and the macula ectopia in this patient are undoubtedly caused by the retinal pucker in the temporal fundus periphery, which is probably a complication secondary to the retinal defect.

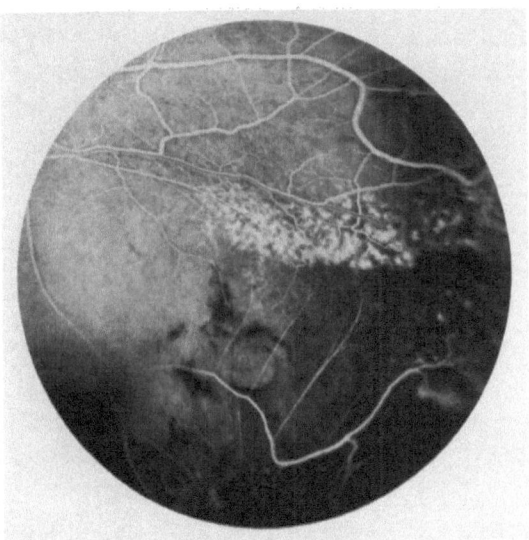

Figure 200. Fluorescein angiogram of the temporal fundus periphery. Retinal vessels stretched due to an epiretinal membrane.

DOMINANT EXUDATIVE VITREORETINOPATHY AND OTHER
VASCULAR DEVELOPMENTAL DISORDERS OF THE PERIPHERAL
RETINA

## SUMMARY

*Chapters 1 and 2*

The vascular development of the normal human neuroretina is a process which
occurs surprisingly late in the course of foetal life, and is not quite complete
even at birth. Vascularization of the peripheral retina, particularly in the temporal half of the fundus, does not take place until the final months of the
intra-uterine period. This implies that vascular developmental disorders in this
part of the retina have a late foetal pathogenesis.

Contact lens biomicroscopy and fluorescein angiography are by far the
most important methods of investigation to demonstrate vascular anomalies
in the peripheral fundus. The possibilities of these techniques are limited by
optical factors. Interpretation of vascular anomalies on a fluorescein angiogram of the peripheral fundus is impeded by optical artefacts and variations
in the vascular configuration of the retina and choroid which occur in this
part of the fundus in normal eyes.

*Chapters 3–6*

Only in the past decade have investigators become more familiar with the
clinical features of dominant exudative vitreoretinopathy (DEVR). Apart
from previous publications from our institute (Nijhuis et al., 1979; Van
Nouhuys, 1981), only about 60 cases of this condition (in fewer than ten
different families) have been reported.

This thesis describes nine families in which DEVR was diagnosed. Some
200 members of these families were ophthalmologically examined by me.
Evident symptoms of DEVR were found in 75, and in 12 others the diagnosis
was plausible but not certain.

The primary lesion in DEVR is a perfusion disorder of the peripheral retina
which manifests itself in the temporal part of the fundus. In uncomplicated
cases it is possible to establish the absence of retinal vessels in the area anterior to the temporal equator by contact lens biomicroscopy. The configuration of blood vessels in the retina posterior to the temporal equator is nearly
always aberrant: this area usually shows an increased number of vascular
ramifications with a strikingly parallel course, while the venous branches are
abnormally tortuous. In many cases the stretched course of the temporal

retinal vessels in the posterior pole is a conspicuous feature. This phenomenon is often associated with some temporal or inferior temporal ectopia of the macula.

Fluorescein angiography of the temporal fundus periphery as a rule clearly reveals the disturbed perfusion of the retina anterior to the equator in DEVR. A typical characteristic of the condition is abrupt termination of the retinal vasculature in the equatorial zone and fluorescein leakage from a zone of small terminal ramifications which demarcates the non-perfused retinal periphery.

The appearance of these aberrant terminal ramifications of retinal vessels and the configuration of the line of demarcation they form, show a marked similarity to the peripheral zone of incompletely developed retinal vasculature in normal foetal eyes during the final months of the intra-uterine period. This similarity implies that DEVR is based on a disturbance in the development of the retinal vasculature which must have occurred during the final months of the period of gestation. This disturbance has caused the temporal retinal periphery (last to be vascularized in the course of development) to remain avascular in DEVR.

Our study has shown that, in a number of cases, there was no fluorescein leakage from the peripheral ramifications in the temporal equatorial zone of the retina, and that these terminal ramifications formed a less clearly defined continuous zone than they did in most other cases of DEVR. This angiographic variant was mainly encountered in one particular family (the H family), which was also characterized by a high incidence of rhegmatogenous retinal detachment. Both the ophthalmoscopic and the fluorescein-angiographic features of this variant of DEVR are very subtle and inconspicuous, and in my opinion this fact has important diagnostic consequences.

In DEVR, the fluorescein angiogram of the posterior pole often discloses dilatations of macular capillaries in the early phase, and hyperfluorescence of the disc and leakage from capillaries in the centre of the posterior pole in the late phase.

In many eyes the symptoms of DEVR are largely confined to the above-mentioned vascular retinal changes. Visual acuity in such eyes is usually good. Of the 144 eyes of persons with evident DEVR, 102 (71%) had a visual acuity of 0.6 or better. This shows that the condition is in most cases compatible with fair-to-good visual function.

Retinal neovascularizations were found only at the demarcation between vascular and avascular retina, but only in a minority of cases. Intraretinal and subretinal exudates of widely varying size were likewise relatively rare (11% of eyes). Various types of pigmentations, whitish degenerative areas in the peripheral retina and atrophic changes of the pigment epithelium and choroid were encountered slightly more frequently.

Vitreous changes of widely varying severity were found in 48% of the eyes examined; in the remaining 52% the vitreous was quite normal. This observation demonstrates that DEVR is not a true vitreoretinopathy, as for example

Wagner's syndrome is. The vitreous changes are most likely a complication secondary to the retinal vascular changes. Classification of DEVR among the (vitreoretinal) dystrophies or degenerations is not consistent with the nature of the condition. The most characteristic feature of this group of conditions is gradual progression of the disease symptoms as a result of cell degeneration. Such a progression, however, was not demonstrated in any of our patients on the basis of history or data obtained by examination.

Visual function is determined largely by the presence or absence of complications. In DEVR, two types of complication are mainly responsible for severe visual impairment: amblyopia and retinal detachment.

Amblyopia was found in 11 of the 75 affected family members, and in most cases could be ascribed to anisometropia. The latter anomaly of refraction was quite common, as were myopia and myopic astigmatism.

Retinal detachment in DEVR can be due to traction exerted by vitreous membranes, formation of subretinal exudates, or the presence of retinal ruptures. The latter (rhegmatogenous) type of retinal detachment can occur as a result of large ruptures caused by traction, but also as a result of very small atrophic defects which are usually localized in the avascular part of the retina.

The fact that it is in particular the abovementioned complications that determine the prognosis, opens some perspectives for preventive and curative measures in cases of DEVR. In the vast majority of cases the complications develop before age 20, and the most severe forms of tractional retinal detachment were in fact found in patients younger than 10 years. This is why ophthalmological examination of young children in families with DEVR is very important.

The histopathological features of DEVR have been recently described. One of the persons I examined had been submitted to enucleation of one eye shortly after birth. The microscopic features of this eye were consistent with a terminal stage of a proliferative retinopathy.

Penetrance of the DEVR gene was found to be very high. Using the diagnostic methods described, I found a gene penetrance of about 90%. The gene is also characterized by very variable expression. It is probable that this variability is largely caused by non-genetic factors.

The mechanism by which the DEVR gene effects the disturbance in retinal vasculogenesis has so far remained obscure. General symptoms possibly related to the ocular changes have not been found.

The deformation of the vasculature of the posterior pole and periphery of the retina, and the often observed macular ectopia, cannot be explained in less severe cases of DEVR by traction resulting from the presence of cicatricial tissue. A hypothesis is advanced which explains these phenomena as direct consequence of the vascular developmental disorder.

The ophthalmological literature includes numerous descriptions of patients whose symptoms are suggestive of DEVR. Such cases are often reported in descriptive diagnostic terms such as macular ectopia or pseudoglioma, or by diagnoses whose correctness seems dubious, e.g. (familial) Coats' disease, (familial) persistent hyperplastic primary vitreous (PHPV) and retrolental fibroplasia (RLF). There are numerous case reports on congenital retinal fold (ablatio falciformis congenita) in which the descriptions of the fundus changes tally exactly with the falciform retinal folds found in several of our patients.

*Chapter 7*

Congenital retinal fold (ablatio falciformis congenita) is a fundus anomaly which can be found in several diseases. DEVR is the primary possibility to be taken into account in patients with unilateral or bilateral congenital retinal folds who show no general symptoms and have no record of neonatal oxygen administration.

In most cases, and certainly in DEVR, a congenital retinal fold is not formed until the final months of the intra-uterine period, and is a result of a retinal vascular developmental disorder.

*Chapter 8*

The symptoms of cicatricial RLF seem to differ hardly, if at all, from those of DEVR. Differential diagnosis between the two conditions is therefore based entirely on the neonatal history and on ophthalmological examination of a patient's family members.

The clinical symptoms are so similar that RLF can be described as a phenocopy of DEVR. Observations on neonates with DEVR have not been sufficiently numerous to establish with certainty whether, like RLF, the condition shows an acute phase.

There are numerous reports on RLF in children not given oxygen administration during the postnatal period. Since most of these publications make no mention of opthalmological examination of near relatives it is possible — and in fact probable — that some of these cases represent manifestations of DEVR.

It has not been established with certainty whether neonates who possess the gene of DEVR run an increased risk at neonatal oxygen administration. This question merits further investigation.

*Chapter 9*

Several syndromes are known to be associated with congenital organizations in the vitreous space and retinal detachment.

In mild manifestations of incontinentia pigmenti (Bloch-Sulzberger syndrome) there are fluorescein-angiographic changes which suggest disturbed vascularization of the peripheral retina. The fact that the acute symptoms of this syndrome develop in the perinatal period supports the postulate of a disturbance in the late phase of development of the retinal vasculature. Unlike DEVR, this syndrome also involves occlusive changes in the retinal vessels of the posterior pole of the fundus. Severe manifestations of the syndrome – e.g. proliferations in the vitreous space and retinal detachment – are probably caused by peripheral neovascularizations from the retina.

Norrie's disease is associated with congenital proliferative changes in the vitreous and retinal detachment. The ocular symptoms of this disease closely resemble those in severe cases of DEVR. It seems quite possible that the symptoms of Norrie's disease may likewise result from a congenital developmental disorder of the retinal vasculature with secondary neovascularization. This hypothesis is supported by the absence of changes suggestive of an early developmental disorder.

Some cerebral anomalies such as microcephaly and hydrocephalus can be associated with ocular symptoms which closely resemble those of RLF and DEVR, and indicate disturbed retinal vascularization. In describing patients with this syndrome, the old term "encephalo-ophthalmic dysplasia" can continue to be used for the time being, although the fundus changes are not based on primary dysplasia of the nerve tissue of the retina.

Unmistakable evidence of disturbed vasculogenesis of the peripheral retina has been found in some neonates with anencephalia. Histological examination of eyes of such neonates by several investigators has demonstrated avascularity of the peripheral retina and neovascularizations in the most peripheral zone of retinal vessels.

In the syndrome described by Reese, Blodi and Straatsma, which in most cases is probably based on trisomy 13, severe changes in the vitreous space have been frequently found at histological examination. These changes may well be a result of a congenital proliferative retinopathy. The syndrome also includes symptoms which indicate an early disorder of foetal development.

*Chapters 10-12*

In several patients with Wagner's syndrome I found fluorescein-angiographic changes in the equatorial region of the fundus which unmistakably suggested disturbed development of retinal vessels in this region. The cause of the disorder seems to lie not so much in the foetal vessels themselves as in the presence of sharply defined areas of dysplasia in choroid, pigmented layer and neuroretina, which have impaired the development of retinal vessels. It seems quite likely that the aberrant configuration of blood vessels in the central retina and the nasal macular ectopia found in some patients with Wagner's syndrome result from this impairment of retinal vascular development in the equatorial zone.

Sex-linked juvenile retinoschisis is associated in incidental cases with symptoms that could be interpreted as indicating a developmental disorder of peripheral retinal vessels. This disorder may have been caused by retinoschisis occurring before completion of retinal vascular development. There are no indications that vascular changes play a role in the aetiology of the retinoschisis in this condition.

Another relatively rare phenomenon in sex-linked juvenile retinoschisis is deformation of retinal vessels in and around the posterior pole and macula ectopia.

There are several reports on fluorescein-angiographic changes of the peripheral retinal vasculature found in usually young persons with non-traumatic rhegmatogenous retinal detachment. The vascular changes described in some of these publications are undoubtedly suggestive of a primary disorder in the vasculogenesis of the peripheral retina, and more specifically DEVR, can play a role in the pathogenesis of rhegmatogenous retinal detachment.

Congenital bilateral arterial anastomosis between the peripheral choroid and retina is a rare vascular malformation. This anastomosis, previously described by Van Nouhuys and Deutman (1980), is probably based on continued growth of a recurrent ciliary artery into the retina through a small colobomatous defect in Bruch's membrane and the retinal pigment epithelium.

Coats' disease and retinal angiomatosis can both be regarded as disorders of retinal vascular development, although it is usually impossible to establish the congenital presence of the lesions. Both conditions can ophthalmoscopically resemble forms of DEVR which are associated with extensive intraretinal and subretinal exudates. Coats' disease differs from DEVR in that hereditary factors are absent, as demonstrated by the case history of monozygotic twins of whom only one child proved to be (bilaterally) affected.

*Chapters 13 and 14*

Several conditions not associated with disturbances in the foetal vasculogenesis of the retina can pose problems of differential diagnosis from DEVR.

Persistent hyperplastic primary vitreous (PHPV) is a condition in which it is uncertain which clinical manifestations may occur in the posterior vitreous space. The hypothesis that a congenital retinal fold as a rule results from persistence of elements of the primary vitreous is untenable.

Our study has shown that DEVR, if associated with large chorioretinal cicatrices, can easily be mistaken for a condition resulting from congenital toxoplasmosis.

Of the acquired disorders of the peripheral retinal circulation, only Eales' disease and sickle cell retinopathy are briefly discussed. The principal difference between such occlusive retinopathies and conditions based on disturbed vascular development, such as DEVR, is the absence of a regular zone of underdeveloped peripheral capillaries in the angiogram, and the absence of distinct deformation of the retinal vasculature.

A few other acquired conditions such as ocular toxocariasis, pars planitis, and vascular retinal changes associated with myopia may lead to confusion with the symptoms of DEVR.

# DOMINANTE EXSUDATIEVE VITREORETINOPATHIE EN ANDERE VASCULAIRE ONTWIKKELINGSSTOORNISSEN VAN DE PERIFERE RETINA

## SAMENVATTING

### Hoofdstuk 1 en 2

De vasculaire ontwikkeling van de normale menselijke neuroretina is een proces, dat zich wonderlijk laat in het foetale leven voltrekt en zelfs bij de geboorte nog niet geheel is voltooid. Vascularisatie van de perifere retina met name in de temporale helft van de fundus geschiedt pas in de laatste maanden van de intra-uteriene periode. Dit impliceert, dat vasculaire ontwikkelingsstoornissen in dit gedeelte van de retina een laat foetale pathogenese hebben.

Voor het aantonen van vasculaire afwijkingen in de perifere fundus zijn contactglasbiomicroscopie en fluorescentie angiografie veruit de belangrijkste methoden van onderzoek. De mogelijkheden van deze technieken worden beperkt door optische oorzaken. De beoordeling van vasculaire anomalieën op het fluorescentie angiogram van de perifere fundus wordt bemoeilijkt door optische artefacten en variaties in de vaatconfiguratie van retina en chorioidea, die in dit deel van de fundus bij normale ogen voorkomen.

### Hoofdstuk 3–6

Dominante exsudatieve vitreoretinopathy (DEVR) is een aandoening, waarvan het klinische beeld pas het laatste decennium enige bekendheid heeft gekregen. Afgezien van eerdere publicaties van ons instituut (Nijhuis et al., 1979; Van Nouhuys, 1981) zijn slechts ongeveer een 60 tal gevallen van de aandoening behorend tot nog geen 10 families onder deze diagnose gerapporteerd.

In deze studie worden 9 families beschreven, waarin de diagnose DEVR gesteld werd. Ruim 200 leden van deze families werden door mij oogheelkundig onderzocht. Bij 75 van hen werden evidente verschijnselen van DEVR gevonden, terwijl bij 12 anderen de diagnose waarschijnlijk was, doch niet zeker.

De primaire afwijking bij DEVR is een perfusiestoornis van de perifere retina, die zich hoofdzakelijk manifesteert in het temporale deel van de fundus. Door contactglasonderzoek is het bij ongecompliceerde gevallen van de aandoening mogelijk de afwezigheid van retinavaten in het gebied voor de temporale equator vast te stellen. De configuratie van bloedvaten in de retina achter de temporale equator is bijna altijd aberrant: doorgaans zijn een toegenomen aantal vaattakken in deze gebieden gelegen met een opvallend parallel verloop en veelal vertonen de venetakken een abnormale tortuositeit. In de achterpool valt dikwijls het gestrekte verloop van de temporale retinavaten op. Dit verschijnsel gaat vaak gepaard met enige ectopie van de macula naar temporaal of naar temporaalonder.

Fluorescentie angiografie van de temporale periferie van de fundus toont bij DEVR meestal duidelijk de gestoorde perfusie van de retina voor de equator. Typisch voor de aandoening is het abrupte eindigen van het vaatbed van de retina in het equatorgebied en lekkage van fluoresceine uit een zoom van kleine terminale vertakkingen, die de niet geperfundeerde periferie van de retina begrenzen.

Het uiterlijk aspect van deze aberrante terminale vertakkingen van retinavaten alsmede de configuratie van de grenslijn die deze vormen, vertoont grote gelijkenis met de perifere zone van de onvolgroeide retina vasculatuur in normale foetale ogen gedurende de laatste maanden van de intrauteriene periode. Deze overeenkomst duidt erop, dat DEVR berust op een stoornis die in de ontwikkeling moet hebben plaats gevonden. Deze stoornis heeft er toe geleid, dat de temporale retinaperiferie, die het laatst in de ontwikkeling gevasculariseerd wordt, bij DEVR avasculair is gebleven.

Bij ons onderzoek is gebleken, dat bij een aantal gevallen geen lekkage van fluoresceine uit de perifere vertakkingen in de temporale equatorstreek van de retina optrad en dat deze terminale vertakkingen veel minder duidelijk een aaneengesloten zoom vormden dan doorgaans het geval was bij DEVR. Deze angiografische variant werd hoofdzakelijk in één familie (fam. H.) aangetroffen, waarin tevens het frequente vóórkomen van rhegmatogene ablatio retinae opviel. Zowel de ophthalmoscopische als fluorescentieangiografische verschijnselen van deze variant van DEVR zijn zeer onopvallend, hetgeen naar mijn mening belangrijke diagnostische consequenties heeft.

Het fluorescentie angiogram van de achterpool toont bij DEVR dikwijls dilataties van maculaire capillairen in de vroege fase en hyperfluorescentie van de papil en lekkage uit capillairen in het centrum van de achterpool in de late fase.

In veel ogen zijn de verschijnselen van DEVR hoofdzakelijk beperkt tot de hierboven genoemde vasculaire afwijkingen van de retina. De meeste van dergelijke ogen hebben een goede gezichtsscherpte. Van de 144 ogen van personen met zekere DEVR werd bij 102 ogen (71%) een gezichtsscherpte van 0.6 of hoger gevonden. Hieruit blijkt, dat de aandoening in de meeste gevallen compatibel is met een redelijke tot goede visuele functie.

Retinale neovascularisaties werden alleen aangetroffen ter plaatse van de grenszone tussen vasculaire en avasculaire retina, doch kwamen slechts in een minderheid van de gevallen voor. Ook intraretinale en subretinale exsudaten, van zeer uiteenlopende omvang waren betrekkelijk schaars (11%). Wat frequenter werden pigmentaties van verschillende aard, wittige degeneratieve gebieden in de perifere retina en atrofische veranderingen van pigmentblad en choroidea waargenomen.

Glasvochtveranderingen van zeer verschillende ernst waren aanwezig in 48% van de ogen. Bij de overige 52% was het glasvocht geheel normaal. Deze observatie toont aan dat DEVR geen echte vitreoretinopathie is, zoals b.v. het syndroom van Wagner. De glasvochtveranderingen treden naar alle waarschijnlijkheid secundair op aan de vasculaire afwijkingen in de retina. De rangschikking van DEVR onder de (vitreoretinale) dystrofieën of degeneraties is niet in overeenstemming met het karakter van de aandoening. Het meest kenmerkende aspect van deze groep aandoeningen is geleidelijke progressie van de ziekteverschijnselen tengevolge van het te gronde gaan van cellen. Een dergelijk beloop hebben wij echter bij geen van onze patiënten op grond van de anamnese of onderzoek kunnen vaststellen. De visuele functie wordt grotendeels bepaald door het al of niet optreden van complicaties. In hoofdzaak zijn twee soorten complicaties bij DEVR verantwoordelijk voor ernstige visusvermindering: amblyopie en ablatio retinae.

Amblyopie werd bij 11 van de 75 familieleden met onmiskenbare ziekteverschijnselen gevonden en kon in de meeste gevallen toegeschreven worden aan een anisometropie. Deze laatste refractieanomalie kwam frequent voor evenals een myopie of een myoop astigmatisme.

Ablatio retinae kan bij DEVR ontstaan door tractie van glasvochtmembranen, vorming van subretinale exsudaten of door rhegmatogene oorzaak. Dit laatste type netvliesloslating kan optreden als gevolg van grote scheuren onder invloed van tractie, maar ook door het ontstaan van zeer kleine atrofische defectjes, die meestal in het niet gevasculariseerde deel van de retina zijn gelegen.

Het feit, dat het met name de hierboven genoemde complicaties zijn die de prognose bepalen, biedt enige perspectieven voor preventieve en curatieve maatregelen bij patiënten met DEVR. De complicaties treden in veruit de meeste gevallen op voor het 20e jaar, terwijl de meest ernstige vormen van tractionele ablatio retinae zelfs beneden de 10 jarige leeftijd voorkomen. Om deze reden is het herkennen van de aandoening alsmede het verrichten van oogheelkundig onderzoek bij jonge kinderen in families, waarin de ziekte geconstateerd is, van grote betekenis.

De histopathologische afwijkingen van DEVR zijn pas onlangs voor het eerst beschreven. Van één van de door mij onderzochte personen had enucleatie van één oog kort na de geboorte plaats gehad. Het microscopische beeld van dit oog paste bij een eindstadium van een proliferatieve retinopathie.

Het gen van DEVR bleek een hoge penetrantie te hebben. Met onze diagnostiek werd een penetrantie van ongeveer 90% gevonden. Voorts kenmerkt het gen zich door een zeer variabele expressie. Het is waarschijnlijk, dat deze variabiliteit voor een belangrijk deel veroorzaakt wordt door niet genetische factoren.

Langs welke weg het gen van de aandoening de storing in de retinale vasculogenese bewerkstelligt is tot nu toe onbekend. Algemene verschijnselen die een relatie met de oogafwijkingen konden hebben, werden niet gevonden.

De vervorming van het vaatbed van achterpool en periferie van de retina, alsmede de vaak aanwezige ectopie van de macula kan bij minder ernstige gevallen van DEVR niet verklaard worden door tractieverschijnselen tengevolge van littekenweefsel. Een hypothese wordt geboden, waarin deze verschijnselen verklaard worden als direct gevolg van de vasculaire ontwikkelingsstoornis.

In de oogheelkundige literatuur komen veel beschrijvingen van ziektegevallen voor, waarvan de verschijnselen suggestief zijn voor DEVR. Dergelijke gevallen zijn vaak aangeduid met descriptieve diagnosen, zoals ectopia maculae, pseudoglioom of met diagnosen, waarvan de juistheid in twijfel getrokken moet worden, zoals: (familiaire) ziekte van Coats, (familiaire) PHPV en RLF. Talrijk zijn de publicaties van gevallen van congenital retinal fold (ablatio falciformis congenita), waarvan de descripties van de fundusafwijkingen exact overeenkomen met de bij verschillende van onze patiënten gevonden falciforme retinaplooien.

*Hoofdstuk 7*

Congenital retinal fold (ablatio falciformis congenita) is een fundusafwijking die bij verschillende aandoeningen kan voorkomen. Bij patiënten met deze afwijking in één of beide ogen, die geen algemene verschijnselen hebben, en waaraan geen zuurstof in de neonatale periode is toegediend, moet in eerste instantie aan DEVR gedacht worden als oorzaak.

De vorming van een falciforme ablatio retinae geschiedt in de meeste gevallen, en zeker bij DEVR, niet voor de laatste maanden van de intrauteriene periode en is het gevolg van een vasculaire ontwikkelingsstoornis van de retina.

*Hoofdstuk 8*

De symptomen van cicatriciële RLF en DEVR lijken niet of nauwelijks te verschillen. De differentiaal diagnose tussen beide aandoeningen berust daarom geheel op de neonatale anamnese en oogheelkundig onderzoek van familieleden van een patiënt.

De klinische verschijnselen komen dermate overeen, dat gezegd kan worden dat RLF een phenocopie is van DEVR. Er zijn te weinig observaties bij zuigelingen met DEVR verricht om te kunnen vaststellen in hoeverre de aandoening evenals RLF gepaard gaat met een acute fase.

Gevallen van RLF bij kinderen die in de postnatale periode geen extra zuurstof hebben ontvangen zijn herhaaldelijk beschreven. Daar in de meeste van deze publicaties geen melding gemaakt is van oogheelkundig onderzoek van naaste familieleden van de patiënten is het mogelijk, en zelfs waarschijnlijk, dat een aantal van deze gevallen manifestaties zijn geweest van DEVR.

Het staat niet vast of pasgeborenen die het gen van de aandoening bezitten een verhoogd risico lopen bij toediening van extra zuurstof. Dit onderwerp verdient verder onderzoek.

*Hoofdstuk 9*

Er zijn verschillende syndromen bekend, die gepaard gaan met congenitale organisaties in de glasvochtruimte en ablatio retinae.

Bij lichte manifestaties van incontinentia pigmenti (syndroom van Bloch-Sulzberger) zijn fluorescentieangiografische verschijnselen aanwezig, die suggestief zijn voor een gestoorde vascularisatie van de perifere retina. Het feit, dat de acute verschijnselen van dit syndroom zich in de perinatale periode voordoen, steunt de veronderstelling van een stoornis gedurende de late fase van ontwikkeling van de retinavasculatuur. In tegenstelling tot DEVR komen bij dit syndroom ook occlusieve veranderingen van retinavaten in de achterpool van de fundus voor. Ernstige manifestaties van het syndroom, zoals proliferaties in de glasvochtruimte en netvliesloslating worden zeer waarschijnlijk veroorzaakt door perifere neovascularisaties vanuit de retina.

De ziekte van Norrie gaat gepaard met congenitale proliferatieve veranderingen in het glasvocht en netvliesloslating. De verschijnselen van de aandoening lijken sterk op die van ernstige gevallen van DEVR. De mogelijkheid dat de symptomen van de ziekte van Norrie eveneens het gevolg zijn van een congenitale ontwikkelingsstoornis van de retinavasculatuur met secundaire neovascularisatie lijkt niet gering. Deze veronderstelling wordt gesteund door het ontbreken van afwijkingen, die op een vroege ontwikkelingsstoornis duiden.

Sommige cerebrale afwijkingen, zoals microcephalie en hydrocephalie kunnen gepaard gaan met oogsymptomen, die grote overeenkomsten vertonen met RLF en DEVR en die duiden op een gestoorde vascularisatie van de retina. Voor de aanduiding van gevallen die tot dit syndroom behoren kan de oude benaming "encephalo-ophthalmic dysplasia" voorlopig gehandhaafd worden, hoewel de fundusafwijkingen niet op een primaire dysplasia van het zenuwweefsel van de retina berusten.

Duidelijke verschijnselen van een storing van de vasculogenese van de perifere retina zijn waargenomen bij sommige pasgeborenen met anencephalie. Histologisch onderzoek van ogen van dergelijke kinderen is door verschillende onderzoekers verricht en heeft avasculariteit van de perifere retina aangetoond en neovascularisaties ter plaatse van de meest perifere zone van retinavaten.

Bij het door Reese, Blodi en Straatsma beschreven syndroom, dat waarschijnlijk in de meeste gevallen berust op trisomie van chromosoom 13, zijn ernstige veranderingen in de glasvochtruimte frequent histologisch waargenomen. Het is mogelijk, dat deze verschijnselen het gevolg zijn vaan een congenitale proliferatieve retinopathie. Bij het syndroom komen ook symptomen voor die duiden op een vroege stoornis in de foetale ontwikkeling.

*Hoofdstuk 10–12*

Bij verschillende patiënten met het syndroom van Wagner werden door ons duidelijke fluorescentieangiografische afwijkingen in de equatoriale gebieden van de fundus gevonden, die duidden op een gestoorde ontwikkeling van retinavaten in dit gebied. De oorzaak van deze stoornis lijkt niet in de foetale vaten zelf gelegen, doch in die aanwezigheid van scherp begrensde arealen, die een dysplasie vertonen van chorioidea, pigmentblad en neuroretina en die een belemmering gevormd hebben voor de ontwikkeling van retinale vaten. Het is waarschijnlijk, dat de aberrante configuratie van bloedvaten in de centrale retina alsmede de nasale ectopie, die bij sommige patiënten met het syndroom van Wagner voorkomt, het gevolg zijn van genoemde belemmering van de ontwikkeling van retinavaten in de equatoriale gebieden.

Geslachtsgebonden juveniele retinoschisis gaat in incidentele gevallen gepaard met verschijnselen, die geduid kunnen worden als een ontwikkelingsstoornis van perifere retinavaten. Het is mogelijk, dat deze stoornissen veroorzaakt zijn door een vroeg opgetreden retinoschisis voor de voltooiing van de retinale vaatontwikkeling. Er zijn geen aanwijzingen dat vasculaire afwijkingen een etiologische rol spelen bij het tot stand komen van de retinoschisis bij deze aandoening.

Een ander eveneens betrekkelijk zeldzaam fenomeen bij geslachtsgebonden juveniele retinoschisis is de deformatie van retinavaten in en om de achterpool en ectopie van de macula.

In verschillende publicaties zijn fluorescentieangiografische afwijkingen van de perifere retinavasculatuur getoond bij meestal jeugdige personen met een niet traumatische, rhegmatogene ablatio retinae. De vasculaire verschijnselen in enkele van deze publicaties duiden zonder twijfel op een primaire storing in de vasculogenese van de perifere retina en zijn niet te onderscheiden van de angiografische symptomen van DEVR. Dergelijke studies verlenen steun aan het concept, dat vasculaire ontwikkelingsstoornissen van de perifere retina, en met name DEVR, een rol kunnen spelen bij de pathogenese van rhegmatogene ablatio retinae.

Een zeldzame vasculaire misvorming is de congenitale bilaterale arteriële anastomose tussen perifere chorioidea en retina. Deze anastomose, die eerder beschreven is (Van Nouhuys en Deutman, 1980) berust waarschijnlijk op een doorgroei van een arteria ciliaris recurrens naar de retina door een klein colobomateus defect van de membraan van Bruch en retinale pigmentblad.

De ziekte van Coats en angiomatosis retinae zijn beide te beschouwen als vasculaire ontwikkelingsstoornissen van de retina, hoewel doorgaans niet vast te stellen is in hoeverre de lesies congenitaal aanwezig zijn geweest. Beide aandoeningen kunnen ophthalmoscopische gelijkenis vertonen met vormen van DEVR, die gepaard gaan met uitgebreide intra en subretinale exsudaten. In tegenstelling tot DEVR ontbreken bij de ziekte van Coats erfelijke factoren, hetgeen gedemonsteerd wordt aan de hand van de ziektegeschiedenis van een ééneiige tweeling, waarvan slechts één kind (bilateraal) aangedaan bleek te zijn.

*Hoofdstuk 13 en 14*

Verschillende aandoeningen, die niet gepaard gaan met storingen van de foetale vasculogenese van de retina, kunnen differentiaaldiagnostische problemen met DEVR opleveren.

Persisterend hyperplastisch primair glasvocht (PHPV) is een aandoening, waarvan het onzeker is met welke klinische manifestaties in de achterste glasvochtruimte deze zich kan presenteren. De veronderstelling, dat een congenital retinal fold doorgaans het gevolg is van persisteren van elementen van het primaire glasvocht is onjuist.

Zoals in onze studie is gebleken kan DEVR, indien de aandoening gepaard gaat met grote chorioretinale littekens, gemakkelijk aangezien worden voor de gevolgen van congenitale toxoplasmose.

Van de verkregen circulatiestoornissen van de perifere retina zijn slechts de ziekte van Eales en sikkelcelretinopathie kort vermeld. Het belangrijkste onderscheid van dergelijke occlusieve retinopathieën met aandoeningen die op een gestoorde vaatontwikkeling berusten, zoals DEVR, is het ontbreken van een regelmatige zoom van onvolgroeide perifere capillairen op het angiogram en de afwezigheid van duidelijke deformatie van het vaatbed van de retina.

Enkele andere verkregen aandoeningen, zoals toxocariasis, pars planitis en vasculaire afwijkingen van de retina bij myopie kunnen verward worden met de verschijnselen van DEVR.

# REFERENCES

Aan de Kerk AL (1973) Photographic aids in ophthalmic practice. Doc Ophthalmologica Proc Series 3:5—42

Adamkin DH, Shott RJ, Cook LN and Andrews BF (1977) Non hyperoxic retrolental fibroplasia. Pediatrics 60:828—829

Addison DJ, Font RL and Manschot WA (1972) Proliferative retinopathy in anencephalic babies. Am J Ophthalmol 74:828—829

Alexander RL and Shea M (1965) Wagner's disease. Arch Ophthalmol 74:310—318

Amalric P (1969) Angiographie fluorescéinique dans le décollement juvenile. Mod Probl Ophthalmol 8:394—406

Amalric P, Cenac P, Norati M (1975) Angiographie fluorescéinique de la périphérie rétinienne. Mod Probl Ophthalmol 15:91—97

Ancona S (1935) Persistentie van het koppelstuk van Von Szily. Ned T Geneesk 79: 135—150

Anderson SR, Warburg M (1961) Norrie's disease. Congenital bilateral pseudotumor of the retina with recessive X-chromosomal inheritance. Arch Ophthalmol 66:614—618

Appelmans M (1947) L'angiomathose de la rétine chez l'enfant. Arch Ophthalmol 7: 489—510

Appelmans M, Michiels J, Roquet P (1965) Uvéite avec hypopyon a éosinophiles par larve de nématode. Bull Soc Belge Ophthalmol 140:505—512

Apple DJ, Fishman GA, Goldberg M (1974) Ocular histopathology of Norrie's disease. Am J Ophthalmol 78:196—203

Apple DJ. Naumann GOH (1980) Spezielle Pathologie der Retina. In: Naumann GOH. Pathologie des Auges 577—666 (Spezielle pathologische Anatomie, part 12) Springer Verlag, Berlin

Archer DB, Krill AE, Newell FW (1970) Fluorescein studies of normal choroidal circulation. Am J Ophthalmol 69:543—554

Archer DB, Nevin NC (1977) Sturge-Weber syndrome. Krill's hereditary Retinal and Choroidal Diseases vol 2. Harper and Row, Hagerstown USA

Asdourian GK, Goldberg MF (1979) The angiographic pattern of the peripheral retinal vasculature. Arch Ophthalmol 97:2316—2324

Ashton N (1954) Pathological basis of retrolental fibroplasia. Brit J Ophthalmol 38: 385—396

Ashton N (1957) Retinal vascularization in health and disease. Am J Ophthalmol 44: 7—17

Ashton N (1966) Oxygen and the growth of retinal vessels. Am J Ophthalmol 62:412—435

Ashton N (1970) Retinal angiogenesis in the human embryo. Br Med Bull 26:103—107

AshtonN (1979) The pathogenesis of retrolental fibroplasia. Ophthalmology 86:1695—1699

Ashton N, Cook C (1955) Studies on developing retinal vessels: II. Influence of retinal oxygen vaso-obliteration. Brit J Ophthalmol 39:457—462

Augsberger JJ, Annesley WH, Sergott RC, Felberg NT, Bowman JH, Raymond LA (1981) Familial pars planitis. Ann Ophthalmol 13:553—557

Ayesh I, Sanders MD, Friedmann AJ (1976) Retinitis pigmentosa and Coats' disease. Brit J Ophthalmol 60:775—777

Babel J (1966) Les malformations pseudotumorales du globe oculaire. Ophthalmologica 151:405—426

Badtke G (1954) Ueber seltene Duplikaturenbildungen in der embryonalen Netzhaut. Graefes Arch Ophthalmol 155:266−283

Badtke G (1960) Zur Frage des entwicklungsphysiologischen Zusammenhangs zwischen der Ablatio falciformis congenita und pathologischen Entwicklungsschritten der Netzhaut im Bereich der embryonalen Augenbecherspalte, insbesondere den typischen Funduskolobomen. Klin Mbl Augenheilk 136:806−815

Badtke G and Domke H (1966) Klinisch-histologischer Beitrag zur normalen Genese und Entwicklungsphysiologie der Ablatio falciformis congenita. Klin Mbl Augenheilk 149:593−609

Balen AThM van, Falger ELF (1970) Hereditary hyaloideoretinal degeneration and palatoschisis. Arch Ophthalmol 83:152−162

Balian JV, Falls HV (1960) Congenital vascular veils in the vitreous. Arch Ophthalmol 63:92-101

Barr CC, Rice TA, Michels RG (1980) Angioma mass in retrolental fibroplasia. Am J Ophthalmol 89:647−650

Barber AN (1955) Embryology of the human eye. Kimpton, London

Barsewisch B von (1968) Ablatio falciformis. Ber Deutsche Ophthalmol Ges 69:481−487

Bec P, Ravault M, Arné, Trepsat C (1980) La périphérie du fond de l'oeil. Masson et cie ed, Paris

Beck de (1890) Persistent remains of the fetal hyaloid artery. Am Ophthalmol Monograph no 1

Bedell AJ (1966) Retinal folds. Am J Ophthalmol 61:60−62

Benedikt O, Ehalt H (1970) Familiär auftretendes Bloch-Sulzberger Syndrom (Incontinentia Pigmenti) mit Augenbeteiligung. Klin Mbl Augenheilk 157:652

Bengtsson B, Linder B (1967) Sex-linked juvenile retinoschisis (presentation of two affected families) Acta Ophthalmol 45:411−422

Best W, Rentsch F (1974) Ueber das "Pseudogliom" bei der Incontinentia pigmenti. Klin Mbl Augenheilk 164:19−32

Bird AC (1981) Personal communication

Bird AC, Lawton-Smith J, Curtin VT (1970) Nematode optic neuritis. Am J Ophthalmol 69:72−77

Blair NP, Albert DM, Liberfahr RM, Hirose T (1979) Hereditary progressive arthro-ophthalmopathy of Stickler. Am J Ophthalmol 88:876−888

Bloch B (1926) Eigentümliche bisher nicht beschriebene Pigmentaffection (Incontinentia pigmenti). Schweiz Med Wochenschr 7:404−405

Blodi F and Hunter W (1969) Norrie's disease in North America. Doc Ophthalmol 26: 434−450

Böringer HR, Dieterle P and Landolt E (1960) Zur Klink und Pathologie der Degeneratio hyaloideo-retinalis hereditaria (Wagner). Ophthalmologica 139:23−31

Brockhurst RJ, Albert DM, Zakov, ZN (1981) Pathologic findings in familial exudative vitreoretinopathy. Arch Ophthalmol 99:2143−2146

Brockhurst RJ, Chishti MI (1975) Cicatricial retrolental fibroplasia: its occurrence without oxygen administration and in full-term infants. Graefes Arch Ophthalmol 195: 113−128

Brockhurst RJ, Schepens CL, Okamura JD (1960) Peripheral uveitis. Clinical description, complications and differential diagnosis. Am J Ophthalmol 49:1257−1266

Bruckner HL (1968) Retrolental fibroplasia associated with intrauterine anoxia? Arch Ophthalmol 80:504−505

Burch JV, Leveille AS and Morse PH (1980) Ichthyosis hystrix (epidermal nevus syndrome) and Coats' disease. Am J Ophthalmol 89:25−30

Busacca A, Goldmann H, Schiff-Wertheimer S (1957) Biomicroscopie du corps vitré et du fond de l'oeil. Masson et cie, Paris (1957)

Busse BJ, Mittelman D (1976) Use of the astigmatism correction device on the Zeiss funduscamera for peripheral retinal photography. Ophthalmic Photography 16:63−74

Byer NE (1974) Prognosis of asymptomatic retinal breaks. Mod Probl Ophthalmol 12: 103−108

Campbell FP (1976) Coats' disease and congenital vascular retinopathy. Trans Am Ophthalmol Soc 74:365−424

Campbell K (1951) Intensive oxygen therapy as a possible cause of retrolental fibroplasia: A clinical approach. Med J Australia 2:48–50

Canny CLB and Oliver GL (1976) Fluorescein angiographic findings in familial exudative vitreoretinopathy. Arch Ophthalmol 94:1114–1120

Carney RG (1976) Incontinentia pigmenti. A world statistical analysis. Arch Dermatol 112:535–542

Chaudhuri PR, Rosenthal AR, Goulstine DB et al (1982) Familial exudative vitreoretinopathy associated with familial thrombocytopathy. (ARVO abstract). Invest Ophthalmol 22:3:9 (suppl)

Chisholm IA, Foulds WS, Christison. (1974) Investigation and therapy of Coats' disease. Trans Ophthalmol Soc UK 94:335–341

Cibis PA (1965) Hereditary hyaloidea-retinopathy with retino-schisis. Vitreo-retinal pathology and surgery in retinal detachment pp 87–95 Mosby, St. Louis

Clark ER (1918) Studies on the growth of blood vessels in the tail of the frog larva by observation and experiment on the living animal. Am J Anat 23:37

Clarke E (1898) "Pseudoglioma" in both eyes. Trans Ophthalmol Soc UK 18:136–138

Coats G (1908) Forms of retinal disease with massive exudation. R London Ophthalmol Hosp Rep 17:440

Coats G (1911) A case of exudative retinitis. Ophthalmol Rev 30:289

Coats G (1912) Ueber Retinitis exsudativa (Retinitis haemorrhagica externa) Graefes Arch Ophthalmol 81:275–327

Cogan DG (1963) Development and senescence of the human retinal vasculature. Doyne memorial lecture. Trans Ophthalmol Soc. UK 83:465–489

Cogan DG, Kuwabara T (1964) Ocular pathology of the 13–15 trisomy syndrome. Arch Ophthalmol 72:246–253

Cohen J, Alfano JE, Boshes LD'et al. (1964) Clinical evaluation of school-age children with retrolental fibroplasia. Am J Ophthalmol 57:41–57

Collins ET (1890) On the development and abnormalities in the zonule of Zinn. R London Ophthalmol Hosp Rep 13:81–96

Collins ET (1908) Developmental deformities of the crystalline lens. J A M A 51:1051–1056

Constantaras J, Dobbie JG, Chromokes EA, Frenkel M (1972) Juvenile sex-linked recessive retinoschisis in a black family. Am J Ophthalmol 74:1166–1178

Conway BP and Welch RB (1977) X-chromosome-linked juvenile retinoschisis with haemorrhagic retinal cyst. Am J Ophthalmol 83:853–855

Criswick VG and Schepens CL (1969) Familial exudative vitreoretinopathy. Am J Ophthalmol 68:578–594

Czermak W (1905) Path.-anat. Befund bei der von E von Hippel beschriebenen sehr seltenen Netzhauterkrankung. Ber Vers D Ophthalmol Ges 32:184–195

Czermak W (1907) Pseudophakia fibrosa, eine faserige Scheinlinse hervorgegangen aus der Tunica vasculosa lentis. Arch Ophthalmol 57:79–96

Daicker B (1972) Anatomie und Pathologie der menschlichen retino-ziliaren Fundusperiferie. Karger, Basel

Daicker B, Guggenheim R and Gywat L (1977a) Raster elektronenmikroskopische Befunde an Netzhautinnenflächen. II. Hintere Glaskörperabhebung. Graefes Arch Ophthalmol 204:19–29

Daicker B, Guggenheim R and Gywat L (1976) Raster elektronenmikroskopische Befunde an Netzhautinnenflächen. III. Epivaskuläre Gliabüschel. Graefes Arch Ophthalmol 204:31–37

Danis M (1921) Congenital anomalies of the fundus of the eye. Am J Ophthalmol 4:233–237

Dejean Ch, Leplat G, Hervouët (1958) L'embryologie de l'oeil et sa tératologie. Masson, Paris

Dekking HM (1949) Toxoplasmosis as a cause of congenital defects. Ophthalmologica 117:1–7

Delaney WV jr, Podedworny W, Havener WH (1963) Inherited retinal detachment. Arch Ophthalmol 69:78–82

Deutman AF (1971) The hereditary dystrophies of the posterior pole of the eye. v Gorcum, Assen

Deutman AF (1977) In: Krill's hereditary retinal and choroidal diseases vol 2 p 1093 Harper and Row, Hagerstown

Doesschate G ten (1916) Canalis Cloqueti. Klin Mbl Augenheilk 57:206

Donders PCM (1958) Eales' disease. Junk, The Hague

Dudgeon J (1979) Familial exudative vitreoretinopathy. Trans Ophthalmol Soc UK 99: 45–49

Duguid IM (1961) Features of ocular infestation by toxocara. Brit J Ophthalmol 4: 789–796

Eisenberg IJ (1948) Congenital retinal fold with vitreous disorganization. Am J Ophthalmol 31:337–338

Eisner G (1973) Biomicroscopy of the peripheral fundus. Springer Verlag, Berlin, Heidelberg

Elliott AJ (1976) Periphlebitis retinae. TD Duane: Clinical Ophthalmology vol 3 chap 16 Harper and Row, Hagerstown

Ellsworth RM (1976) Retinoblastoma. TD Duane: Clinical Ophthalmology vol 3 chap 35 Harper and Row, Hagerstown

Engerman RL, Meyer RK (1965) Development of retinal vasculature in rats. Am J Ophthalmol 60:628–641

Ewing CC, Yves EJ (1969) Juvenile hereditary retinoschisis. Trans Ophthalmol Soc UK 89:29–39

Faris BM and Brockhurst RJ (1969) Retrolental fibroplasia in the cicatricial stage. Arch Ophthalmol 82:60–65

Favre M (1958) A propos de deux cas de dégénérescence hyaloideo-rétinienne. Ophthalmologica 135:604–609

Felberg NT, McFall R and Shields JA (1977) Aqueous humor enzyme patterns in retinoblastoma. Invest Ophthalmol 16:1039–1046

Findlay EK (1925) Congenital membraneous cataract. Am J Ophthalmol 8:216–218

Findlay GH (1952) On the pathogenesis of incontinentia pigmenti with observations on an associated eye disturbance resembling retrolental fibroplasia. Brit J Dermatol 64:141–146

Fletcher MC (1955) Retrolental fibroplasia, role of oxygen. Report of the 16th Rosse Pediatric Research Conferences, Columbus, Ohio

Fletcher MC and Brandon S (1955) Myopia of prematurity. Am J Ophthalmol 40:474–481

Flynn JT, Cassady J, Essner D, Zeskind J, Meritt J, Flynn R and Williams MJ (1979) Fluorescein angiography in retrolental fibroplasia: experience from 1969–1977. Ophthalmology 86:1700–1723

Flynn JT, O'Grady GE, Herrera JA, Kusher BJ, Cantolino S and Milam W (1977) Retrolental fibroplasia: I. Clinical observations. Arch Ophthalmol 95:217–223

Foos RY (1972) Vitreoretinal juncture; topographical variations. Invest Ophthalmol 11:801–808

Foos RY (1975) Acute retrolental fibroplasia. Graefes Arch Ophthalmol 195:87–100

Foos RY (1977) Vitreoretinal juncture over retinal vessels. Graefes Arch Ophthalmol 204:223–234

Foos RY and Kopelow S (1973) Development of retinal vasculature in paranatal infants. Survey Ophthalmol 18:117–127

Forsius H, Eriksson AW and Vainio-Mattila BA (1963) Geschlechtsgebundene erbliche Retinoschisis in zwei Familien in Finnland. Klin Mbl Augenheilk 143:806–816

Franceschetti A, Babel J and Francois J (1963) Les hérédo-dégénérescences choriorétiniennes: vol 2 Masson, Paris

Francois JA, Neetens A and Colette JM (1955) Microangiographie oculaire. Ophthalmologica 129:145–159

Frandsen E (1966) Hereditary hyaloideo-retinal degeneration (Wagner) in a Danish family. Acta Ophthalmol 44:223–233

Fried M and Meyer-Schwickerath G (1980) Incontinentia pigmenti (Bloch-Sulzberger syndrom) mit Ablatio falciformis congenita: eine Langzeitbeobachtung über 18 jahre. Klin Mbl Augenheilk 176:44–49

Friedenwald JS, Owens WC and Owens EU (1951) Retrolental fibroplasia in premature infants, III: The pathology of the disease. Trans Am Ophthalmol Soc 49:207–230

Friedman B (1939) Familial retinal degeneration leading to detachment and cataract formation. Arch Ophthalmol 22:271–273

Fujita S, Fujiwara N and Ohba N (1980) Norrie's disease; report of cases in two japanese families. Jpn J Ophthalmol 24:22–28

Fulton AB, Craft JL, Howard RO and Albert DM (1978) Human retinal dysplasia. Am J Ophthalmol 85:690–698

Galinos SO, McMeel W, Trempe CL and Schepens CL (1976) Chorioretinal anastomoses after argon laser photocoagulation. Am J Ophthalmol 82:241–245

Gans B (1959) The pupillary membrane in premature infants. Arch Dis Child 34:292–297

Gartner S (1941) Congenital retinal folds and microcephaly. Arch Ophthalmol 25:93–100

Gärtner J (1962a) Klinische Beobachtungen über den Zusammenhang der Glaskörpergerüst und Netzhautgefässen in der Ora-Aequator-Gegend. Klin Mbl Augenheilk 140:524–545

Gärtner J (1982b) Histologische Beobachtungen über physiologische vitrovaskuläre Adherenzen. Klin Mbl Augenheilk 141:530–545

Gärtner J (1964) Ueber persisterende Netzhautadhärente Glaskörperstränge und vitreoretinal Gefässanastomosen. Graefes Arch Ophthalmol 167:103–121

Gärtner J (1966) Electron-microscopic observations of the relationships between vitreous body and retina. Mod Probl Ophthalmol 4:67–75

Gitter KA, Rothschild H, Waltmann D, Scott B and Azar P (1978) Dominantly inherited peripheral retinal neovascularization. Arch Ophthalmol 96:1601–1605

Gloor BP (1975) Persistierende hyperplastischen primären Glaskörper. Klin Mbl Augenheilk 166:293–297

Godel V, Romano A, Stein R, Adam A and Goodman RM (1978) Primary retinal dysplasia transmitted as X-chromosome linked recessive disorder. Am J Ophthalmol 86:221–227

Goldberg MF (1976a) Chorioretinal vascular anastomoses after blunt trauma to the eye. Am J Ophthalmol 82:892–895

Goldberg MF (1976b) Sickle cell retinopathy. TD Duane: Clinical Ophthalmoloy vol 3 chap 17

Goldberg MF and Duke JR (1968) v Hippel-Lindau disease. Am J Ophthalmol 66:693–705

Goldberg MF and Koenig S (1974) Argon laser treatment of von Hippel-Lindau retinal angiomas. I. Clinical and angiographic findings. Arch Ophthalmol 92:121–125

Goldmann H (1964) Senile changes of the lens and the vitreous. Am J Ophthalmol 57:1–13

Goldschmidt R (1935) Gen und Ausseneigenschaft I und II. Z Vererbungslehre 69:38–69; 70–131

Gonvers M, Faggioni R, Zografos L and Gailloud C (1977) Persistance et hyperplasie du vitré primaire. Adv Ophthalmol 34:74–92

Gorlin RG and Knobloch WH (1972) Syndromes of genetic juvenile retinal detachment. Z Kinderheilk 113:81–92

Gow J and Oliver L (1971) Familial exudative vitreoretinopathy. Arch Ophthalmol 86:150–155

Graham Scott J, Friedmann AJ, Chitters AJ and Pepler WJ (1955) Ocular changes in the Bloch-Sulzberger syndrome (incontinentia pigmenti). Brit J Ophthalmol 39:276–282

Green WR and Gass JDM (1971) Senile disciforme degeneration of the macula. Arch Ophthalmol 86:487–494

Grolman W von (1889) Microphthalmus und Cataracta congenita vasculosa. Arch J Ophthalmol 35:187–198

Grüneberg T (1955) Zur Frage der Incontinentia pigmenti (Bloch-Sulzberger) Arch Klin Exp Derm 201:218–254

Guerrier CWJ and Wong CK (1974) Ultrastructural evolution of the skin in incontinentia pigmenti (Bloch-Sulzberger). Dermatologica 149:10–22

Hamburg A (1963) Pseudoglioma. Ophthalmologica 146:355–357

Hamburg A (1970) Norrie's disease. Ophthalmologica 160:375–377

Hanscom T and Machemer R (1980) Scleral resection in combination with vitrectomy. Int Ophthalmol 2:23–26

Hansen AH (1968) Norrie's disease. Am J Ophthalmol 66:328–332

Harris GS (1976) Retinopathy of prematurity and retinal detachment. Can J Ophthalmol 11:21–25

Heimann K (1972) The development of the choroid in man. Ophthalmol Res 3:257–273

Heine L (1904) Klinisches und Anatomisches über eine bisher unbekannte Missbuldung des Auges: angeborene Cystenretina. Graefes Arch Ophthalmol 58:38–44

Henkind P and de Oliveira LF (1967) Development of retinal vessels in the rat. Invest Ophthalmol 6:520–530

Heydenreich A (1959) Zur Pathogenese des Pseuodoglioms. Klin Mbl Augenheilk 134:465–481

Hindle NW and Leyton J (1978) Prevention of cicatricial retrolental fibroplasia by cryotherapy. Can J Ophthalmol 13:277–281

Hippel E v (1895) Vorstellung eines Patienten mit einem sehr ungewöhnlichen Netzhaut-bzw Aderhautleiden. Ber Deutsche Ophthalmol Ges 24:p 269

Hippel E v (1904) Ueber eine sehr seltene Erkrankung der Netzhaut. Graefes Arch Ophthalmol 59:83–106

Hirose T, Lee Y and Schepens CL (1973) Wagner's hereditary vitreo-retinal degeneration and retinal detachment. Arch Ophthalmol 89:176–185

His W (1880) Abbildungen über das Gefässsystem der menschlichen Netzhaut und derjenigen des Kaninchens. Arch Anat Entwicklungsg 5:224

Hittner HM, Rhodes RL and McPherson AR (1979) Anterior segment abnormalities in cicatricial retinopathy of prematurity. Ophthalmology 86:803–816

Hoepner J and Yanoff M (1972) Ocular anomalies in trisomy 13–15. Am J Ophthalmol 74:729–737

Hoffman H (1926) Ueber eine seltene Strangbildung im Augenhintergrund (arteria hyaloidea persistens). Klin Mbl Augenheilk 77:370–379

Hogan MJ and Kimura SJ (1961) Cyclitis and peripheral chorioretinitis. Arch Ophthalmol 66:667–677

Holmes LB (1971) Norrie's disease. An X-linked syndrome of retinal malformation, mental retardation and deafness. N Eng J Med 234:367–368

Howard GM and Ellsworth RM (1965) Differential diagnosis of retinoblastoma. I. Relative frequency of the lesions which simulate retinoblastoma. Am J Ophthalmol 60:610–616

Huggert A (1954) Appearance of the fundus oculi in prematurely born infants treated with and without oxygen. Acta Paediatr Scan 43:327–336

Hulsbus R, Malbran E and Dodds R (1972) Retinal detachment and Eales' syndrome. Mod Probl Ophthalmol 10:262–268

Hunter WS and Zimmerman LE (1965) Unilateral retinal dysplasia. Arch Ophthalmol 74:23–30

Ingalls TH (1948) Congenital encephalo-ophthalmic dysplasia. Pediatrics 1:315–325

Jacklin HN (1980) Falciform fold, retinal detachment and Norrie's disease. Am J Ophthalmol 90:76–80

Jager GM (1953) A hereditary retinal disease. Tr Ophthalmol Soc UK 73:617–619

Jakobiec FA, Abramson D and Scher R (1978) Increased aqueous lactate dehydrogenase in Coats' disease. Am J Ophthalmol 85:686–689

Jampol LM and Goldbaum MH (1980) Peripheral proliferative retinopathies. Survey Ophthalmol 25,1:1–14

Jansen LMAA (1966) Het syndroom van Wagner. v Gorcum, Assen, the Netherlands (1966)

Jarmas AL, Weaver DD, Ellis FD and Davis A (1981) Microcephaly, microphthalmia, falciform retinal folds and blindness. A new syndrome. Am J Dis Child 135:930–933

Jesberg DD, Spencer WH and Hoyt WF (1968) Incipient lesions of von Hippel-Lindau disease. Arch Ophthalmol 80:632–640

Joannidès Th and Protonotarios P (1965) Décollement falciforme de la rétine chez un frère et une soeur. Ann Oculist 198:904–911

Jones HE (1963) Hyaloid remnants in the eyes of premature babies. Brit J Ophthalmol 47:39–44

Joseph N, Ivry M and Oliver M (1972) Persistent hyperplastic primary vitreous at the optic nervehead. Am J Ophthalmol 73:580–583

Kalina RE (1980) Treatment of retrolental fibroplasia. Surv. Ophthalmol 24:229–236

Kalina RE, Hodson WA and Morgan BC (1972) Retrolental fibroplasia in a cyanotic infant. Pediatrics 50:765–768

Kaplan C, Sayre GP and Greene CF (1961) Bilateral nephrogenic carcinomas in Lindau-Von Hippel disease. J Urol 86:26–42

Karlsberg RC, Green R and Patz A (1973) Congenital retrolental fibroplasia. Arch Ophthalmol 89:122–123

Kaufman SJ, Goldberg MF, Orth DH et al. (1982) Autosomal dominant vitreoretino-choroidopathy. Arch Ophthalmol 100:272–278

Kelley JS and Danzinger P (1979) Rhegmatogenous retinal detachment with retinal telangiectasia. Am J Ophthalmol 88:52–54 (1979)

Kimura C and Uemura Y (1977) Congenital angiodysplastic exudative vitreoretinopathy. Jpn J Clin Ophthalmol 31(11):1327–1334

Kindler P (1970) Morning glory syndrome:unusual congenital disk anomaly. Am J Ophthalmol 69:376–384

King MJ (1950) Retrolental fibroplasia. Arch Ophthalmol 43:694–711

Kingham JD (1977) Acute retrolental fibroplasia. Arch Ophthalmol 95:36–47

Kingham JD (1978) Acute retrolental fibroplasia. II. Treatment by cryosurgery. Arch Ophthalmol 96:2049–2053

Kinsey VE (1956) Retrolental fibroplasia. Cooperative study of retrolental fibroplasia and the use of oxygen. Arch Ophthalmol 56:481–529

Kinsey VE, Kalina RE, Stern L, Stahlman M et al (1977) PaO2 levels and retrolental fibroplasia. Pediatrics 60:655–688

Kinsey VE and Hemphill FM (1955) Etiology of retrolental fibroplasia: Preliminary report of a cooperative study of retrolental fibroplasia. Am J Ophthalmol 40:166–173

Klein S, Pilz D and Marré (1974) Zur Spaltlampphotografie der Netzhautrandzone, Ora Serrata und Pars plana corporis ciliaris. Jenaer Rundschau 119–120

Klien BA (1949) Histopathological aspects of retrolental fibroplasia. Arch Ophthalmol 41:553–561

Knobloch WH (1975) Inherited hyaloideoretinopathy and skeletal dysplasia. Trans Am Soc Ophthalmol 73:417–450

Krause AC (1946) Congenital encephalo-ophthalmic dysplasia. Arch Ophthalmol 36:387–444

Krey HF (1981) Distribution of arterioles, capillaries and venules in the equatorial choroid of the human eye. Ophthalmologica 183:20–23

Krey HF and Laux U (1974) Netzhautgefässveränderungen bei Incontinentia pigmenti (Bloch-Sulzberger Syndrom). Klin Mbl Augenheilk 164:138–142

Krümmel H and Rausch L (1955) Anomalien des Auges bei der sogenannten Incontinentia pigmenti. Ophthalmologica 130:31–53

Kushner BJ, Essner D, Cohen IJ and Flynn JT (1977) Retrolental fibroplasia. Arch Ophthalmol 95:29–38

Kuwabara T and Cogan DG (1960) Studies on retinal vascular patterns. I. Normal architecture. Arch Ophthalmol 64:904–911

Lahav M and Albert DM (1973) Clinical and histopathological classification of retinal dysplasia. Am J Ophthalmol 75:648–667

Laqua H (1980) Familial exudative vitreoretinopathy. Graefes Arch Ophthalmol 213:121–133

Leber TH (1916) In: Graefe-Saemisch: Handbuch der gesamten Augenheilkunde. Part 7, pp 1267–1319. 2nd ed. Engelmann, Leipzig

Lemmingson W (1966) Vitalmikroscskopische Untersuchungen zur Morphogenese des retinalen Gefässsystems bei der Katze. Graefes Arch Ophthalmol 171:271–286

Lieb WA and Guerry D (1958) Fundus changes in incontinentia pigmenti. Am J Ophthalmol 45:265–271

Lindau A (1927) Zur Frage Angiomatosis retinae und ihrer Hirnkomplikationen. Acta Ophthalmol 4:193–226

Lisch K (1968) Idiopathische hereditäre retinoschisis. Klin Mbl Augenheilk 153 (2):204–210

408

Loewer-Seiger DH, de Keizer RWJ and de Jong PTVM (1980) Persisterend hyperplastisch primair glasvocht. Ned T Geneesk 124:2202

Lorijn RWH (1980) Fetal oxygen consumption and placental oxygen exchange. pp 66–71. Thesis. Krips Repro, Meppel, The Netherlands

Lorijn RWH (1981) Personal communication

Lotmar W (1971) Theoretical eye model with aspherics. J Opt Soc Am 61:1522–1529

Luciano L, Spitznas M and Reale E. (1977) Electron-microscopy histochemistry of the most peripheral retinal vessels. Graefes Arch Ophthalmol 203:231–236

Lyon MF (1961) Gene action in the X-chromosome of the mouse (Mus musculus L) Nature 190:372–373

Mackensen G (1953) Angeborene Netzhautfalten und Persistenz der Glaskörpergefässe. Klin Mbl Augenheilk 123:417–433

Magnus H (1927) Doppelseitiges Pseudogliom, vorgetäuscht durch Bindegewebsbildung hinter der Linse mit Arteria hyaloidea persistens bei Mikrophthalmus. Graefes Arch Ophthalmol 18:359–368

Manen JG van (1944) Décollement rétinienne falciforme congénital et anomalies congenitales connexes. Ophthalmologica 107:122–147

Mann I (1935) Congenital retinal fold. Brit J Ophthalmol 19:641–658

Mann I (1957) Developmental abnormalities of the eye. 2nd ed. Brit Med Assoc, London

Mann I (1964) The development of the human eye. 3rd ed. Grune and Stratton, New York

Manschot WA (1958) Persistent hyperplastic primary vitreous. Arch Ophthalmol 59:188–203

Manschot WA (1971) Pathology of hereditary conditions related to retinal detachment. Ophthalmologica 162:223–234

Manschot WA (1972) Pathology of hereditary juvenile retinoschisis. Arch Ophthalmol 88:131–138

Manschot WA and de Bruijn WC (1967) Coats' disease: definition and pathogenesis. Brit J Ophthalmol 51:145–157

Masuda Y (1962) Two cases of ablatio falciformis congenita and two other cases of ocular congenital anomalies, which appeared in a pedigree with consanguineous marriages. Jpn J Clin Ophthalmol, Tokyo 16:325–331

Maumenee, IH (1979) Vitreoretinal degeneration as a sign of generalized connective tissue diseases. Am J Ophthalmol 88:432–449

McCormick A (1977) The retinopathy of prematurity in the newborn. Curr Probl Pediatr 7(11):1-28

McPherson A and Hittner HM (1979) Scleral buckling in $2\frac{1}{2}$–11 month-old premature infants with retinal detachment associated with acute retrolental fibroplasia. Ophthalmology 86:819–835

Mensheha-Manhart O, Rodrigues MM, Shields JA, Cannon GM and Mirabelli RP. Retinal pigment epithelium in incontinentia pigmenti. Am J Ophthalmol 79:571–577

Michaelson IC (1948) The mode of development of the vascular system of the retina with some observations on its significance for certain retinal diseases. Trans Ophthalmol Soc UK 68:137–180

Michaelson IC (1954) Retinal circulation in man and animals. Thomas, Springfield

Michaelson IC (1965) Intertissue vascular relationships in the fundus of the eye. Invest Ophthalmol 5:1004–1015

Miller RF and Dowling JE (1970) Intracellular response of the Müller (glial) cells of the mudpuppy retina: their relation to b-wave of electroretinogram. J Neurophysiol 33:323–341

Miller MM, Fisher R, Medeais R and Rosenthal J (1963) A case of 13–15 trisomy. Am J Ophthalmol 55:901–910

Minoda K and Kanagami S (1976) Fluorography of the fundus periphery with rhegmatogenous retinal detachment. Doc Ophthalmol Proc Series 9:573–581

Miyakubo H, Numaga T (1980) Vascular pattern in the extreme peripheral retina. Acta-Soc Ophthalmol Jpn 84:1765–1776

Morgan WE and Crawford JB (1968) Retinitis pigmentosa and Coats' disease. Arch Ophthalmol 79:146–149

Müller L (1903) Eine neue operative Behandlung der Netzhautabhebung. Klin Mbl Augenheilk 41:459–462

Mutlu F and Leopold JH (1964) Structure of the retinal vascular system. Am J Ophthalmol 58:261–270

Nagata M (1977) Treatment of acute proliferative retrolental fibroplasia: Its indications and limitations, Jpn J Ophthalmol 21:436–459

Nagata M and Tsuruoka Y (1972) A new indirect method of fundus photography. Jpn J Ophthalmol 16:131–143

Nagata M, Tsuruoka Y and Yamamoto Y (1972) Photocoagulation therapy of acute retrolental fibroplasia. Jpn J Clin Ophthalmol 26:271–280

Naiman J, Green WR and Patz A (1979) Retrolental fibroplasia in hypoxic new-born. Am J Ophthalmol 88:55–58

Naumann GOH (1980) Pathologie des Auges (Spezielle pathologische Anatomie, part 12) 569–570 Springer Verlag, Berlin

Nicholson DH, Green WR and Kenyon KR (1976) Light- and electronmicroscopic study of early lesions in angionathosis retinae. Am J Ophthalmol 82:193–204

Nichols RL (1956) The etiology of visceral larva migrans. I. Diagnostic morphology of infective second stage larvae. J Parasitol 42:349

Niessel P (1977) Untersuching der Fundusperipherie. Dtsch Ophthalmol Ges 74:49–60

Nilausen K (1958) The vasoformative tissue in the foetal retina with particular reference to the histochemical demonstration of alkaline phosphatase activity. Acta Ophthalmol 36:65–70

Nishimura M (1980) Clinical studies on falciform retinal folds. Jpn J Clin Ophthalmol 34:325–333

Nishimura Y, Oshima K and Otaguro S. Clinical study and photocoagulation upon the retinopathy of prematurity. Folia Ophthalmol Jpn 26:1027–1035

Nouhuys CE v (1981a) Congenital retinal fold as a sign of dominant exudative vitreoretinopathy. Graefes Arch Ophthalmol 217:55–67

Nouhuys CE v (1981b) Chorioretinal dysplasia in young subjects with Wagner's hereditary vitreoretinal degeneration. Int Ophthalmol 3:67:67–77

Nouhuys CE v and Aan de Kerk AL (1982) Dominante exsudative vitreoretinopathie:een aandoening met vele gezichten. Ned T Geneesk 126(3):129

Nouhuys CE v and Deutman AF (1980) Congenital bilateral anastomosis between the choroid and peripheral retina. Am J Ophthalmol 90:154–159

Numaga T and Miyakubo H (1981) Developmental vascular abnormality in the peripheral retina in juvenile retinal detachment. Jpn J Ophthalmol 35:65–77

Nijhuis FA, Deutman AF and Aan de Kerk AL (1979) Fluorescein angiography in mild stages of dominant exudative vitreoretinopathy. Mod Probl Ophthalmol 20:107–112

Ober RR, Bird AC, Hamilton AM and Sehmi K (1980) Autosomal dominant exudative vitreoretinopathy. Brit J Ophthalmol 64:112–120

O'Connor PR (1972) Visceral larva migrans of the eye: subretinal tube information. Arch Ophthalmol 88:526–529

Ohba N, Watanabe S and Fujita S (1981) Primary vitreoretinal dysplasia transmitted as an autosomal recessive disorder. Brit J Ophthalmol 65:631–635

Oliveira LNF de (1968) A origem e o desenvolvimento dos vasos da retina. Thesis, Lisboa

Orts Llorca F and Geniz Gálvez JM (1961) Pliegues congénitos de la rétina, "retinal septa", "ablatio falciformis retina". Mécanismo patogénico. Zbl Ges Ophthalmol 82: 141

Otuki H (1939) Zwei Fälle von "Ablatio falciformis congenita Weve's" Acta Soc Ophthalmol Jpn 43:68

Owens WC (1955) Symposium retrolental fibroplasia. AM J Ophthalmol 40:159–162

Pagenstecher HE (1913) Ueber eine unter dem Bilde der Netzhautablösung verlaufende, erbliche Erkrankung der Retina. Arch J Ophthalmologie (Leipzig) 86:457–462

Pagenstecher, HE (1916) Strahlenwirkung auf fötale Auge. Ber Ophthalmol Ges Heidelberg. 40:447

Pajtas J (1950) Cas de pseudogliome familial héréditaire dans trois générations (retinitis exsudativa Coats). Ophthalmologica 120:411:415

Palich-Szántó O (1958) Beitrage zum Krankheitsbild der Ablatio falciformis retinae. Klin Mbl Augenheilk 132:574–575

Parsons JH (1903) - Fleming. Arteria hyaloidea persistens. Klin Mbl Augenheilk 41(2): 490

Patau K, Dmith DW, Therman E, Inhorn SL and Wagner HP (1960) Multiple congenital anomaly caused by an extra autosome. Lancet 1:790–793

Patz A (1965) The effect of oxygen on immature retinal vessels. Invest Ophthalmol 4: 988–999

Patz A, Hoeck LE and de la Cruz E (1952) Studies on the effect of high oxygen administration in retrolental fibroplasia: I. Nursery observations. Am J Ophthalmol 35: 1248–1253

Pau H (1957) Zur Entwicklung der Glaskörperstrukturen und der Zonula. Ophthalmologica 134:320–331

Payne JW and Patz A (1972) Treatment of acute proliferative retrolental fibroplasia. Am Acad Ophthalmol and Otolar 76:1234–1246

Payne JW and Patz A (1977) Fluorescein angiography in retrolental fibroplasia. Int Ophthalmol Clin 17:121–135

Pederson JE, Kenyon KR, Greem WR, Maumenee AE (1978) Pathology of pars planitis. Am J Ophthalmol 86:762–774

Pelláthy B v (1931) Ablatio retinae und Uveitis congenita bei drei Geschwistern. Z Augenheilk 73:249–254

Perkins ES (1966) Pattern of uveitis in children. Brit J Ophthalmol 50:169–185

Petersen HP (1968) Persistence of the Bergmeister Papilla with glial overgrowth. Acta Ophthalmol 46:430–440

Pflüger E (1885) Microcephalie und microphthalmie. Archiv für Augenheilk 14:1–11

Philips CI, Leighton DA and Forrester RM (1973) Congenital hereditary bilateral nonattachment of the retina. Acta Ophthalmol 51:425–433

Pinckers AJLG (1970) Le syndrome de Wagner, electro-oculographie et sens chromatique. Ann Oculist 203:569–578

Pollard ZP, Jarrett WH. Hagler WS, Allain DS and Schantz PM (1979) ELISA for diagnosis of ocular toxocariasis. Ophthalmology 86:743–752

Pomerantzeff O (1975) Equator-plus camera. Invest Ophthalmol 14:401–406

Poulsen G (1947) Ablatio falciformis congenita atypica. Acta Ophthalmol 25:447–453

Pruett RC (1975) The pleomorphism and complications of posterior hyperplastic primary vitreous. Am J Ophthalmol 80:625–629

Raskind RH (1966) Persistent hyperplastic primary vitreous. Am J Ophthalmol 62: 1072–1076

Reese AB (1949) Persistence and hyperplasia of primary vitreous; retrolental fibroplasia – two entities. Arch Ophthalmol 41:527–552

Reese AB (1955) Persistent hyperplastic primary vitreous. Am J Ophthalmol 40:317–331

Reese AB and Blodi FC (1950) Retinal dysplasia. Am J Ophthalmol 33:23

Reese AB and Stepanik J (1954) Cicatricial stage of retrolental fibroplasia. Am J Ophthalmol 38:308–316

Reese AB and Straatsma BR (1958) Retinal dysplasia. Am J Ophthalmol 45:199–211

Ricci A (1960) Clinique et transmission génétique des differentes formes des dégénérescences vitréo-rétiniennes. Ophthalmologica 139:338–343

Ricci A (1961) Clinique et transmission héréditaire desdégénérescences vitréo-rétiniennes. Bull Soc Ophthalmol 61:618–662

Ricci A (1969) Les dysplasies hyaloideo-rétiniennes congénitales et leur diagnostic différentiel. J Génétic hum (suppl) 17:20–53

Ring HG and Fujino T (1967) Observations on the anatomy and pathology of the choroidal vasculature. Arch Ophthalmol 78:431–444

Röhrs K (1963) Ueber kongenitale Pseudogliome an Hand von 4 Beobachtungen innerhalb einer Familie. Klin Mbl Augenheilk 142:809–827

Rosen ES (1968) A photographic investigation of simple retinal detachment. Trans Ophthalmol Soc UK 88:331–342

Rosen DA and Yamashita T (1964) Persistent hyperplastic primary vitreous. Am J Ophthalmol 57:1002–1007

Roth AM (1977) Retinal vascular development in premature infants. Am J Ophthalmol 84:636–640

Rubinstein K (1980) Posterior hyperplastic primary vitreous. Brit J Ophthalmol 64: 105–111

Rutnin U (1967) Fundus appearance in normal eyes. I. The choroid. Am J Ophthalmol 64:821–839

Rutnin U and Schepens CL (1967) Fundus appearance in normal eyes. II. The standard peripheral fundus and developmental variation. Am J Ophthalmol 64:840–852

Saari M, Mietinnen R and Raisanen S (1975) Retinochoroidal vascular anastomosis in toxoplasmic chorioretinitis. Acta Ophthalmol 53:44–51

Sabates F (1966) Juvenile retinoschisis. AM J Ophthalmol 62:683–688

Saga U and Uemura Y (1977) Histology and histochemistry of developing vessels and choroid in premature infants. Acta Soc Ophthalmol Jpn 81/1:6–12

Salffner O (1902) Bulbus sepatus. Graefes Arch Ophthalmol 59:552–562

Sasaki K, Yamashita Y, Maekawa T and Adachi T (1976) Treatment of retinopathy of prematurity in active stage by cryocautery. Jpn J Ophthalmol 20:384–395

Sato K (1972) Fluorography of the peripheral retina in normal ocular fundus. In: Shimizu: Proceedings Int Symp Fluorescein Angiography. Shoin, Tokyo

Scarlett HW (1922) Opaque canal of Cloquet with persistent hyaloid artery. Am J Ophthalmol 5:941–943

Schaffer DB, Johnson L, Quinn GE, Boggs TR (1979) A classification of retrolental fibroplasia to evaluate vitamin E therapy. Ophthalmology 86:1749–1760

Schantz PM, Glickman LT (1978) Toxocaral visceral larva migrans. N Engl J Med 298:436–439

Schappert-Kimmijser J, Hansen E, Haustrate-Gosset MF, Lindstadt E. Skydsgaard H and Warburg M (1975) Causes of severe visual impairment in children and their prevention. Doc Ophthalmol 39:213–342

Schlaegel TF (1976) Toxoplasmosis. In: Duane: Clinical Ophthalmology vol 4 chap 51 Harper and Row, Hagerstown

Schlaegel TF and Knox DL (1976) Uveitis and parasitoses. In: Clinical Ophthalmology vol 4 chap 52, Harper and Row (1976)

Schmidt D and Faulborn J (1972) Familiäres Vorkommen von Coats'-Syndrom kombinierty mit Retinopathia pigmentosa. Klin Mbl Augenheilk 160:158–163

Schulman J, Jampol LM and Schwartz H (1980) Peripheral proliferative retinopathy without oxygen therapy in a full term infant. Am J Ophthalmol 90:509–513

Scialdone D and Artifoni E (1962) L'ablation falciforme congenita. G Ital Oftal 15:256–274

Scott JG, Friedmann AJ and Chitters M (1955) Ocular changes in the Bloch-Sulzberger syndrome (incontinentia pigmenti). Brit J Ophthalmol 39:276–282

Seedorff T (1968) Retrolental fibroplasia as the cause of blindness. Nord Med 79:269–274

Seefelder R (1909) Ueber Anomalien im Bereich des Sehnerven und der Netzhaut normaler fötaler Augen, ein Beitrag zur Gliomfrage. Graefes Arch Ophthalmol 69:463–478

Serpell G (1954) Polysaccaride granules. Brit J Ophthalmol 38:460–471

Shakib M, Oliveira LF de and Henkind P (1968) Development of retinal vessels II. Earliest stages of vessel formation. Invest Ophthalmol 7:689–699

Shimizu K and Ujiie K (1976) Intern symp fluorescein angiography. In: JJ de Laey. International symposium on fluorescein angiography. Doc Ophthalmol Proc series vol 9:pp 187–200. Junk, The Hague

Silverstein AM (1974) Retinal dysplasia and rosettes induced by experimental intrauterine trauma. Am J Ophthalmol 77:51–58

Silverstein AM, Osburn BI and Prendergast R (1971) The pathogenesis of retinal dysplasia. Am J Ophthalmol 72:13–21

Slezak H and Kenyeres P (1977) Photographische Dokumentation des extremen Fundusperipherie. Dtsch Ophthamol Ges 74:71–74

Slusher MM, Hutton WE (1979) Familial exudative vitreoretinopathy. Am J Ophthalmol 87:152–156

Slusher MM, Tyler ME (1980) Choroidoretinal vascular anastomoses. Am J Ophthalmol 90:217–222

Snell AC (1965) Retinal dysplasia. Am J Ophthalmol 60:621–627

Sorsby A, Klein M, – Hurndalt, Gann J and Siggins G (1951) Unusual retinal detachment possibly sex-linked. Brit J Ophthalmol 35:1–10

Spaulding AG, Naumann GOH (1957) Persistent hyperplastic primary vitreous in an adult. Arch Ophthalmol 77:666–671

Spitznas M and Bornfield N (1977) The architecture of the most peripheral retinal vessels Graefes Arch Ophthalmol 203:217–229

Spitznas M, Joussen F and Wessing A (1976) Treatment of Coats' disease with photocoagulation. Graefes Arch Ophthalmol 199:31–37

Spitznas M, Meyer-Schwickerath G and Stephan B (1975) The clinical picture of Eales' disease. Graefes Arch Ophthalmol 194:73–85

Stefani FH and Ehalt H (1974) Non oxygen induced retinitis proliferans and retinal detachment in full-term infants. Brit J Ophthalmol 58:490–513

Stefani FH and Laszczyk WA (1976) Vitreoretinal reactions and persistent hyaloid vessels. Brit J Ophthalmol 60:829–834

Stickler GB, Belau PG, Farrell FJ, Jones JD, Pugh DG, Steinberg AG and Ward CE. (1965) Hereditary progressive arthro-ophthalmopathy. Mayo Clin Proc 40:433–455

Straub W (1951) Beitrag zur Klinik der persisterenden Glaskörperarterie. Ophthalmologica 121:194–200

Stübel A (1927) Ueber Schlauchbildungen im Glaskörper. Klin Mbl Augenheilk 79:393–396

Stübel A (1928) Zur Frage des fötalen Augenentzündung. Archiv für Augenheilk 48:184–191

Sulzer – (1888) Gefässhaltige Ueberreste des hinteren Abschnittes der Gefässhaltigen fötalen Linsenkapsel beim Erwachsenen an einem Auge mit Membrana Pupillaris perserverans und anderen Entwicklungsanomalien. Klin Mbl Augenheilk 29:425–429

Svedberg B (1975) Retrolental fibroplasia or congenital encephalo-ophthalmic dysplasia? Acta Paediatr Scan 64:891–894

Takei Y (1976) Origin of ghost cells in Coats' disease. Invest Ophthalmol 15:677–681

Tanabe Y and Ikema M (1972) Retinopathy of prematurity and photocoagulation therapy. Acta Soc Ophthalmol Jpn 76:260–266

Tasman W (1970) Vitreoretinal changes in cicatricial retrolental fibroplasia. Tr Am Ophthalmol Soc 68:548–549

Tasman W (1975) Retinal detachment in retrolental fibroplasia. Graefes Arch Ophthalmol 195:129–139

Tasman W (1979) Late complications of retrolental fibroplasia. Graefes Arch Ophthalmology 86:1724–1740

Tasman W and Shields JA (1980) Disorders of the peripheral fundus. Harper and Row, New York

Tatsuyama C and Shimizu K (1972) Fluorography of the fundus periphery with detached retina. In: Fluorescein angiography. Proc Int Symp fluorescein angiography. Tokyo

Terry TL (1942) Extreme prematurity and fibroplastic overgrowth of persistent vascular sheath behind each crystalline lens. I. Preliminary report Am J Ophthalmol 25:203–204

Theodore FH and Ziporkes J (1940) Congenital retinal fold. Arch Ophthalmol 23:1188–1197

Thiel HJ (1968) Beitrag zur Klinik und Genese des Ablatio falciformis congenita. Klin Mbl Augenheilk 152:46–50

Thuránsky K (1957) Der Blutkreislauf der Netzhaut. Verlag der Ungarischen Akademie der Wissenschaften Budapest

Thijssen JM, Pinckers AJLG and Otto AJ (1974) A multipurpose optical system for ophthalmic diagnosis. Ophthalmologica 168:308–314

Tillema A (1937) Infantile and congenital retinal fold. Brit J Ophthalmol 21:94–98

Tolentino FI, Schepens CL and Freeman HM (1976) Vitreoretinal disorders. Diagnosis and management. Saunders, Philadelphia

Toussaint D and Danis P (1970) Vascular density coefficients in normal human relationship to distance from disc. Arch Ophthalmol 83:281–286

Toussaint D, Kuwabara T and Cogan D (1961) Retinal vascular patterns. Part II: Human retinal vessels studied in three dimensions. Arch Ophthalmol 65:575–581

Townes PL and Roca PD (1973) Norrie's disease (hereditary oculo-acoustic-cerebral degeneration). Am J Ophthalmol 76:797–803

Treister G and Machemer R (1977) Results of vitrectomy for rare proliferative and hae-morrhagic diseases. Am J Ophthalmol 84:394–412

Triebenstein O (1919) Ueber Heterotopie des Sehnverven und der Fovea centralis. Klin Mbl Augenheilk 62:442–455

Tripathi R and Ashton N (1971) Electron microscopical studies of Coats' disease. Brit J Ophthalmol 55:289–301

Uebel H, Ludwig A and Korting GW (1950) Zur Kenntnis der Incontinentia pigmenti (Bloch-Sulzberger). Arch Dermatol Syph 190:114–124

Uemura Y, Akiya S, Ogata T et al (1977) Experimental approach to the pathogenesis of retrolental fibroplasia. Jpn J Ophthalmol 21, 4:460–476

Velhagen C (1912) Bindegewebsbildung an der hinteren Linsenfläche unter dem Bilde des Glioma retinae. Klin Mbl Augenheilk 14:580–586

Vergex A, Dhermy P and Cosson C (1966) Syndrome de Seckel s'accompagnant d'un décollement rétinienne bilatéral du type fibroplasia rétrolental. Arch Ophthalmol (Paris) 26:355–364

Versari R (1904) La morfogenesi dei vasi sanguigni della retina umana. Richerche Fatti nel Laboratorio di Anatomia Normale della Regia Universita di Roma. 10:25–62

Vries, WM de (1904) Ueber eine Missbildung des menschlichen Auges (Coloboma iridis Katarakt, Stränge und Gefäss im Glaskörper). Graefes Arch Ophthalmol 57:544–570

Waardenburg PJ, Franschetti A and Klein D (1963) Genetics and Ophthalmology. vol I and II van Gorcum, Assen

Wagner H (1938) Ein bisher unbekanntes Erbleiden des Auges (degeneratio hyaloide-retinalis hereditaria), beobachtet im Kanton Zürich. Klin Mbl Augenheilk 100:840–856

Wang MK and Phillips CJ (1973) Persistent hyperplastic primary vitreous in non-identical twins. Acta Ophthalmol 51:434–437

Warburg M(1966) Norrie's disease. A congenital progressive oculo-acoustico-cerebral de-generation. Acta Ophthalmol suppl 89: E Munksgaard Copenhagen

Warburg M (1974) Norrie's disease and falciform detachment of the retina. In: Genetic and Metabolic Eye disease. M Goldberg, Little, Brown & Co, Boston

Warburg M (1976) Heterogeneity of congenital retinal non-attachment, falciform folds and retinal dysplasia. Hum Hered 26:137–148

Warburg M (1978) Hydrocephaly, congenital retinal non-attachment and congenital falci-form fold. Am J Ophthalmol 85:88–94

Watzke RC, Stevens ThS and Carney RG (1976) Retinal vascular changes of incontinentia pigmenti. Arch Ophthalmol 94:743–746

Welch RB, Maumenee AE, Wahler HE (1960) Peripheral posterior segment inflammation, vitreous opacities and edema of the posterior pole. Arch Ophthalmol 64:540–549

Wessing A (1967) Zehn Jahre Lichtkoagulation bei Angiomathosis retinae. Klin Mbl Augenheilk 150:57–71

Wessing A (1974) New aspects of angiographic studies in retinal detachment. Mod probl Ophthalmol 12:202–206

Wessing A and Schlicke B (1976) Equatorial degeneration with atypical vessels. Doc Ophthalmol Proc Series vol. 9:613–616

Weve H (1933) Ueber Ablatio falciformis congenita. Archiv für Augenheilk 109:371–394

Weve H (1938) Ablatio falciformis congenita (retinal fold). Brit J Ophthalmol 22:456–470

Weve H (1953) The origin and relationship between anterior dialysis, retinal cysts, retinal folds and retrolental fibroplasia. Tr Ophthalmol Soc Australia 13:35–46

Wien S van and Sullivan WB (1955) Congenital retinal fold. Am J Ophthalmol 39:643–647

Wilkinson CP and Welch RB (1971) Intraocular Toxocara. Am J Ophthalmol 71:921–930

Willets GS (1966) Heterotopia of the macula. Brit J Ophthalmol 50:595–598

Wilson WMG (1949) Congenital blindness (Pseudoglioma) occurring as a sex-linked devel-opment anomaly. Can Med Ass J 60:580–584

Winning CHOM von (1952) Retrolental fibroplasia. Drukkerij Trio, Den Haag

Wise GN (1957) Coats' disease. Am Arch Ophthalmol 58:735–746

Wise GN (1961) Factors influencing retinal new vessel formation. Am J Ophthalmol 52:637–650

Wise GN, Dollery CT and Henkind P (1971) The retinal circulation. 1st ed. Harper & Row, New York

Wolff JR, Goerz Ch, Bärr Th and Güldner FH (1975) Common morphogenetic aspects of various organotypic microvascular patterns. Microvascular research 10:373−395

Wolter JR (1957) Perivascular glia of the blood vessels of the human retina. Am J Ophthalmol 44:766−773

Wolter JR (1957) Das Verhalten der Astrologia bei fortgeschrittener Degeneration der Netzhaut. Klin Mbl Augenheilk 130:498−511

Wolter JR and Flaherty NW (1959) Persistent hyperplastic primary vitreous. Am J Ophthalmol 47:491−503

Wollensak J (1959) Karakteristische Augenbefunde beim Syndroma Bloch-Sulzberger (incontinentia pigmenti). Klin Mbl Augenheilk 134:692−706

Woods AC and Duke JR (1963) Coats' disease. I. Review of the literature, diagnostic criteria, clinical findings, and plasma lipid studies. Brit J Ophthalmol 47:385−411

Wybar KC (1954) Vascular anatomy of the choroid in relation to selective localization of ocular disease. Brit J Ophthalmol 38:513−527

Yamana T, Nishimura M, Oishi J and Yamana Y (1981) Exudates in the peripheral retina in the newborns. Fol Ophthalmol Jpn 32:254−261

Yanoff M, Kertesz Rahn E and Zimmerman LE (1968) Histopathology of juvenile retinoschisis. Arch Ophthalmol 79:49−53

Zollinger HU (1944) Die Beziehungen zwischen Gefässsystem und peripherer zystoider Degeneration der Netzhaut. Graefes Arch Ophthalmol 146:403−423

## CURRICULUM VITAE

Christiaan Erik van Nouhuys werd op 6 mei 1946 te Leeuwarden geboren. Na de voltooiing van de gymnasium B opleiding te Arnhem studeerde hij één jaar chemie aan de Universiteit van Groningen. Van 1965 tot 1972 studeerde hij geneeskunde aan dezelfde universiteit. Van 1973 tot 1976 was hij als huisarts in gouvernementsdienst werkzaam te Curaçao (Ned. Antillen). Van 1976 tot 1980 specialiseerde hij zich in de oogheelkunde in de oogheelkundige kliniek van het St. Radboudziekenhuis van de Universiteit van Nijmegen (hoofd: Prof. Dr. A.F. Deutman). Tijdens deze periode werd het onderzoek, dat in dit proefschrift beschreven wordt, aangevangen. Door een subsidie van het Praeventiefonds werd het mogelijk gemaakt het onderzoek voort te zetten tot eind 1981. Vanaf 1 februari 1982 is hij werkzaam als oogarts in het Canisius-Wilhelmina Ziekenhuis te Nijmegen.